# Health Information Technology and Management

# Health Information Technology and Management

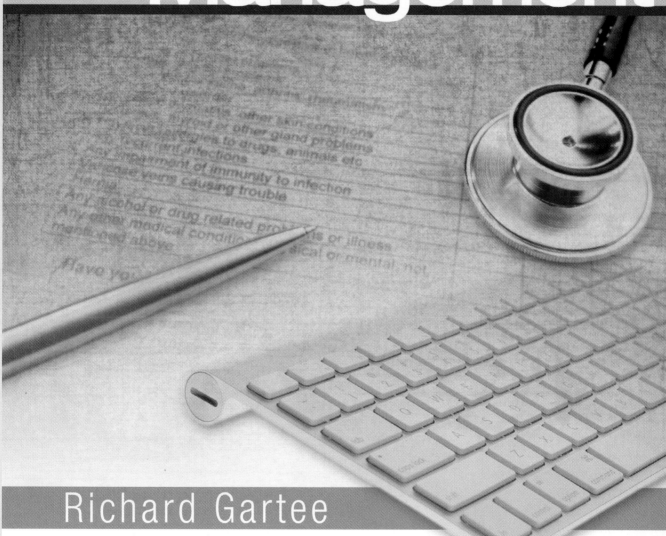

## Richard Gartee

**Pearson**

Boston   Columbus   Indianapolis   New York   San Francisco   Upper Saddle River
Amsterdam   Cape Town   Dubai   London   Madrid   Milan   Munich   Paris
Montreal   Toronto   Delhi   Mexico City   São Paulo   Sydney
Hong Kong   Seoul   Singapore   Taipei   Tokyo

**Library of Congress Cataloging-in-Publication Data.**
Gartee, Richard.
  Health information technology and management/Richard Gartee.
    p. cm.
  Includes bibliographical references and index.
  ISBN-13: 978-0-13-159267-4 (alk. paper)
  ISBN-10:   0-13-159267-X (alk. paper)
1.  Medical records—Data processing.   I. Title.
  [DNLM:   1. Medical Records Systems, Computerized.   2. Forms and Records Control—methods.
WX 173 G244h 2011]
  R864.G374 2011
  610'.285—dc22

                                                                2009035087

**Publisher:** Julie Levin Alexander
**Publisher's Assistant:** Regina Bruno
**Editor-in-Chief:** Mark Cohen
**Executive Editor:** Joan Gill
**Associate Editor:** Bronwen Glowacki
**Developmental Editor:** Jill Rembetski, Triple SSS Press
  Media Development.
**Editorial Assistant:** Mary Ellen Ruitenberg
**Director of Marketing:** Karen Allman
**Senior Marketing Manager:** Harper Coles
**Marketing Specialist:** Michael Sirinides
**Marketing Assistant:** Judy Noh
**Managing Production Editor:** Patrick Walsh
**Production Liaison:** Julie Boddorf
**Production Editor:** Peggy Kellar
**Senior Media Editor:** Amy Peltier
**Media Project Manager:** Lorena Cerisano

**Manufacturing Manager:** Ilene Sanford
**Manufacturing Buyer:** Pat Brown
**Senior Art Director:** Maria Guglielmo
**Art Director:** Kristine Carney
**Interior Designer:** Nesbitt Graphics, Inc.
**Cover Designer:** Koala Bear Design
**Cover Images:** Istockphoto.com and Shutterstock
**Director, Image Resource Center:** Melinda Reo
**Manager, Rights and Permissions:** Zina Arabia
**Manager, Visual Research:** Beth Brenzel
**Manager, Cover Visual Research
  and Permissions:** Karen Sanatar
**Image Permission Coordinator:** Debbie Latronica
**Composition:** Aptara®, Inc.
**Printing and Binding:** Quebecor
**Cover Printer:** Phoenix Color Corporation

10 9 8 7 6 5 4 3 2 1

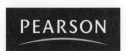

www.pearsonhighered.com

ISBN 13: 978-0-13-159267-4
ISBN 10:   0-13-159267-X

*for Dad*

# Brief Contents

# Contents

# Chapter 3 Accreditation, Regulation, and HIPAA    42

# Chapter 4 Fundamentals of Information Systems  74

# Chapter 5 Healthcare Records  98

# Preface

## Introduction

Welcome to the Information Age! We live in a century when the flow of information increases with every leap in technology. This book introduces students to the fundamentals of the healthcare delivery system, health information management, and health information systems based on the *core competencies* defined by AHIMA[1] of what students need to know.

Health information is the backbone of healthcare delivery. The medical record is the essential component for maintaining continuity of care for the patient and the prevention of medical errors. The abstracted and aggregate data from health records is essential to the financing and operation of the facility.

Yet it may surprise you that the concept of creating and maintaining complete and accurate medical records as a necessity of healthcare is less than a century old. The year 1918 is considered the starting point of health information management. It was the first time hospitals were required by the American College of Surgeons to keep "accurate and complete medical records for all patients, filed in an accessible manner."

There followed the creation of occupations, professions, and an organization concerned with the processing and handling of patient charts. Standardization made the information in those records more useful. The profession evolved from record filing to managing health information, but until recently a lot of the information was on paper.

Health information management in the 21st century differs from health information management just 10 years ago, and the reason for that is technology. The old world of managing paper health records is giving way to computerized records. Here are indicators of that change:

> AHIMA, the leading organization for Health Information Technicians and Health Information Management professionals is focusing its membership toward the implementation of electronic health records.

> President Barack Obama, in the first month of his presidency, signed into law an act to promote the widespread adoption of electronic health records and eventually penalize those providers who don't make the change.[2]

To prepare for 21st century health information occupations, students need to understand not only the principles and practices of health information management, but the technology of it as well.

While this text thoroughly covers traditional concepts of organizing and filing paper charts, it goes further than previous books on the subject in helping the student understand the connectivity and applications that make up the health information systems of today and of tomorrow.

---

[1] American Health Information Management Association.
[2] H.R. 1 American Recovery and Reinvestment Act of 2009, Title XIII Health Information Technology for Economic and Clinical Health, February 17, 2009.

# AHIMA Competencies

The AHIMA Education Strategy Committee has created a list of entry-level competencies for associate degree students. This book familiarizes students with the concepts and subject matter in each of the 5 domains and 15 subdomains recommended by AHIMA. Listed beneath each domain and subdomain is the material covered in this book:

## I. Domain: Health Data Management

**A. Subdomain: Health Data Structure, Content and Standards** **This book covers:** data elements, data sets, and databases; record analysis; the application of policies and procedures to ensure the accuracy of health data; the use of clinical vocabularies and terminologies; the importance of timeliness, completeness, accuracy, and appropriateness of data and data sources; records management; billing; and reports, registries, and indexes.

**B. Subdomain: Healthcare Information Requirements and Standards** **This book covers:** documentation guidelines; policies and procedures to ensure organizational compliance with internal and external regulations and standards; and healthcare organization accreditation, licensing, and certification.

**C. Subdomain: Clinical Classification Systems** **This book covers:** electronic applications and work processes that support clinical classification and coding including diagnosis/procedure codes using ICD-9-CM, CPT/HCPCS, DRG, APC, ICD-10; medical nomenclatures such as SNOMED-CT and MEDCIN; and ethics, regulations, guidelines, and penalties related to code assignment and billing.

**D. Subdomain: Reimbursement Methodologies** **This book covers:** healthcare reimbursement; inpatient and outpatient prospective payment systems; coding, billing, claims management, and billing workflow processes; and reporting requirements such as the National Correct Coding Initiative.

## II. Domain: Health Statistics, Biomedical Research, and Quality Management

**A. Subdomain: Healthcare Statistics and Research** **This book covers:** clinical indices; disease, implant, and transplant registries; research databases; quality management; utilization management; risk management; and clinical trial studies and healthcare statistics.

**B. Subdomain: Quality Management and Performance Improvement** **This book covers:** quality management and performance improvement programs; and the analysis of data to identify trends that improve quality, safety, and effectiveness of healthcare.

## III. Domain: Health Services Organization and Delivery

**A. Subdomain: Healthcare Delivery Systems** **This book covers:** the structure and organization of various healthcare provider entities, and the laws, accreditation, licensure, and certification standards under which they operate; how the policies, procedures, and regulations of Medicare, Medicaid, managed care, and other insurers affect healthcare providers and facilities; the roles of various providers and disciplines throughout the continuum of healthcare and their information needs.

**B. Subdomain: Healthcare Privacy, Confidentiality, Legal, and Ethical Issues** **This book covers:** the legal and regulatory requirements that govern healthcare providers, facilities, and their employees including a thorough exploration of HIPAA privacy and security regulations that govern the handling and disclosure of personal health information. The book also includes and promotes ethical standards of health information management.

## IV. Domain: Information Technology and Systems

**A. Subdomain: Information and Communication Technologies** **This book covers:** technology commonly used in the healthcare setting; differentiates hardware, software, and data; the different forms of data storage, acquisition, analysis, and reporting; the various software applications used in the creation, tracking, coding, imaging, billing, and quality improvement of paper and electronic health records; computer networks; the intranet; and electronic health records, personal health records and public health records.

**B. Subdomain: Data, Information, and File Structures** **This book covers:** database architecture including data dictionaries and data types.

**C. Subdomain: Data Storage and Retrieval** **This book covers:** document and diagnostic imaging; image formats; and archival and retrieval systems for patient information stored as digital images.

**D. Subdomain: Data Security** **This book covers:** HIPAA security measures; protection of electronic health information; data integrity and validity using software or hardware technology; security policies and procedures; and audit trails, data quality monitoring programs, risk management, contingency planning, and data recovery procedures.

**E. Subdomain: Healthcare Information Systems** **This book covers:** how healthcare facilities implement, integrate, interface, test, and support health information systems; and ergonomics and workflow process design.

## V. Domain: Organizational Resources

**A. Subdomain: Human Resources** **This book covers:** the various functions of the human resources department and continuing education and training programs in healthcare organizations.

**B. Subdomain: Financial and Physical Resources** **This book covers:** administrative systems and processes necessary to healthcare organizations including the coding and revenue cycle process, accounting, ordering and purchasing, accounts receivable, accounts payable, budgets, and provider contracts.

# The Development and Organization of the Text

The text is drawn from the author's extensive experience in the field of health systems design and implementation, from health information professionals from numerous hospitals across the country, and from the resources of the leading health information nonprofit organizations including AHIMA, HIMSS,[3] and the Joint Commission. In areas where government regulations are explained, the text draws directly from the rules and guidance documents published by various agencies of the U.S. Department of Health and Human Services.

The book has been organized to provide a comprehensive understanding of the history, theory, and potential benefits of health information management systems. Each chapter is designed to build on the knowledge acquired in previous chapters. The 12 chapters are arranged in three units designed to guide the learner through increased levels of understanding. A *Comprehensive Evaluation* after each unit can be used to evaluate the students' mastery of the material.

## Healthcare Fundamentals

To understand healthcare information and how it is managed, it is first necessary to be familiar with the environments where it is gathered, by whom it is used, and the technology behind health information systems. The first four chapters provide a foundation for student learning, introducing concepts that are developed more extensively in subsequent chapters.

**Chapter 1, Healthcare Delivery Fundamentals,** defines the types of healthcare facilities; explains the differences between ambulatory, acute care, and subacute care facilities; and compares the workflows in an inpatient versus outpatient setting. Students learn about healthcare facility ownership models, how they are organized, and how to read an organizational chart. This chapter introduces direct care providers, clinical allied professions, and several organizations important to medical professionals.

**Chapter 2, Health Information Professionals,** acquaints the student with the history of health information management, the many occupations available in the health information field, the skills necessary to succeed, and the professional and standards setting organizations working to improve health information.

**Chapter 3, Accreditation, Regulation, and HIPAA,** introduces students to the Joint Commission, the fundamental concepts of accreditation, and how healthcare entities are regulated. The chapter provides an in-depth explanation of HIPAA's Privacy and Security Rules. The HIPAA transactions, code sets, and uniform identifiers introduced in this chapter are more fully explained in subsequent chapters as the learner progresses.

**Chapter 4, Fundamentals of Information Systems,** is intended to familiarize even the computer novice with the basic terminology and ideas underpinning the computer technology used in healthcare. These include the fundamental concepts of computers, hardware, software, communications, and networks. Information technology is fully explained from the smallest bit to the largest relational database in a manner that every student will grasp. Concepts of data elements, data sets, and image data are amply illustrated. Health system interoperability and standards setting organizations are also discussed.

## Healthcare Information Systems

With the fundamentals of the healthcare and computer systems complete, the next section fully explores the core subject matter: health information. With a focus on primary health records, the next four chapters cover in detail both paper and electronic health records.

**Chapter 5, Healthcare Records,** begins to develop the student's understanding of health records, the different forms they take, the functions that healthcare records serve, and how health records assist with continuity of care for patients. The topics of data elements and data sets introduced in the previous chapter are further developed and the concepts of primary and secondary health records are introduced. Sharing of health information by regional health information organizations (RHIO), telemedicine, personal health records, and E-visits are also covered.

---

[3]Healthcare Information Management Systems Society.

**Chapter 6, Organization, Storage, and Management of Health Records,** describes how paper charts are organized, filed, and tracked. Students learn the source-oriented, problem-oriented, and integrated method of organizing charts. Students also learn the differences among alphanumeric, sequential numeric, terminal digits, middle digits, and color-coded filing systems. Various chart numbering schemes are explained. Students learn to calculate storage requirements for paper records and the legal and ethical rules of record circulation, retention, destruction, and release of information. Technological changes to health information management are introduced with discussions of document imaging systems, electronic views, and automated chart tracking systems.

**Chapter 7, Electronic Health Records,** begins with the history and social forces driving the transition from paper to electronic health records (EHRs). The chapter defines the EHR and describes the functional benefits derived from its use. Students then learn about the various forms of EHR data, the concepts of codified records, and medical nomenclatures. With this foundation, the learner is then introduced to a broad range of EHR concepts including health maintenance, trend analysis, alerts, decision support, protocols, point-of-care documentation, patient-entered data, preventive health screening, flow sheets, and electronic signatures.

**Chapter 8, Additional Health Information Systems,** covers departmental systems that contribute documents and data to the primary health record. This chapter includes discussions of patient registration, radiology, pathology, laboratory information systems, pharmacy, digital pathology, digital radiology, speech recognition, and dictation and transcription systems. The chapter also discusses emergency departments, biomedical devices, surgical departments, implant registries, transplant registries, medical research and clinical trials.

## Healthcare Billing and Management

Having covered the many aspects of primary health records and the functional benefits derived from the patient record, the final section explores the uses of secondary health records to operate healthcare facilities and improve patient care.

**Chapter 9, Healthcare Coding and Reimbursement,** shifts the focus to the creation and use of secondary health records for the business aspects of healthcare. Students learn patient account, registration, and insurance terminology and concepts. Different reimbursement methodologies by which providers are paid are compared and prospective payment systems are explained in detail. Standardized codes used for billing such as CPT-4, HCPCS, procedure modifier codes, ICD-9-CM, ICD-10, DRGs, and MS-DRGs are covered as well as examples of billing fraud and abuse.

**Chapter 10, Healthcare Transactions and Billing,** furthers the student's understanding of the practical business aspects of health information management and technology. A billing workflow discussion provides an overview of the charge posting, insurance billing, payment posting, and patient billing processes. This is followed by a more detailed examination of the HIPAA transaction coding standards first introduced in Chapter 3. Examples of paper and electronic insurance forms are compared as students learn about electronic data interchange, electronic claims, electronic remittance, clearinghouses, claim scrubbers, claim status, claim attachments, insurance eligibility, referrals, and authorizations.

**Chapter 11, Health Statistics, Research, and Quality Improvement,** covers the processing and maintenance of secondary health records for internal and external uses such as cancer registries and clinical trials research. The chapter then explores how secondary health records are used and reported to outside entities for quality improvement performance measures such as ORYX, HEDIS, and the National Hospital Quality Measures. Data analysis and statistics are explained using easy-to-understand diagrams and the National Hospital Quality Measures in the examples.

**Chapter 12, Management and Decision Support Systems,** introduces students to the numerous information systems used to support healthcare operations. Some of the systems discussed in this chapter include administrative, financial accounting, human resources, quality management, case management, risk management, and comparative performance measures.

# Learning Made Easy

## Learning About Health Information Technology and Management

This book makes learning about health information technology and management easy. It reinforces theoretical material, with first-hand experience of professionals working in the areas discussed in each chapter, and includes many other helpful features.

## Learning Outcomes

Each chapter begins with a list of learning outcomes that highlights the key concepts contained in that chapter.

---

### LEARNING OUTCOMES

After completing this chapter, you should be able to:

- Describe the history of health information management and organizations
- Differentiate the roles of health information professionals
- Describe the organizational hierarchy of HIM and IT departments
- Compare various nonclinical allied healthcare occupations
- Explain the role of a project manager
- Understand how skill sets from multiple disciplines can help you in your career

---

## Acronyms

Students need to master the numerous acronyms that are used extensively in both medicine and computers. To facilitate learning, each chapter includes a list of the acronyms and their definitions to provide learners with a quick reference.

---

### ACRONYMS USED IN CHAPTER 6

Acronyms are used extensively in both medicine and computers. The following are those which are used in this chapter.

| | | | |
|---|---|---|---|
| **AHIMA** | American Health Information Management Association | **HIPAA** | Health Insurance Portability and Accountability Act |
| **ALOS** | Average Length of Stay | **OCR** | Optical Character Recognition |
| **CD** | Compact Disk | **OSHA** | Occupational Safety and Health Administration |
| **CMS** | Centers for Medicare and Medicaid Services | **PACS OR PAC SYSTEM** | Picture Archiving and Communication System |
| **COP** | Conditions of Participation | **PDF** | Portable Document Format |
| **DVD** | Digital Video Disk | **PHI** | Protected Health Information |
| **EHR** | Electronic Health Record | **SOAP** | Subjective, Objective, Assessment, Plan |
| **EPHI** | Electronic Protected Health Information | **VPN** | Virtual Private Network |
| **ER** | Emergency Room | | |
| **FTE** | Full-Time Equivalent Employee | | |

---

## Highlights

Boxes found within the chapters call additional attention to key concepts or terms to familiarize learners with common health information management terminology and prepare them to communicate effectively with others in a clinical setting.

### COVERED ENTITY

HIPAA documents refer to healthcare providers, insurance plans, and clearinghouses as *covered entities*. A clearinghouse is a business that converts nonstandard HIPAA transactions into the correct format required by HIPAA.

As a future HIM employee, think of a covered entity as a healthcare organization and all of its employees.

## Real-Life Stories

Each chapter features one or more *Real-Life Stories* told by health information professionals, healthcare providers, administrators, technicians, and project managers about their experiences with different aspects of health information management. These vignettes help learners connect chapter content to real life in a healthcare facility or medical office.

### A REAL-LIFE STORY

#### Automating HIM Workflow

*By Shannon Welchi and Shelly Wymer*

*Shannon Welchi, RHIA, is HIM department manager, and Shelly Wymer, RHIT, CCS, is electronic records coordinator at Allegiance Health Hospital in Jackson, Michigan.*

Our Health Information Management department is pretty well computerized, though a portion of our records are still in paper; these are scanned into a document imaging system. About 70% of our inpatient record is now imported data; therefore, it does not have to be scanned.

We usually receive the patient's chart the same day the patient is

For example, when a physician signs in to complete his discharge summary, he receives a subset that will give him a list of documents pertinent to dictating his discharge summary. Generally these subsets are task or role based. For example, a billing coder would see what billing would typically need, but our system allows subsets to be customized by user, so a particular user can set up subsets specific to them.

## Chapter Summary

Detailed summaries at the end of each chapter synthesize key points for students.

## Chapter 5 Summary

### Understanding Healthcare Records

Healthcare records have many purposes, the most important of which is the patient's care.

- The patient health record is the repository of data and information about a patient, the condition of the patient's health, the care and treatments the patient received, and the outcome of that care.
- The term *patient health record* has replaced the term *patient medical record* because it encompasses a holistic view of patient care. Though the terms are

- Data and information is not the same thing. Data are records of facts. Information is data in a useful form that conveys meaning.

### Functions of Healthcare Records

- A patient's health record serves as the principal communication document among various providers who might care for the patient at different times in different departments.
- The patient record provides the basis for all billing and reimbursement. Medical claims will not be paid

# Figures and Tables

Ample color photographs, tables, and drawings throughout the text help learners visualize various aspects of health information, including workflow scenarios and technical concepts.

| Sample Health Record Retention Schedule | |
|---|---|
| **Hospital Health Information** | **Recommended Retention Period** |
| Adult Patients' health records | 10 years after the most recent encounter |
| Children's health records | 10 years after child reaches the age of majority (or longer if required by state law) |
| Fetal heart monitor records | 10 years after child reaches the age of majority (or longer if required by state law) |
| Registers of births and deaths | Permanently |
| Register of surgical procedures | Permanently |
| Master patient/person index | Permanently |
| Disease index | 10 years |
| Comprehensive outpatient rehabilitation facilities (CORF) | 5 years after patient discharge |
| Laboratory Pathology tests | 10 years after date of results report |
| Diagnostic images (such as x-ray film) | 5 years |
| Mammography | 5 years if subsequent mammograms performed on the patient at the fac 10 years if no additional mammogra performed |

## Critical Thinking Exercises

Each chapter includes questions that challenge students to apply critical thinking to solve a problem or explore a scenario, encouraging the student to learn by doing.

### Critical Thinking Exercises

1. You have a job in the HIM department. A friend of yours works for a lawyer. She comes to your facility to pick up copies of records for one of her boss's clients. She has forgotten to bring the client's authorization form. She is in a hurry and doesn't have time to go back to her office. You have known her for many years and are good friends. Do you give her the records
2. If you decide to give your friend the employer?
3. Is there a way to help your friend get to her office?

### Critical Thinking Exercises

1. CMS takes the position that "if it isn't documented, it wasn't done." What does this mean and why would it matter to CMS?
2. Chapters 4 and 5 discussed data sets. Design a basic demographic data set. Make a list of just the fields you would need for the patient information. (You do not need to include insurance information.)

## Test Your Knowledge

The end of every chapter includes a variety of question types, including short answer, true/false, and multiple choice, to allow learners to test their knowledge and think critically.

### Testing Your Knowledge of Chapter 2

1. What does the acronym HIM stand for?
2. What does the acronym HIT stand for?
3. Give an example of how the fields of HIM and IT are merging.
4. In what year did the American College of Surgeons establish standards for hospital records?
5. What is forms control?
6. How would understanding medical terminology help a billing clerk?

*For each of the following allied health professions, indicate if the job is clinical or nonclinical by circling the correct answer:*

7. Clinical applications coordinator

   *Clinical       Nonclinical*
8. Lab technician

   *Clinical       Nonclinical*
9. Coding specialist

   *Clinical       Nonclinical*

10. Cancer registrar

    *Clinical       Nonclinical*
11. In the HIM profession what is *abstracting*?
12. What are two requirements to become a Registered Health Information Administrator?

*For each of the following statements circle true if it is correct, or false if the statement is not true:*

13. Diagnosis-related groups are used for Medicare billing and reimbursement.

    *True       False*
14. A Registered Health Information Technician is required to implement and train users on imaging systems.

    *True       False*
15. A security officer is a position found exclusively at inpatient facilities or very large medical practices.

    *True       False*

## Comprehensive Evaluations

Learners will have an opportunity to test their mastery of the material through three comprehensive evaluations found at the conclusion of Chapters 4, 8, and 12.

# Comprehensive Evaluation of Chapters 9–12

This comprehensive evaluation will enable you and your instructor to determine your understanding of the material covered so far.

1. Which Medicare plan pays for professional services?
   a. Part A
   b. Part B
   c. Part C
   d. P

7. Which of the following hospital types is exempt from IPPS?
   a. children's hospitals
   b. cancer hospitals
   c. critical access hospitals
   d. all of the above

8. Which central tendency value is the midpoint in a

# About the Author

Richard Gartee is the author of four college textbooks on health information technology, computerized medical systems, managed care, and electronic health records. Prior to becoming a full-time author and consultant, Richard spent 20 years in the design, development, and implementation of the preeminent practice management and electronic health records systems.

Richard also served as a liaison to other companies in the medical computer industry as well as Blue Cross/Blue Shield, a U.S. Department of Commerce International Trade Mission, and various universities.

Richard is a current or past member of many of the professional organizations and national standards groups recommended in this book:

- American Health Information Management Association (AHIMA)
- Healthcare Information Management Systems Society (HIMSS)
- American National Standards Institute (ANSI) X12n committee for development of electronic claims standards
- Health Level Seven (HL7) committee for development of claims attachment standards
- Workgroup for Electronic Data Interchange (WEDI) task force for development of electronic remittance guidelines
- A faculty member/speaker at the Medical Records Institute international Electronic Health Records Conference (TEPR) for 12 years.

# Acknowledgments

This book was made possible by the contributions of many individuals and several of the most prominent commercial vendors whom I would like to personally thank and acknowledge here.

I would first like to thank the many individuals who provided me with helpful interviews and firsthand experiences. I would especially like to thank Rick Warren, Sharyl Beal, John Bachman, M.D., and Dave Schinderle who set up countless interviews with the staff at their respective facilities.

I am also grateful to the following people many of whom contributed the real-life stories for the book and for their assistance: Henry Palmer, M.D.; Sharron Carr, ARNP-BC; Thomas Rau; Marvin P. Mitchell; Ron Rea; Tanya Townsend; Shannon Welchi, RHIA; Shelly Wymer, RHIT, CCS; Judy Cullen, RHIA; Wesley McCann, BA, MA, RT-R; David Goldbaum; Craig Gillespie; Mary E. Bazan; Jayme Stewart; Jeanne Wymer; Allen Wenner, M.D.; and William Moody, M.D.

I am also indebted to the following businesses, which provided photographs and images of computer screens to allows students to see actual examples of real-world applications. I thank them for allowing their copyrighted work to be reprinted herein. Listed in alphabetical order:

Allscripts, LLC

Ames Color-File

Aperio, Inc.

Carestream Health, Inc

Clinipace, Inc.

Digital Identification Solutions, LLC

GE Healthcare

Good Health Network, Inc.

Imaging Business Machines, LLC.

Kaiser Permanente

Massachusetts General Hospital

McKesson Corporation

MidasPlus, Inc.

Midmark Diagnostics Group

NextGen

Nuance, Inc.

Primetime Medical Software & Instant Medical History

Sage Software

Shands Healthcare and Teaching Hospital

Sunquest Information Systems

Finally, I would like to acknowledge the help of all my editors who assisted me with this work, but especially Joan Gill, my executive editor. Thanks again, Joan!

# Reviewers

Susan R. Collins, MHSA, CPC, CCA, CPMA

*Senior Healthcare Consultant–Coding/Reimbursement*
*Altarum Institute*
*Alexandria, VA*

Marie T. Conde, MPA, RHIA, CCS

*Health Information Technology Program Director and Instructor*
*City College of San Francisco*
*San Francisco, CA*

Kirstie DeBiase, MAED/CI

*Academic Dean*
*San Joaquin Valley College*
*Rancho Cordova, CA*

Suzanne B. Garrett, MSA, RHIT

*Associate Professor*
*HIT Program Facilitator*
*Central Florida Community College*
*Ocala, FL*

Cindy Glewwe, MEd, RHIA

*Health Science Curriculum Manager*
*Rasmussen College*
*Eagan, MN*

Janice C. Hess, MS, RMT

*Coordinator, Health Information Management Systems*
*Metropolitan Community College*
*Omaha, NE*

and *Vice President*
*Nebraska State AHDI*
*Omaha, NE*

Deborah Honstad, MA, RHIA

*Assistant Professor*
*San Juan College*
*Farmington, NM*

Jacqueline L. Keller, ASN, CPC, NCMA

*Instructor*
*Wichita Technical Institute*
*Wichita, KS*

Margie Konik, MA, RHIA

*Program Director/Instructor*
*Health Information Technology*
*Chippewa Valley Technical College*
*Eau Claire, WI*

Timothy McCall

*Director Medical Billing/Coding Program*
*Four D College*
*Colton, CA*

Sandra K. Rains, MBA, RHIA

*Chairperson Health Information Technology*
*DeVry University*
*Columbus, OH*

Sulea Rucker, RPT/CMA (AAMA)

*Health Studies Division Manager*
*San Joaquin Valley College*
*Modesto Campus*
*Salida, CA*

M. Beth Shanholtzer, MAEd, RHIA

*Director, Health Information Management Programs*
*Kaplan College*
*Hagerstown, MD*

Juan Troy, MBA

*Program Director*
*Health Information Technology*
*Western Career College*
*Antioch, CA*

# Healthcare Delivery Fundamentals

## LEARNING OUTCOMES

After completing this chapter, you should be able to:
- Differentiate ambulatory and acute care facilities
- Read an organizational chart
- Explain the difference between rehabilitation and long-term facilities
- Compare the workflows in an inpatient versus outpatient setting
- Understand the roles of various direct care providers
- Identify the various organizations associated with the healthcare professions

## ACRONYMS USED IN CHAPTER 1

Acronyms are used extensively in both medicine and computers. The following acronyms are used in this chapter.

| | | | |
|---|---|---|---|
| **AHA** | American Hospital Association | **HIM** | Health Information Management |
| **ALOS** | Average Length of Stay | **HIT** | Health Information Technician; Health Information Technology |
| **AMA** | Against Medical Advice; also American Medical Association | **ICU** | Intensive Care Unit |
| **ANA** | American Nurses Association | **IT** | Information Technology |
| **ASHA** | American Speech-Language-Hearing Association | **JAMA** | *Journal of the American Medical Association* |
| **CAT** | Computerized Axial Tomography | **LPN** | Licensed Practical Nurse |
| **CCC** | Certificate of Clinical Competence | **LVN** | Licensed Vocational Nurse |
| **CEO** | Chief Executive Officer | **LOS** | Length of Stay |
| **CFO** | Chief Financial Officer | **MD** | Medical Doctor |
| **CIO** | Chief Information Officer | **MRI** | Magnetic Resonance Imaging |
| **CNO** | Chief Nursing Officer | **MSO** | Management Service Organization |
| **COO** | Chief Operating Officer | **OT** | Occupational Therapist |
| **CRNA** | Certified Registered Nurse Anesthetist | **PA** | Physician Assistant |
| | | **PT** | Physical Therapist |
| **DRG** | Diagnosis-Related Group | **RD** | Registered Dietitian |
| **EHR** | Electronic Health Record | **RN** | Registered Nurse |
| **EMT** | Emergency Medical Technician | **RT** | Respiratory Therapist |
| **ER** | Emergency Room or Emergency Department | **SA** | Surgeon Assistant |
| | | **SNF** | Skilled Nursing Facility |
| **HCA** | Home Care Aide | | |
| **HHA** | Home Health Aide | | |

## Understanding Healthcare Facilities

Healthcare is provided in a variety of locations and facilities. To understand healthcare information and how it is managed, it is first necessary to be familiar with the environments where it is gathered and used. This chapter discusses and compares different types of healthcare service facilities, their organization charts, and the diverse professions of the healthcare workers employed in them.

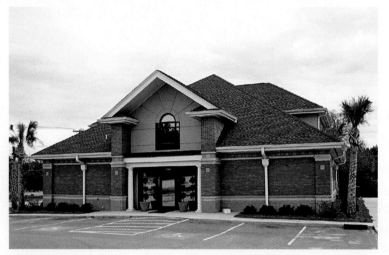

**FIGURE 1-1**

**A physician's office in South Carolina.**

(Photo courtesy of Allen Wenner, M.D.)

**FIGURE 1-2**

**Kaiser Permanente medical offices in Otay Mesa, California.**

(Photo courtesy of Kaiser Permanente.)

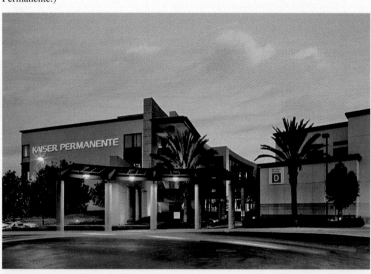

### Ambulatory Care Facilities

*Ambulatory care* is defined as care received by the patient that does not require or involve an overnight stay. This type of care is also called *outpatient care*. The healthcare provider's office is by far the most prevalent location for outpatient services. These providers include physicians, osteopaths, physical therapists, chiropractors, dentists, and all others who treat patients in their offices. In addition, ambulatory care facilities also include medical clinics provided by schools and employers, public health departments, walk-in clinics, and urgent care centers. Figure 1-1 shows the office of a private medical practice.

The majority of ambulatory care facilities are privately owned. Medical, dental, and chiropractic practices are usually owned and managed by the clinicians themselves. Large group medical practices are typically owned by the physicians within the group, but may be managed by professional administrators.

In the 1990s hospitals and management service organizations (MSOs) attempted to acquire and merge multiple physician practices with hospitals in an ownership model that has since gone out of favor. However, universities with teaching hospitals often own or operate medical offices and other freestanding ambulatory care facilities as part of their mission to train physicians and serve the community.

A small number of health insurance plans own and operate ambulatory clinics and medical practices. Not many insurance plans take this approach, but two examples of those that do it well include Urban Health Plan in New York and Kaiser Permanente in California (Figure 1-2).

Increasingly, *inpatient* hospitals have begun offering ambulatory care through outpatient clinics, surgery centers, and diagnostic centers. Medical advances in surgical techniques have resulted in a greater number of procedures that can be performed safely without the need to keep the patient overnight. This has resulted in the development of outpatient surgery centers, including those that are *freestanding* (meaning not attached to a hospital) as shown in Figure 1-3. Ambulatory surgery centers offer surgeries lasting less than two hours, after which the patient can be expected to return home following a few hours of recovery. Ambulatory surgery centers are usually privately owned, either by a hospital, as mentioned, or by a group of physicians.

**DIAGNOSTIC AND THERAPY FACILITIES**   Other types of ambulatory facilities include those that provide diagnostic testing, radiation therapy, or physical therapy on an outpatient basis.

Reference laboratories test blood and other body fluids. Tests are performed on specimens obtained from patients who come to the laboratory facility and on specimens received by courier from doctors' offices.

The mammogram is another common ambulatory test that uses radiographic images to screen for breast cancer. Mammograms are most frequently performed in freestanding diagnostic imaging centers or in a radiologist's office. In larger cities, computerized axial tomography (CAT) scans or magnetic resonance imaging (MRI) may be available from ambulatory facilities called diagnostic imaging centers, although these large diagnostic devices are more frequently found in acute care facilities (described in the next section).

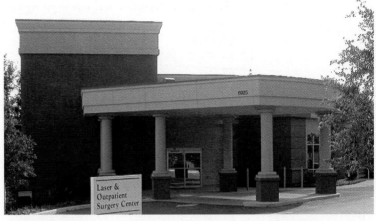

**FIGURE 1-3**

**Freestanding ambulatory surgery center in Florida.**

Radiation is one of the methods used to treat cancer. Patients undergoing radiation therapy utilize either a freestanding or hospital-based radiation therapy center one or more times a week for treatment.

Physical therapy is frequently prescribed as a follow-up treatment after hospital discharge for patients suffering serious injuries, a debilitating disease, or a stroke. Outpatient physical therapy is performed at an ambulatory facility or as a home care service. Inpatient physical therapy is performed in a rehabilitation hospital as described later in the chapter.

## Acute Care Facilities

When most people use the word *hospital* they are usually referring to an acute care facility (though the term *hospital* applies to other types of facilities as well.) Acute care facilities typically serve patients who have an illness or injury that is severe enough to require them to stay overnight for one or more days. Because the patients stay in the hospital, the term *inpatient* is also used for these facilities and the services they provide.

Acute care hospitals offer many therapeutic and diagnostic services, often organized as separate departments within the hospital. Some examples of separate departments include the surgical, radiologic, and emergency departments and the laboratory. Larger hospitals may also have trauma centers, where lifesaving procedures are performed, and intensive care units (ICUs), where critical patients are monitored continuously by highly trained nurses. Hospitals may also provide several outpatient services such as renal dialysis, oncology or radiation therapy clinics, and ambulatory surgery, as discussed previously. Figure 1-4 shows one of the first acute care hospitals in the United States.

Acute care hospitals have many possible ownership models. These include not-for-profit (or nonprofit) organizations, religious organizations, universities, city and county governments, military, the Veterans Administration, and for-profit corporations. However, the majority of hospitals are owned by nonprofit organizations or governments.[1] The ownership of the hospital influences not only its goals, but its management and financial structure.

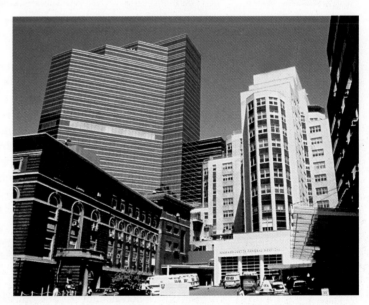

**FIGURE 1-4**

**Massachusetts General Hospital is the nation's third oldest hospital.**

(Photo courtesy of Massachusetts General Hospital.)

---

[1]Anthony R. Kovner and James R. Knickman, eds., *Jonas and Kovner's Health Care Delivery in the United States*, 8th ed. (New York: Springer, 2005).

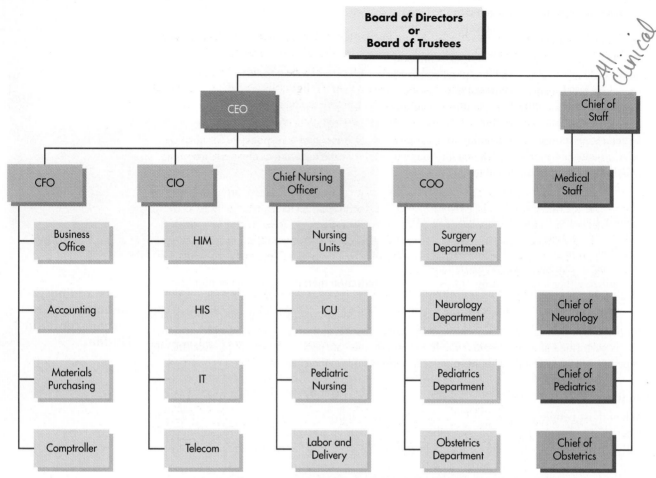

**FIGURE 1-5** **Organizational chart for an acute care hospital.**

For-profit hospitals are owned by investors. Profits are the monies earned minus the costs of operating the hospital. These are paid to the investors as dividends or reinvested in expansion or improvement of the business.

Not-for-profit hospitals are typically owned by another not-for-profit organization such as a church or university. Any money remaining after paying the expenses of operating the hospital is used to improve the facility or to provide healthcare services to the community.

Both for-profit and not-for-profit hospitals are organized similarly. Figure 1-5 is an organizational chart that could represent the hierarchy of either a for-profit or not-for-profit hospital. Note that Figure 1-5 represents only a few of the jobs and departments that make up a modern hospital.

## UNDERSTANDING AN ORGANIZATIONAL CHART

Organizational charts are used in business and other organizations to illustrate the managerial relationship between the various jobs shown in the boxes on the chart. In an organizational chart the most responsible position is listed at the top, the next level of management below that, then the next, and so forth. A given position is responsible for the management of persons in the jobs connected to the vertical line below it. For example, Figure 1-5 indicates that the chief financial officer (CFO) is responsible for the business office, accounting, purchasing, and comptroller functions. A horizontal line indicates two or more persons report to the same manager above them, but not to each other. For example, in Figure 1-5 the CFO, CIO, CNO, and COO all report to the CEO, but not to each other.

An acute care hospital is usually organized as follows:

- A governing board is responsible for the organization's by-laws, policies, and legal obligations and also appoints and governs the hospital's administrative and medical staff.

  The governing board for a nonprofit hospital will typically be a Board of Trustees selected from the local community, the university, or a religious organization associated with the hospital. The governing board of a for-profit hospital is a Board of Directors whose members are elected by the investors or stockholders of the corporation.

- The hospital administration reports to the governing board and is responsible for hospital finances, management of the facility, daily operations, and ensuring compliance with hospital policies and state and federal laws.

  The head of hospital administration is the president or chief executive officer (CEO). The president or CEO is assisted by vice presidents who manage different aspects of the organization such as operations, finance, and human resources. Larger hospitals may also have a chief financial officer (CFO), chief information officer (CIO), and chief operating officer (COO). These executives report to the CEO, and the respective vice presidents report to these officers.

- The hospital's medical staff and clinical services are the responsibility of the chief of staff and other officers of the medical staff. They report to the governing board and are responsible for ensuring the quality of patient care.

  The medical staff creates policies and by-laws that govern the standards of care and the qualifications a provider must have to provide services at the hospital (called *clinical privileges*). Medical staff members also elect the officers that govern them.

  As discussed earlier, hospitals may be divided into different departments such as cardiology, neurology, obstetrics, pediatrics, and many more. These departments may be headed by exceptionally qualified physicians who are referred to as the *chiefs* of the department (chief of cardiology, chief of neurology, etc.). Department chiefs report to the chief of staff.

- Hospitals also have a head of nursing services, sometime called chief nursing officer (CNO) or vice president of nursing who has administrative responsibility for all nurses and to whom all nurse supervisors report. Although nurses provide most of the patient care in a hospital, the CNO or VP of nursing usually reports to the CEO, not to the chief of staff.

**DECLINING NUMBERS OF ACUTE CARE HOSPITALS** According to the American Hospital Association, the number of acute care hospitals has been declining in recent years. The graph in Figure 1-6 shows the number of hospitals in operation during the past 100 years. The number of hospitals peaked in the 1970s and has steadily declined since. Some of the reasons for this decline are related to improvements in surgical techniques, such as laparoscopic surgery, that shorten or eliminate the need for patients to stay overnight. These and other advances in medicine allow the same number of beds to serve more patients because patient stays are shorter. Thus, fewer hospitals are needed.

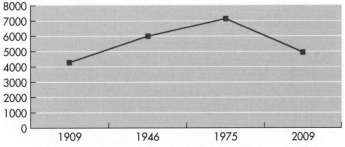

**FIGURE 1-6** **Growth and decline of the number of hospitals in the United States.**

Shorter stays and increased outpatient services are also the result of efforts by Medicare, managed care, and health insurance plans to reduce health costs. One example of this is the DRG, which stands for diagnosis-related group. DRGs will be discussed further in Chapter 9, but essentially DRG reimbursement is determined by the medical diagnosis for the patient, not the length of stay. The implementation of DRGs discouraged facilities from keeping patients longer than necessary. Medicare and other insurance programs also encouraged the use of outpatient services, rather than inpatient, for various treatments and surgeries.

## Emergency Department

The hospital emergency department has historically been referred to as the ER, which stands for emergency room. Though emergency departments are almost exclusively found in acute care hospitals, they are considered ambulatory settings. Why? Because patients do not stay in the ER—they are not inpatients. ER patients are either admitted to the hospital or sent home. Therefore, the emergency department is not an inpatient facility even though it is usually in the hospital building.

This complication is furthered when a patient who is sent home from the emergency department then returns and is admitted to the hospital for the same condition. Just as a doctor's office cannot bill for two visits by the same patient on the same day, an emergency department cannot bill for an ER visit if the patient is admitted to the hospital within 72 hours.

## Subacute Care Facilities

Physical rehabilitation facilities, long-term care facilities, and home care are sometimes referred to as providing *subacute care*. Subacute care facilities and home care services are appropriate for patients whose nursing care needs are less frequent and less intensive than the care offered in an acute care facility.

**REHABILITATION FACILITIES**   Rehabilitation facilities strive to help patients return to their maximum possible functionality. Different facilities help patients with different conditions. Some specialize in physical medicine, physical therapy, and occupational therapy, helping patients recover from the effects of accidents, severe injuries or illnesses, strokes, or serious surgery.

Other rehabilitation facilities help patients detoxify and recover from dependence on alcohol or drugs. Treatment includes counseling and therapy by psychiatrists, psychologists, and other mental health workers.

Rehabilitation facilities can be privately owned, not-for-profit, or affiliated with a hospital or university.

## Long-Term Care Facilities

Long-term care facilities offer medical care to patients who need inpatient services, but at a less intense level than that provided at an acute care facility. Long-term care patients generally have a length of stay greater than 30 days and, although these patients are technically inpatients, they are generally referred to as residents. Examples of long-term care facilities include skilled nursing facilities (SNFs), nursing homes, residential care facilities, and rehabilitation hospitals.

Residential care facilities provide residents with a living environment that is more apartment-like than a nursing home. Residents are independent, yet have access to the level of assistance they need. Group meals, activities, and transportation are often provided by the facility. Residents have the ability to notify management of a medical or other emergency at the touch of a button.

## Home Care

Though not an actual facility, home care, as the name implies, allows patients to remain in their homes, yet receive the services of nurses, physical therapists, occupational therapists, or other healthcare providers. The home care provider visits the patient's home on a regularly scheduled basis and provides services based on a physician's orders. The visiting nurse or therapist carries with him or her a small portion of the patient's record. Home care providers then record all notes concerning the home care visit, the patient's progress, and any measurements taken such as vital signs, range of motion, and so forth.

Home care provides an important component of healthcare delivery, but tracking the records of the visits provides a challenge to health information management, especially with regard to integration of home care visit notes into a comprehensive health record.

Home care is provided by agencies that are independently owned or affiliated with a hospital.

## Comparing Inpatient and Outpatient Facilities

To further understand healthcare facilities, we will explore some of the differences between inpatient and outpatient facilities. These are by no means the only differences between the two settings, but they are major areas that impact health records, data collection, billing, and patient flow—all topics of concern for health information managers.

Unless it is owned by a hospital, an ambulatory facility such as a doctor's office usually has a much simpler management structure than an acute care facility. Figure 1-7 shows the organizational chart for a group medical practice in which the doctors own the practice. In this organizational chart the office manager has responsibility for most of the staff, the exceptions being the nurse practitioners and physician assistants, who report directly to the doctor, and the accountant. Note that in some practices the nurses report to the doctors instead of to the office manager (as indicated by the dashed line.) The accountant is typically not an employee of the practice, but rather an outside firm contracted to provide accounting services. Compare Figure 1-7 with the organizational chart of an inpatient facility presented in Figure 1-5.

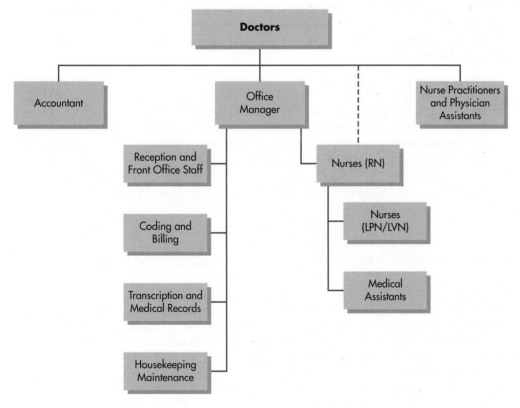

**FIGURE 1-7**

**Organizational chart for a group medical practice.**

As mentioned earlier, the type of facility is determined by the duration of the patient's stay. In an ambulatory care facility, the patient does not stay overnight. In an acute care facility the average length of stay (ALOS) is less than 30 days. In a long-term care facility the ALOS is greater than 30 days.

The capacity of an inpatient facility is measured differently than that of an outpatient facility. Although the size of an outpatient facility, such as a group medical practice, is often measured by the number of patient *visits* or *encounters* per day, the size of inpatient facilities is measured by the number of *beds*. Note, however, that the number of beds determined by inpatient facilities may be measured in two different ways. These are the number of *licensed beds* and the *bed count*.

States license hospitals for a specific capacity, or number of licensed beds; in other words, *capacity* refers to the maximum number of patients a hospital can have as inpatients at one time. When the hospital is not at maximum capacity, the administration may close certain floors or wings of the hospital to save the costs associated with maintenance and medical staff. Thus, the bed count (the number of beds staffed and available for patients) may be less than the number of licensed beds. The size of the facility is usually measured by the number of licensed beds. However, daily operations at the facility are usually more concerned with the bed count.

### Differences That Affect Health Information Management

One difference between inpatient and outpatient care that affects health information management (HIM) is the amount of information gathered about each patient and the number of individuals who will need access to it. To better understand this, let us compare the charts used in the ambulatory setting of a primary care physician's office with those of the acute care setting of a typical hospital. Figure 1-8 highlights some of the differences between inpatient and outpatient charts.

In an ambulatory setting such as a physician's office, the patient visits the physician's office a number of times over a period of months or years. While items produced outside of each visit, such as lab results and consult reports, are integrated into the patient's chart, the most important element of the outpatient chart is the clinician's brief notes about each visit. The clinician reviews previous notes on each subsequent visit using them to follow up on past ailments and to measure the patient's progress in managing chronic problems.

The medical chart is primarily used by the physician and nurse, but is also used briefly by the administrative staff to prepare billings following each visit. The focus of the chart is the

**FIGURE 1-8**

**Comparison of outpatient versus inpatient charts.**

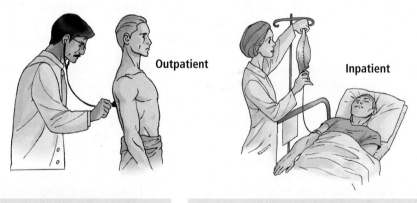

Outpatient

Inpatient

| Most physician offices have a single chart for the patient. Notes for each visit, test results, and any other reports are added to the chart. | Most hospitals start a new chart each time a patient is admitted. Information from previous stays in the hospital is linked to the patient ID, but the current chart contains only information related to the current stay. |
| --- | --- |
| The quantity of data in an outpatient chart is relatively low by comparison. | The quantity of data in an inpatient chart is likely to be much larger. Vital signs are taken and nurses' notes are added numerous times per day; dietitians, respiratory therapists, and other providers add to the chart; there are typically many more orders for labs, medications, and so on. |
| The central element in the chart is the physician's exam note. | Physician exams tend to be brief; the main focus of the chart is the physician orders and nurse's notes indicating the patient's response. |

longitudinal care of the patient. As such, it usually contains all records of the patient's visits and any reports or results received from other providers.

The inpatient chart, however, focuses on the treatment of a specific ailment or condition for which the patient was hospitalized. Data are gathered more frequently during the inpatient's stay, resulting in a substantially large amount of information gathered during a short period of time. In most hospitals, a new chart or medical record is started for each hospital stay. Although records from previous hospitalizations are available for reference, they are not incorporated into the current chart, except as described in the admitting physician's history and physical notes.

Because a large number of caregivers are involved with the patient's stay in an acute care facility, there are a larger number of individuals with a legitimate need to access a patient's record than in an ambulatory care setting. These caregivers include not only nurses and physicians, but other specialists that may consult on the case, radiologists, respiratory therapists, dietitians, and in many hospitals, even the hospital pharmacists have access to records when consulting with the ordering physicians about the medications being prescribed.

## Admission and Discharge

Another key difference between inpatient and outpatient facilities is apparent in the processes of admission and discharge. In a physician's office, patient registration occurs only at the first visit. On subsequent visits patients simply "check in" by informing the receptionist that they have arrived for their appointment. If it has been a while since the patients' last visit, the receptionist will ask them to verify that their insurance is still current and to update their medical history.

New patients are given a complete history and physical, to help the clinician understand the patient's health and background. Special billing codes differentiate a *new* patient visit from a visit by an *established* patient. The billing for a new patient visit occurs only once. All subsequent visits are billed as "established patient" visits.

After the patient has seen the clinician, a check-out clerk collects a payment or copay for the visit, schedules a follow-up appointment if one is needed, and provides the patient with copies of any paperwork. This might include patient education material, referral form, receipt, or appointment reminder. Although check-in and check-out processes are used, medical offices do not have the formal admission and discharge processes that occur in hospital setting.

Hospitals, on the other hand, do have formal admission and discharge processes. Figure 1-9 illustrates the flow of an inpatient from admission through discharge. Although some patients are admitted to the hospital through the emergency department or by transfer from another facility, most patient admissions begin in the registration department. As depicted in Figure 1-9, the steps involved in an inpatient admission and discharge include the following:

1. When the patient arrives, patient demographic and insurance information is collected or updated, and an account is set up for the patient stay. Even if the patient has been an inpatient previously, a new account is created (although previous patients will use their existing medical record number).

2. An *admitting* and/or *attending* doctor is assigned to the patient. A physician is required to perform a complete history and physical on an inpatient within 24 hours of the admission. In an outpatient facility no such time limit is imposed on when or what type of physical is performed.

3. The doctor orders tests, medications, and procedures.

4. The doctor reviews the results of tests and diagnostic procedures when they are ready.

5. Nurses provide most of the patient care, administer medications, take samples for tests, measure vital signs, perform evaluations and nursing interventions, and enter nursing notes into the chart.

6. When a patient leaves an inpatient facility there is also a formal discharge process. Normally, the physician performs a final examination of the patient and writes a discharge order. Discharge does not necessarily mean the patient goes home. Patients may be discharged to a skilled nursing facility or a rehabilitation facility for further care. Patients who leave without a doctor's order, are discharged *AMA* (*against medical advice*).

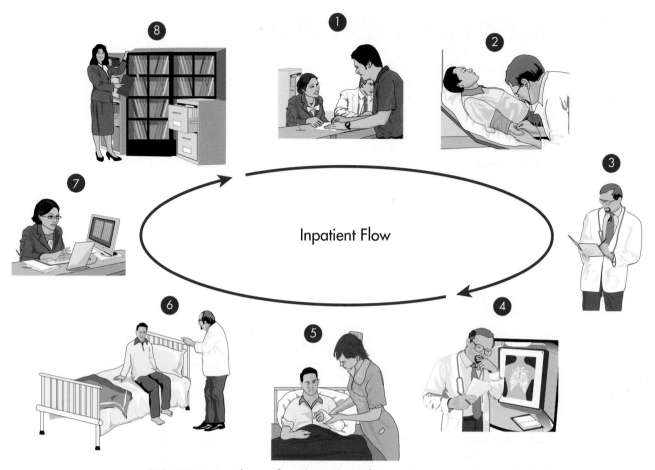

**FIGURE 1-9    Flow of an inpatient from admission through discharge.**

7. Following discharge, the HIM department examines the patient's chart to determine if it has any missing or unsigned documents (called chart deficiencies). When the chart is complete, it is sent to the billing department where the proper billing codes are assigned.

8. In a facility using paper charts, the last step is to file the chart. (Paper and electronic charts will be discussed further in subsequent chapters.)

Several elements of the inpatient process are required by billing rules and/or by law. The length of stay is determined by the admission and discharge dates, without regard to the number of actual hours involved. The date of admission is the calendar date on which the patient was admitted, and the discharge date is the calendar date on which the patient was discharged or left the facility. Even if a patient arrived at 11:00 P.M. and was discharged at 5:00 in the morning, the records would show admission and discharge on different dates.

Admission and discharge dates are important in an inpatient facility because they are used to calculate the length of stay (LOS) and the average length of stay (ALOS) for billing and reporting purposes. To calculate the LOS or ALOS, count the date of admission, but not the date of discharge. For example, if the patient is admitted February 1, and discharged February 3, count the first and second of February, but not the third; this equals a LOS of two days.

In contrast, if a patient arrived at an outpatient facility, such as a doctor's office, for an appointment in the morning, but returned a second time later in the day for the same or a different problem, the physician would only be paid for one visit. Insurance plans consider multiple encounters at an outpatient facility on a single calendar date to be one visit.

Another difference is the amount of time spent with a patient. Although time spent with the patient is not a factor in inpatient billing, the number of minutes spent with the patient can be an overriding factor in outpatient billing.

### USING DISCHARGES TO MEASURE CAPACITY

Earlier in this chapter we discussed measuring the capacity of an acute care hospital by the number of licensed beds. Another method for measuring capacity is to compare the ALOS and resulting number of discharges. For example, consider two competing hospitals that have the same number of licensed beds, but different ALOSs:

- Hospital A has an average length of stay of three days and discharges 32,000 patients a year.
- Hospital B has an average length of stay of six days and discharges 16,000 patients a year.

In this scenario, hospital A has the greater capacity because it makes better use of the same number of beds and thereby serves more patients per year.

## Healthcare Providers and Professions

Having examined the various facilities that make up the healthcare delivery system, we now discuss the professionals who provide and support healthcare services. Their professions may be classified as those who provide care directly to the patient and those who serve the healthcare system but do not provide direct patient care.

### Direct Care Providers

The first groups of healthcare professionals we discuss are those who provide care directly to the patient. In all states, these professionals must have a license and are typically regulated by professional or licensing boards.

**DOCTORS**   Several types of healthcare professionals have the title *doctor*. Some examples are chiropractors, dentists, psychologists, and of course osteopathic and medical doctors. These various types of doctors have different educational backgrounds and different modes of treating patients. What they have in common is that they are the responsible entities in the healthcare continuum; that is, the doctor has a legal and ethical responsibility not only for the treatments they provide, but for treatments provided by other caregivers under their orders.

Because all of these types of doctors keep health records, many of which are becoming computerized, you may find yourself working as a health information professional in a chiropractic or dental office or a behavioral health practice. However, the most prevalent opportunities by far are in traditional medical practices and facilities. Therefore, let us discuss the role of the doctor in terms of the medical doctor (MD).

After completing college and medical school, medical doctors each select an area of medicine in which they wish to specialize. A few examples of these are general or family practice, pediatrics, obstetrics, gynecology, radiology, surgery, or internal medicine. There are 24 American boards of specialties that certify doctors for their specialties and subspecialties. A subspecialist focuses on a particular body system or disease. For example, within the specialty of internal medicine three subspecialties are gastroenterology, cardiovascular disease, and hematology. There are 14 more subspecialties just in internal medicine. The table in Figure 1-10 lists the specialties and subspecialties.

To perfect their areas of specialization, medical doctors practice medicine as *residents* under the supervision of established experienced physicians in their field of specialization. Although residents are licensed medical doctors, their medical licenses are limited and they cannot open their own practices until they have completed the period of residency.

In addition to tests given by state boards for medical licensing, each specialty has a medical board that sets standards of education and offers certification in that specialty and its various subspecialties. Doctors can take additional examinations to become *board certified* in their chosen

| Specialty | Subspecialty |
|---|---|
| Allergy and Immunology | |
| Anesthesiology | |
| | Critical Care Medicine |
| | Pain Medicine |
| Colon and Rectal Surgery | |
| Dermatology | |
| | Clinical & Laboratory Dermatological |
| | Immunology |
| | Dermatopathology |
| | Pediatric Dermatology |
| Emergency Medicine | |
| | Medical Toxicology |
| | Pediatric Emergency Medicine |
| | Sports Medicine |
| | Undersea and Hyperbaric Medicine |
| Family Medicine | |
| | Adolescent Medicine |
| | Geriatric Medicine |
| | Sleep Medicine |
| | Sports Medicine |
| Internal Medicine | |
| | Adolescent Medicine |
| | Cardiovascular Disease |
| | Clinical Cardiac Electrophysiology |
| | Critical Care Medicine |
| | Geriatric Medicine |
| | Gastroenterology |
| | Hematology |
| | Infectious Disease |
| | Interventional Cardiology |
| | Endocrinology, Diabetes and Metabolism |
| | Medical Oncology |
| | Nephrology |
| | Pulmonary Disease |
| | Rheumatology |
| | Sleep Medicine |
| | Sports Medicine |
| | Transplant Hepatology |
| Clinical Biochemical Genetics | |
| Clinical Cytogenetics | |
| Clinical Genetics (MD) | |
| | Medical Biochemical Genetics |
| Clinical Molecular Genetics | |
| | Molecular Genetic Pathology |
| PhD Medical Genetics | |
| Neurological Surgery | |
| Nuclear Medicine | |
| Obstetrics and Gynecology | |
| | Critical Care Medicine |
| | Gynecologic Oncology |
| | Maternal and Fetal Medicine |
| | Reproductive Endocrinology/Infertility |
| Ophthalmology | |
| Otolaryngology | |
| | Neurotology |
| | Pediatric Otolaryngology |
| | Sleep Medicine |
| | Plastic Surgery Within the Head and Neck |
| Pathology—Clinical | |
| Pathology—Anatomic | |
| Anatomic Pathology and Clinical Pathology | |
| | Blood Banking/Transfusion Medicine |
| | Chemical Pathology |
| | Cytopathology |
| | Dermatopathology |
| | Forensic Pathology |
| | Hematology |
| | Medical Microbiology |
| | Molecular Genetic Pathology |
| | Neuropathology |
| | Pediatric Pathology |

| Specialty | Subspecialty |
|---|---|
| Orthopaedic Surgery | |
| | Orthopaedic Sports Medicine |
| | Surgery of the Hand |
| Pediatrics | |
| | Adolescent Medicine |
| | Child Abuse Pediatrics |
| | Developmental-Behavioral Pediatrics |
| | Medical Toxicology |
| | Neonatal-Perinatal Medicine |
| | Neurodevelopmental Disabilities |
| | Pediatric Cardiology |
| | Pediatric Critical Care Medicine |
| | Pediatric Emergency Medicine |
| | Pediatric Endocrinology |
| | Pediatric Gastroenterology |
| | Pediatric Hematology-Oncology |
| | Pediatric Infectious Diseases |
| | Pediatric Nephrology |
| | Pediatric Pulmonology |
| | Pediatric Rheumatology |
| | Pediatric Transplant Hepatology |
| | Sleep Medicine |
| | Sports Medicine |
| Physical Medicine and Rehabilitation | |
| | Neuromuscular Medicine |
| | Pain Medicine |
| | Pediatric Rehabilitation Medicine |
| | Spinal Cord Injury Medicine |
| | Sports Medicine |
| Plastic Surgery | |
| | Plastic Surgery Within the Head and Neck |
| | Surgery of the Hand |
| Aerospace Medicine | |
| Occupational Medicine | |
| Public Health and General Preventive Medicine | |
| | Medical Toxicology |
| | Undersea and Hyperbaric Medicine |
| Psychiatry | |
| | Addiction Psychiatry |
| | Child and Adolescent Psychiatry |
| | Forensic Psychiatry |
| | Geriatric Psychiatry |
| Neurology | |
| | Clinical Neurophysiology |
| | Neurodevelopmental Disabilities |
| | Neuromuscular Medicine |
| | Pain Medicine |
| | Psychosomatic Medicine |
| | Sleep Medicine |
| | Vascular Neurology |
| Neurology with Special Qualifications in Child Neurology | |
| Diagnostic Radiology | |
| Radiation Oncology | |
| | Neuroradiology |
| | Nuclear Radiology |
| | Pediatric Radiology |
| | Vascular and Interventional Radiology |
| Radiologic Physics | |
| Surgery | |
| | Pediatric Surgery |
| | Surgery of the Hand |
| | Surgical Critical Care |
| Vascular Surgery | |
| Thoracic Surgery | |
| | Congenital Cardiac Surgery |
| Urology | |
| | Pediatric Urology |
| (Subspecialty certificate offered by many Boards) | |
| | Hospice and Palliative Medicine |

**FIGURE 1-10   Medical specialties and subspecialties[2]**

[2]American Board of Medical Specialties, Evanston, IL.

field. Board certification adds to the doctor's credentials and may be helpful in getting hospital privileges, malpractice insurance, and the respect of peers.

In any medical practice or healthcare facility, the doctor is in charge of the patient's care. For example, we noted earlier in the chapter that a patient can neither be admitted nor normally discharged from an inpatient hospital without a doctor's order. Doctors order medications, therapy, diagnostic tests, referrals, and consults with other physicians. With the exception of nurse practitioners and physician assistants (discussed in later sections), every medical order must be authorized by a doctor.

In addition to the responsibility for the patient's care, the doctor is also responsible for a great many documents concerning that patient. Doctors must sign manually or electronically the records of their examination of the patient. Doctors also manually or electronically sign off on test results and reports to indicate that they have reviewed them. Even the insurance claim submitted for the doctor's services must be authorized by the doctor. (Although claims are not usually signed physically by the physician, a signature form authorizing billing in the physician's name must be on file, and the physician is liable for all claims submitted by his or her office.)

Now that we understand the doctor is the source of almost all medical orders, as well as a substantial portion of the result reports and exam documentation, we can discuss their impact on the HIM profession. From a health information perspective, the doctor is both your customer and your supplier.

The doctor is a chief customer of HIM services because the patient health record is a vital reference tool on which the clinician relies to make decisions. Missing or incomplete health records can cause the physician to miss something important in the patient's condition or to create orders that conflict with the patient's other health conditions or allergies.

The doctor is also a key supplier of the information in the health record. In a medical practice the doctor's exam note is the primary focus of the chart. It not only represents the patient's past medical history and treatments, but is the required source document to substantiate the outpatient billing. Similarly, the doctor's orders are key elements in the chart for both inpatient and outpatient settings. Finally, it is the doctor's review and acceptance of documents within the chart that allow the HIM department to close and file the patient chart after discharge.

Healthcare organizations of every size and type are moving toward the use of electronic health records (EHRs). The concept of making sure providers remain happy customers of the HIM department is important to the HIM process. Nothing will stymie the process of computerizing patient records faster than a system in which the clinician cannot quickly find what he or she wants. Similarly, real-time electronic records require systems that work with the physician's workflow process, making it easy for the doctor to record exam notes and orders quickly and efficiently (Figure 1-11).

Finally, it is a mistaken belief that doctors are reluctant to embrace technology. In a modern medical office, you will see all sorts of electronic medical and diagnostic devices in use. What doctors are cautious about is anything that wastes their time without clear benefit to the patient and the practice.

It is important to understand that a doctor's practice is an unusual business model. For the most part, the only money earned by the practice is the amount reimbursed for the doctor's encounter with the patient. The entire cost of the building, insurance, supplies, and the salaries of the nurses, office staff, even the janitor must be paid from that single point of income. As you work with physicians in healthcare information technology and management, bear in mind this is one reason behind their demands for efficient systems.

**FIGURE 1-11**
**Physician examining a patient and recording the exam in an EHR.**

(Photo courtesy of GE Healthcare.)

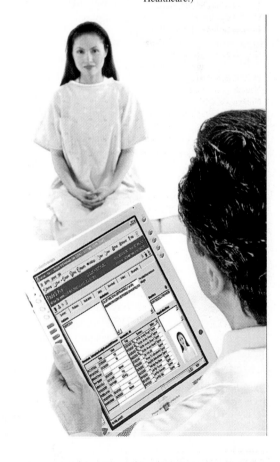

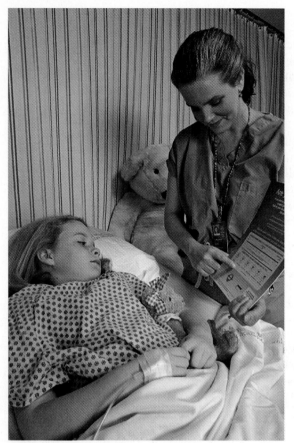

**FIGURE 1-12  A nurse uses a chart to help the patient determine her level of pain.**

**NURSES**   The larger portion of time spent delivering care to the patient is provided by nurses. Nurses are licensed professionals who have received training in patient care (Figure 1-12). The nursing profession offers several different nursing degrees and consequently different levels of nursing licensure with different levels of authority and responsibility, as discussed next.

**Licensed Practical Nurse**  Licensed practical nurses (LPNs) typically graduate from a vocational school or nonacademic nursing program where they have learned how to provide routine care for patients. LPNs are licensed only to work under the direct supervision of registered nurses or physicians. Nurses at this level are sometimes known as licensed vocational nurses (LVNs).

**Registered Nurse**  Registered nurses (RNs) receive academic training in hospital-based nursing schools, two-year community college nursing programs, or four-year baccalaureate degrees in nursing. RNs must pass state board examinations and be licensed by the state. Some nurses take postgraduate studies, earning master of science degrees or otherwise qualifying for higher levels of licensing that are discussed in a later section.

Registered nurses are licensed to administer medications, perform various medical procedures, and render care to the patient. RNs are trained to constantly assess the patient's condition, perform nursing interventions, and record extensive nursing notes about the patient's progress. Nurses may also specialize; some examples are surgical, intensive care, or psychiatric nurses.

With additional study and certification, RNs may qualify for licenses that allow them to perform some duties normally reserved for physicians. Here are three examples:

- Nurse practitioners, working in collaboration with a primary care physician, are permitted to provide a level of services similar to those offered by physicians, including diagnosing the patient and writing prescriptions.

- Certified Registered Nurse Anesthetists (CRNAs) administer anesthesiology during surgery, under the supervision of a medical doctor (an anesthesiologist.) This allows anesthesiologists to supervise multiple concurrent surgeries by having trained nurses acting in their place in the actual operating rooms.

- Nurse midwives receive additional training and are qualified in pregnancy, childbirth, and postpartum care. Midwives typically have a relationship with a medical doctor specializing in obstetrics should a medical emergency arise, but in cases of normal births, they do not need to be supervised or have a doctor present during delivery.

**PHYSICIAN ASSISTANTS**   Physician assistants (PAs) and surgeon assistants (SAs) work under the supervision of physicians to ease the physician's workload. PAs conduct physical exams, diagnose and treat illnesses, order and interpret tests, counsel on preventive healthcare, assist in surgery, and in virtually all states can write prescriptions. PA education consists of a 26-week intensive medical education program. Many PAs were nurses, emergency medical technicians (EMTs), or paramedics before entering the PA program.[3] PAs generally work in primary care offices and SAs work in hospitals or outpatient surgery facilities.

The difference between PAs and nurse practitioners is that PAs can only see patients while the doctor is in the facility; nurse practitioners, however, can practice on their own.

---

[3]Information about PAs and the PA profession, American Academy of Physician Assistants, www.aapa.org.

## *A REAL-LIFE STORY*

## A Nurse Practitioner Talks about Her Profession

*By Sharron Carr, ARNP-BC*

A nurse practitioner is a provider of healthcare. We provide healthcare and prevention in different primary care settings as well as specialized offices. Our duties are very similar to those of a physician. We can prescribe medications; order, perform, and interpret different diagnostic tests; provide treatment plans; and perform minor office procedures—we essentially do the same job that the physician does with the exception of the prescription of controlled substances. There are currently five states that don't allow that, but that will change.

Each state governs the way a nurse practitioner can operate within the state and the scope of practice that is available to that nurse practitioner. The requirement in my state is that I have a collaborating physician with whom I am associated. I file with the board each year a letter of agreement between my collaborating physician and myself, but I can be a private practitioner; I do not need to practice under the care of a physician or in the same office. That is one of the main differences between the role of a nurse practitioner and a physician assistant. The nurse practitioner can practice independently; a physician assistant can never practice without the physician on the premises.

Educationally, the training for a nurse practitioner and physician assistant is very similar, but the program requirements are not. Most people who enter the physician assistant program have their bachelor degree in some aspect of healthcare, but that is not mandatory. Then they progress on through their master's degree and graduate as a physician assistant. A nurse practitioner enters with a nursing degree (either an associate or bachelor degree in nursing) and the experience that goes along with that. We then advance into the master's degree level and graduate as a nurse practitioner.

Many types of nurse practitioner degrees are available and you can specialize within the practice as well. The Board of Nursing, the American Nursing Association, and the various societies are trying to adopt even higher levels of education and standards for nurse practitioners. In the future a doctorate degree may be required in order to practice as a nurse practitioner.

There is also a clinical component to our training. Anytime you obtain a nursing degree, there is always a clinical component that is assigned to provide you the skills you will need to practice at that level. So for the nurse practitioner level you are assigned within the type of care setting that you wish to work in when you leave school. For me it was a primary care office. We had four different semesters during which we were required to do clinical rotations. The number of hours that are required differed each semester. You rotate through different clinical settings. We started out on campus at the health science center and then spread out into community as the semesters progressed. The settings depend on what your specialty is. If you're in pediatrics, you would stay in the pediatric field; if you're into family medicine, you would be exposed to both pediatric and adult practices.

Nursing in general is a field that has many avenues to explore and you can choose many paths. If one is not the right fit for you, you can choose another path. As a nurse practitioner I feel like I have been able to make a difference in people's lives and promote healthcare and health in general to the population.

I started out in the world of nursing as an LPN, so I started out at the most basic level. As life allowed, I advanced my degree and advanced through the ranks of nursing. I went from LPN to an associate degree RN, and from that I went back to school and earned my bachelor and master's degrees. I am currently working on my doctorate.

As an RN I worked in a hospital setting on a renal intensive care unit and also did a little bit of management through that hospital. Subsequently, I began doing home infusion nursing, which I did for eight years. This is a very specialized, highly technological service for a registered nurse. I also assumed the director of nursing position and the director of professional services position within that company, giving me managerial experience as well.

My employer was eventually purchased by another company and was downsized. Though I was given a new job with the new company, after two years I decided I wanted to have more control over my working environment. I wanted to have responsibility for my own actions and to provide quality care. So I decided to go back to school and get my degree as a nurse practitioner. Now, by working on my doctorate, I hope to expand my knowledge and provide better care to my patients.

I am also involved in clinical trials research. My current family practice office participates in pharmaceutical clinical trials for new medications. I also continue my affiliation with a university where a few times each year I participate in their clinical trials research.

I think what makes a nurse practitioner different from a physician is the component of prevention. We bring that provision to healthcare; we take a more holistic approach. I am concerned with how the patient arrived at this point in their health when they present in front of me. What brought them to this level of illness? I look at environmental factors, their health behaviors, what their attitudes and beliefs are, and what their personal involvement is in their scheme of wellness. These are important concepts in the disease process. We look at a whole person rather than just treat the symptom.

The more knowledge that I receive and the more that I am exposed to in the healthcare industry, the more eager I am to know. It is a continually evolving field that I'm practicing in and I try to keep up with the latest technological advances to provide even better care to the patients that I serve.

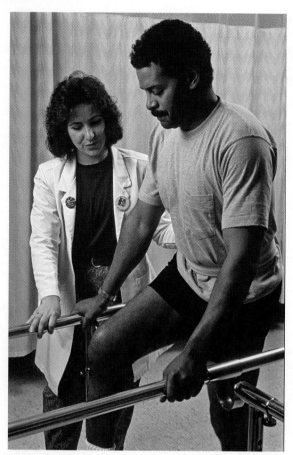

**FIGURE 1-13**

**A physical therapist assists a patient who is learning to walk again.**

(Mira.com/John Greim)

## Allied Healthcare Professions

Allied healthcare represents the categories of occupations involved in healthcare beyond those of doctors, nurses, and physician assistants. Allied healthcare professionals may be divided into two groups: those who provide clinical care services for the patient and those who provide nonclinical services to the healthcare organization or clinicians. Various HIM and information technology (IT) professions are examples of the latter group. In this chapter we discuss some of the clinical allied health professionals.

**CLINICAL ALLIED HEALTH PROFESSIONALS**  The American Medical Association (AMA) lists more than 60 allied health occupations in their annual publication *Health Professions Career and Education Directory*. These health professionals treat patients or perform tests based on the orders of doctors, nurse practitioners, or PAs. Most allied health occupations of a clinical nature require a degree or certification in the area of specialty, and many require examination and licensing by the state. The following sections discuss only a few examples of the many clinical allied health professions:

**Physical Therapists**  Physical therapists (PTs) work with many medical specialties to help patients regain strength, range of motion, and return to maximal functioning in daily activities. Patients include those with cardiovascular problems, neurological and congenital conditions, and those recovering from accidents, surgery, severe burns, or other types of wounds. PTs have a master's degree in physical therapy and work in acute care hospitals, rehabilitation hospitals, and physical therapy practices or provide home care visits. Figure 1-13 shows a physical therapist working in a rehabilitation facility.

**Occupational Therapists**  Occupational therapists (OTs) use work and play therapy to help patients improve their physical abilities, thereby reducing their level of disability and increasing their independence. Occupational therapists work under the direction of a physician. The OT begins by evaluating the patient, designing a program of therapy, and then working with the patient to meet the therapeutic goals. OTs have a bachelor or master's degree in occupational therapy.

**Respiratory Therapists**  Respiratory therapists (RTs) assess and treat patients with breathing disorders such as emphysema and asthma, as well as patients who have had a stroke, heart failure, embolism, or other pulmonary condition. RTs work in both inpatient and home care settings. In hospitals, RTs are an essential part of the ICU, emergency department, and cardiac arrest teams. They also provide therapy to hospitalized patients. RTs have an associate, bachelor, or master's degree and pass a certification exam.

**Clinical Laboratory Technicians**  Clinical laboratory technicians (also sometimes referred to as medical technicians or laboratory technicians) perform a wide variety of tests to analyze blood, urine, and other body fluids. This area is called clinical pathology and the technician works under a physician specialist called a pathologist. A related area of pathology called anatomic pathology is the study of human tissue samples from surgery, autopsy, and cytology.

**Phlebotomists**  Phlebotomists draw blood from patients. They are most often employed at hospitals, reference laboratories, and blood banks, though some larger medical practices and clinics may employ them as well. Phlebotomists receive training through a vocational program offered by a school or hospital.

**Diagnostic Technologists**  Diagnostic technologists operate various types of equipment used to capture diagnostic images for the physician. These allied health professionals include x-ray technicians, radiology technicians, sonographers, cardiovascular technologists, and MRI technicians.

**Pharmacists** Pharmacists not only formulate and dispense medications, but in many hospitals and some medical practices, they provide consultation to the physician as to the drugs being prescribed. In all settings, including retail drugstores, pharmacists check for conflicts and dangerous interactions with other medications the patient may be taking and advise the prescribing physician. Pharmacists complete four years of graduate school training and have a doctorate of pharmacy (also called a PharmD) degree.

**Dietitians** Nutritionists and dietitians are experts in nutrition. They have a bachelor degree in dietetics and hands-on experience in clinical practice, and they pass an examination to become a registered dietitian (RD). They evaluate patients' nutritional needs, plan diets, oversee food services in hospitals, and counsel patients in outpatient services.

**Audiologists** Audiologists measure how well patients hear and recommend and fit hearing aids for those with hearing problems.

**Speech Pathologists** Speech pathologists evaluate and provide treatment for patients with speech problems. Speech pathologists have a graduate degree (master's or doctorate) in speech or speech-language pathology. The American Speech-Language-Hearing Association (ASHA) offers a Certificate of Clinical Competence (CCC). State licensure boards may require the CCC, its equivalent, or waive certain requirements for CCC holders.

**Social Workers** Social workers evaluate patients to determine what social factors need to be addressed and help the patient obtain the proper assistance. In a hospital social workers participate in the patient's care plan and prior to discharge help facilitate services or care the patient may need at home. Social workers are also employed in many nonhospital, public health, and behavioral settings. In settings other than hospitals the term *client* is used instead of *patient* for persons receiving a social worker's services. The minimum educational requirement is a bachelor degree, although a master's degree in social work or a related field has become the standard for many positions.

**Medical Assistants** Medical assistants perform administrative and clinical tasks to keep the offices of physicians, podiatrists, chiropractors, and other health practitioners running smoothly. About 62 percent of medical assistants work in physicians' offices.[4]

The duties of medical assistants vary from office to office, depending on the location and size of the practice and the practitioner's specialty. In small practices, medical assistants usually do many different kinds of tasks, handling both administrative and clinical duties and reporting directly to an office manager, physician, or other health practitioner. Those in large practices tend to specialize in a particular area, under the supervision of department administrators. The administrative duties of medical assistants will be discussed in Chapter 2.

Clinical medical assistants' duties vary according to what is allowed by state law. Some common tasks include taking medical histories and recording vital signs, explaining treatment procedures to patients, preparing patients for examinations, and assisting physicians during examinations. Medical assistants collect and prepare laboratory specimens and sometimes perform basic laboratory tests on the premises, dispose of contaminated supplies, and sterilize medical instruments. They might instruct patients about medications and special diets, prepare and administer medications as directed by a physician, authorize drug refills as directed, telephone prescriptions to a pharmacy, draw blood, prepare patients for x-rays, take electrocardiograms, remove sutures, and change dressings.

Medical assistants also may arrange examining room instruments and equipment, purchase and maintain supplies and equipment, and keep waiting and examining rooms neat and clean.

Medical assistants are projected by the U.S. Department of Labor to be one of the fastest growing occupations during the next decade. Some medical assistants are trained on the job, but many complete one- or two-year programs. Ophthalmic medical assistants, optometric assistants, and podiatric medical assistants are examples of specialized assistants who have additional training and duties.

---

[4]*Occupational Outlook Handbook, 2008–09 Edition* (Washington, DC: U.S. Department of Labor Bureau of Labor Statistics, 2008).

Ophthalmic medical assistants help ophthalmologists provide eye care. They conduct diagnostic tests, measure and record vision, and test eye muscle function. They also show patients how to insert, remove, and care for contact lenses, and they apply eye dressings. Under the direction of the physician, ophthalmic medical assistants may administer eye medications. They also maintain optical and surgical instruments and may assist the ophthalmologist in surgery.

Optometric assistants also help provide eye care, working with optometrists. They provide chair-side assistance, instruct patients about contact lens use and care, conduct preliminary tests on patients, and otherwise provide assistance while working directly with an optometrist.

Podiatric medical assistants make castings of feet, expose and develop x-rays, and assist podiatrists in surgery.

**Home Health Aides**  A home health aide (HHA), also called a home care aide (HCA), provides assistance to patients in their home with tasks such as getting in or out of bed, bathing, or dressing. With additional training, HCAs can provide more extensive services in collaboration with a supervising registered nurse.

There are many other allied health professions, too numerous to describe here.

**NONCLINICAL ALLIED HEALTH PROFESSIONALS**    The term *nonclinical* applies to those occupations in healthcare that do not involve medical or diagnostic services to the patient. However, nonclinical jobs can involve substantial contact with patients. For example, medical office managers and registration and scheduling clerks may be some of the most familiar faces to regular patients at a clinic. They are often the first and last persons the patient sees. Though nonclinical, these allied health professionals impact the ability of the clinic to care for the patient by their attention to accuracy and detail. A similar impact on patient care can be caused by those who have little or no patient contact. Health information technicians (HITs), transcriptionists, computer system analysts, IT managers, and billing and coding specialists are examples of nonclinical personnel who have little direct contact with the patient but who ensure successful operation of the healthcare delivery system. Nonclinical allied health professionals will be covered in detail in Chapter 2.

## Organizations of Importance to Clinical Professionals

Most of the clinical professionals described in this chapter have an association or organization that is dedicated to improving their profession and providing support to their members. Though they are too numerous to describe all of them, three of them are well known and have a strong influence on the American healthcare system: the American Medical Association, the American Nurses Association, and the American Hospital Association.

### American Medical Association

The American Medical Association (AMA) is a voluntary association of physicians in the United States that sets standards for the medical profession and advocates on behalf of physicians. In line with its mission to promote the science and art of medicine and to improve public health, the AMA governs the accreditation of medical schools and residency programs.

The AMA also publishes numerous books and publications useful to its members. The most prestigious of these is the *Journal of the American Medical Association* (JAMA), a highly cited weekly medical journal that publishes peer-reviewed original medical research.

Founded in 1847, the AMA currently has approximately 300,000 members and wields tremendous influence in legislation and policy decisions affecting the practice of medicine with state and federal governments.[5]

### American Nurses Association

The American Nurses Association (ANA) advances the nursing profession by fostering high standards of nursing practice, promoting the rights of nurses in the workplace, projecting a positive and realistic view of nursing, and lobbying the Congress and regulatory agencies on healthcare issues affecting nurses and the public.

---

[5]American Medical Association, www.ama-assn.org.

Founded in 1897, the ANA currently represents the interests of approximately 2.9 million registered nurses.[6]

## American Hospital Association

Founded in 1898, the American Hospital Association (AHA) provides education for healthcare leaders and is a source of information on healthcare issues and trends. It currently has almost 5,000 members.

AHA advocacy efforts strive to ensure that members' perspectives and needs are heard and addressed in national health policy development, legislative and regulatory debates, and judicial matters.[7]

# Chapter 1 Summary

## Understanding Healthcare Facilities

Healthcare is provided in a variety of locations and facilities:

*Ambulatory care facilities* provide care to the patient that does not require or involve an overnight stay. This type of care is also called *outpatient care*. Because doctor offices are ambulatory facilities, ambulatory care vastly outnumbers other types of healthcare facilities. Ambulatory facilities may be owned by the physicians themselves or by a hospital or other healthcare organization.

*Acute care facilities* care for patients who have an illness or injury that is severe enough to require them to stay overnight one or more days. The term *inpatient* is also used for these facilities and the services they provide. When the average person uses the word *hospital* they usually mean an acute care facility. However, some other facilities where patients stay are also called hospitals. Most stays in an acute care facility do not exceed 30 days.

Acute care hospitals are often organized as separate departments within the hospital; for example, the surgical, radiologic, pediatric, and emergency departments, trauma center, intensive care unit, and the laboratory.

The emergency department or emergency room is a special exception. Although usually housed within the hospital building, ER services are considered outpatient services because patients do not stay more than a day before they are sent home or admitted to the hospital.

Hospitals may be owned by for-profit corporations or not-for-profit organizations, but are generally organized along similar lines:

- A Board of Directors or Board of Trustees establishes policy and manages the hospital by hiring a CEO or president who then manages other executives and all of the staff except the doctors.
- The doctors on the hospital medical staff are managed separately by a doctor who is called the chief of staff.
- Nurses are supervised by a chief of nursing who reports to the CEO.

*Subacute care facilities* include physical rehabilitation facilities, long-term care facilities, and home care. Subacute care facilities and home care services are appropriate for patients whose nursing care needs are less frequent and less intensive than the care offered in an acute care facility.

*Rehabilitation facilities* provide inpatient care while helping the patient return to the maximum functionality possible. Rehab facilities specialize in physical medicine, physical therapy, and occupational therapy, helping patients recover from the effects of accidents, severe injuries or illnesses, strokes, or serious surgery. Other rehabilitation facilities help patients detoxify and recover from dependence on alcohol or drugs.

Long-term care facilities provide care to patients who need inpatient services but at a less intense level than that provide at an acute care facility. Long-term care patients generally have a length of stay of greater than 30 days. Examples of long-term care facilities include skilled nursing facilities, nursing homes, residential care facilities, and rehabilitation hospitals.

*Home care* provides an important component of healthcare delivery, because it allows patients to remain in their homes rather than become inpatients. Home care is provided by home health agencies that send nurses, physical therapists, occupational therapists, or other healthcare providers to patients' homes on a regularly scheduled basis to provide care based on a physician's orders.

## Organizational Charts

Organizational charts are used in business and other organizations to illustrate the managerial relationship between the various jobs shown in the chart. In an organizational chart the most responsible position is listed at the top, the next level of management below that, then the next, and so forth. A given position is responsible for persons in the jobs connected to the vertical line below it. A horizontal line indicates two or more persons report to the same manager above them, but not to each other.

---

[6]American Nurses Association, www.nursingworld.org.

[7]American Hospital Association, www.aha.org

## Comparing Inpatient and Outpatient Facilities

There are many differences between inpatient and outpatient (ambulatory) facilities, including the following:

- In an ambulatory care facility, the patient does not stay overnight. In an acute care facility, the average length of stay (ALOS) is less than 30 days. In a long-term care facility, the ALOS is greater than 30 days.
- The size of an outpatient facility is measured by the number of patient *visits* or *encounters* per day. The size of inpatient facilities is measured by the number of *beds*. However, beds are counted in two ways: number of *licensed beds* and the *bed count*. The size of the facility is usually measured by the number of licensed beds. Daily operations at the facility are usually more concerned with the bed count.
- Ambulatory facilities do not have a formal admission/discharge procedure. Hospitals do have a formal admission process; a physical examination must be performed within 24 hours of admission. Normal hospital discharge requires a doctor's order.
- The date and time of hospital admission and discharge determine the LOS and the number of days for billing.

Another difference between inpatient and outpatient care is the amount of information gathered about each patient and the number of individuals who will need access to it.

Consider these characteristics of charts in an ambulatory setting such as a physician's office:

- The patient has a single chart that contains all records of the patient's visits and any reports or results received from other providers.
- The focus of the chart is the longitudinal care of the patient.
- The medical chart is primarily used by the physician and nurse, although it is also used briefly by the billing staff.
- The central element of the outpatient chart is the physician's notes about each visit.
- The quantity of data in an outpatient chart is usually much less than an inpatient chart.

Compare the ambulatory chart characteristics to the following characteristics of charts in an acute care hospital:

- Most hospitals start a new chart each time the patient is admitted.
- The focus of the chart is information related to the current stay.
- The inpatient chart is used extensively by a wide number of caregivers (doctors, nurses, therapists, pharmacists) as well as ward clerks and other administrative personnel.
- Physician exam notes tend to be brief; the main elements of the chart are the doctor's orders and the nurses' notes.

- The quantity of data is much greater for an inpatient chart. Vital signs and nurses notes are entered numerous times day and night, and there are typically many more orders for tests and medications.

## Healthcare Providers and Professions

Healthcare professions may be broadly categorized into two groups:

- *Direct care providers* provide healthcare services directly to the patient.
- Nonclinical allied health professionals serve the healthcare system but do not provide direct patient care. This group will be discussed in Chapter 2.

Doctors, nurses, and PAs provide care directly to the patient. In all states, these professionals must have a license and are typically regulated by professional or licensing boards. The time they spend with a patient and the actions they take and what they observe about the patient must be documented in the patient chart. As such, these providers are the chief contributors of information to the health record. They are also the principal user of the health record and depend on its accuracy and completeness to make accurate decisions about the patient. Clinical allied healthcare professionals also provide care directly to the patient. They perform tests or provide therapy and treatments based on the orders of a licensed provider such as a doctor, nurse practitioner, or PA. A few examples of these professionals include the following:

- Physical therapists (PTs) work with many medical specialties to help patients regain strength, range of motion, and return to maximal functioning in daily activities.
- Occupational therapists (OTs) evaluate the patient, design a program of therapy, and then using work and play therapy to help patients improve their physical abilities, thereby reducing their level of disability and increasing the patient's independence.
- Respiratory therapists (RTs) assess and treat patients with breathing problems caused by diseases such as emphysema or asthma or resulting from a stroke, heart attack, pulmonary embolism, or other trauma. In hospitals, they are an essential part of the ICU, emergency department, and cardiac arrest teams. They also provide therapy to hospitalized patients.
- Clinical laboratory technicians, medical technicians, and laboratory technicians work under a physician specialist called a pathologist, performing a wide variety of tests to analyze blood, urine, and other body fluids.
- Phlebotomists draw blood from persons who need blood tests or are donating blood or plasma.
- Diagnostic technologists include x-ray technicians, radiology technicians, sonographers, cardiovascular technologists, and MRI technicians. They operate various types of instruments to capture images that help the physician diagnose the patient.

- Pharmacists formulate and dispense medications, consult with the physician prescribing the drugs, and check for conflicts and dangerous interactions with other medications the patient may be taking.
- Registered dietitians (RDs) and nutritionists are experts in nutrition. They evaluate patients' nutritional needs, plan diets, oversee food services in hospitals, and counsel patients in outpatient services.
- Audiologists measure how well patients hear and recommend and fit hearing aids for those with hearing problems.
- Speech pathologists evaluate and provide treatment for patients with speech problems.
- Social workers determine what social factors need to be addressed and help their clients obtain the proper assistance. Hospital social workers participate in the patient's care plan and prior to discharge help facilitate services or care the patients may need at home.
- Medical assistants perform administrative and clinical tasks. In small practices, medical assistants usually do many different kinds of tasks, handling both administrative and clinical duties and reporting directly to an office manager, physician, or other health practitioner. Those in large practices tend to specialize in a particular area, under the supervision of department administrators.
- Clinical medical assistants take medical histories, record vital signs, explain treatment procedures to patients, prepare patients for examinations, and assist physicians during examinations.
- Home health aides provide assistance to patients in their home with tasks such as getting in or out of bed, bathing, or dressing.

## Organizations of Importance to Clinical Professionals

Organizations of importance to clinical professionals are the American Medical Association (AMA), the American Nurses Association (ANA), and the American Hospital Association (ANA), plus numerous others.

## Critical Thinking Exercises

1. Which department discussed in this chapter is located in an inpatient hospital, but is considered an outpatient facility?
2. If a patient seen in this department is sent home but is admitted as an inpatient in three days or less how does that affect the hospital's billing?

## Testing Your Knowledge of Chapter 1

1. What is the difference between an ambulatory care and an acute care facility?
2. What is the difference between an acute care and a long-term care facility?
3. An inpatient is admitted June 10 and discharged June 14. What was the LOS?
4. What type of nurse can diagnose patients and write orders?
5. What does the acronym CIO stand for?
6. Is a hospital emergency department an inpatient or ambulatory facility?
7. What is a subacute facility?
8. Name three clinical allied health professions.
9. Explain the difference between the number of licensed beds and a hospital's bed count.
10. Why would the bed count and number of licensed beds be different?

11. How can the number of discharges be used to measure a hospital's capacity?

*For each of the following statements circle true if it is correct, or false if the statement is not true:*

12. Hospitals have a formal admission and discharge process.

   *True*          *False*

13. A physical exam must be performed on a patient within 72 hours of a hospital admission.

   *True*          *False*

14. The hospital CEO is in charge of all medical staff.

   *True*          *False*

15. Hospitals start a new chart each time a patient is admitted.

   *True*          *False*

# 2 Health Information Professionals

## LEARNING OUTCOMES

After completing this chapter, you should be able to:

- Describe the history of health information management and organizations
- Differentiate the roles of health information professionals
- Describe the organizational hierarchy of HIM and IT departments
- Compare various nonclinical allied healthcare occupations
- Explain the role of a project manager
- Understand how skill sets from multiple disciplines can help you in your career

## ACRONYMS USED IN CHAPTER 2

Acronyms are used extensively in both medicine and computers. The following acronyms are used in this chapter.

| | | | |
|---|---|---|---|
| **AAPC** | American Academy of Professional Coders | **CTR** | Certified Tumor Registrar |
| **ACMPE** | American College of Medical Practice Executives | **DISA** | Data Interchange Standards Association (within ANSI) |
| **ACS** | American College of Surgeons | **DRG** | Diagnosis-Related Group |
| **AHDI** | Association for Healthcare Documentation Integrity | **EDI** | Electronic Data Interchange |
| | | **EHR** | Electronic Health Record |
| **AHIMA** | American Health Information Management Association | **EMR** | Electronic Medical Record |
| | | **HCPCS** | Healthcare Common Procedure Coding System |
| **AMIA** | American Medical Informatics Association | **HIM** | Health Information Management |
| **ANSI** | American National Standards Institute | **HIMSS** | Healthcare Information and Management Systems Society |
| **APC** | Ambulatory Payment Classification | **HIPAA** | Health Insurance Portability and Accountability Act |
| **ARLNA** | Association of Record Librarians of North America | **HIS** | Health Information System |
| | | **HIT** | Health Information Technology; Health Information Technician |
| **CCOW** | Clinical Context Object Workgroup | **HL7** | Health Level 7 (within ANSI) |
| **CEO** | Chief Executive Officer | **ICD-9-CM** | International Classification of Diseases, Ninth Revision, Clinical Modification |
| **CIO** | Chief Information Officer | | |
| **CIS** | Clinical Information System | | |
| **CMT** | Certified Medical Transcriptionist | **IOM** | Institute of Medicine |
| **COO** | Chief Operating Officer | **IT** | Information Technology |

| | | | |
|---|---|---|---|
| **JCAHO** | Joint Commission on Accreditation of Healthcare Organizations (now referred to simply as the Joint Commission) | **PHI** | Protected Health Information |
| | | **PRO** | Peer Review Organization (now Quality Improvement Organization) |
| **MGMA** | Medical Group Management Association | **QIO** | Quality Improvement Organization (Formerly Peer Review Organization) |
| | | **RFID** | Radio-Frequency Identification |
| **NAHQ** | National Association for Healthcare Quality | **RHIA** | Registered Health Information Administrator |
| **NCRA** | National Cancer Registrars Association | **RHIT** | Registered Health Information Technician |
| **OR** | Operating Room | **SDO** | Standards Developing Organization (within ANSI) |
| **PDF** | Portable Document Format | | |

# History of Health Information Management and Organizations

Thus far we have discussed facilities and locations where healthcare is delivered and the roles of the doctors and clinical allied healthcare workers who provide *direct care* to the patient. These direct care professionals create and use the health information record. In this chapter we explore some of the nonclinical healthcare professions involved in managing health information once it is recorded. We will also discuss a few of the professional associations and standards setting organizations that have been created to improve healthcare information systems and support those who work in the field of health information.

The concept of creating and maintaining complete and accurate medical records as a necessity of healthcare is less than a century old. When the American College of Surgeons (ACS) sought to improve the results of surgery by establishing minimum standards for hospitals, they included requirements that hospitals keep records of the care and treatment of their patients. Prior to the ACS initiative in 1918, records of hospitalized patients were the responsibility of the attending physician and were filed "as is" upon the patient's discharge. These early records generally consisted of nurses' notes and often did not include admitting or discharge diagnoses.

The ACS addressed this issue by including record-keeping requirements in its Hospital Standardization Program:

> "Accurate and complete medical records [must] be written for all patients and filed in an accessible manner in the hospital, a complete medical record being one which includes identification data; complaint; personal and family history; history of the present illness; physical examination; special examinations such as consultations, clinical laboratory, x-ray and other examinations; provisional or working diagnosis; medical or surgical treatment; gross or microscopical pathological findings; progress notes; final diagnosis; condition on discharge; follow-up; and, in case of death, autopsy findings."[1]

In complying with the program, hospitals soon created positions for medical records clerks to examine the medical records for missing reports, ensure their completion, and store them by some logical filing method.

A decade after the ACS initiated its program, an organization was formed by records clerks and named the Association of Record Librarians of North America. This was the precursor of the health information profession. The organization changed its name to the American Association of Record Librarians in 1941 and to the American Medical Record Association in 1970. In 1991 the name was updated to reflect an evolution from record keeping to managing health information.

---

[1]*Bulletin of the American Association of Medical Record Librarians* (March 1941): 101.

Today the organization is the American Health Information Management Association (AHIMA). AHIMA will be discussed further later in this chapter.

From its inception, the early organization sought to improve the profession by formulating a curriculum of study and accrediting schools to provide training for medical record librarians. AHIMA continues that process today by sponsoring the Commission on Accreditation for Health Informatics and Information Management Education.

## From Record Systems to Information Systems

During its first 60 years, members of the medical records profession improved the processing and handling of patient records. Charts were analyzed for deficiencies and missing items were obtained. Charts were tracked, stored, retrieved, and indexed in various ways.

Chart contents were standardized somewhat through the creation of specific forms for specific purposes. For example, admission, discharge, physical exams, doctor's orders, and nurses' notes were recorded on forms designed by a forms committee and maintained by the medical records department. This process is called *forms control* and is still used today.

However, there was little standardization of medical information in the reports, except that it appeared in the appropriate box on the form. In other words medical records did not use a standard data set or clinical vocabulary. (Data sets and clinical vocabulary will be explained in Chapters 4 through 7.)

Medical records departments were focused and organized around the chart as a physical object to be moved around the hospital with the patient, then moved to the abstracting and billing departments, and finally stored for the long term. Medical records departments became better at chart handling, but at a cost estimated to be from 25 to 40 percent of a hospital's operating budget.[2]

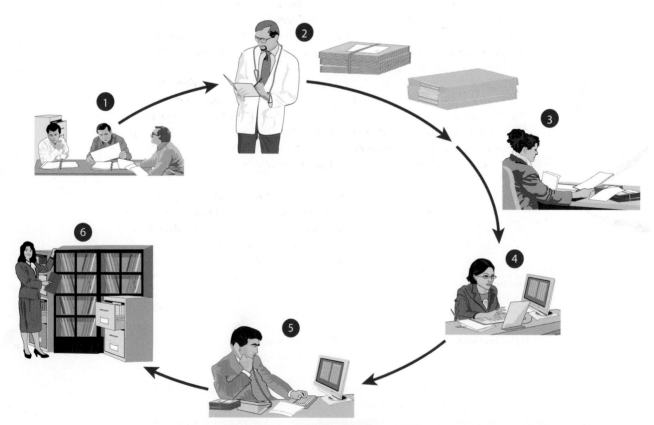

**FIGURE 2-1   Flow of inpatient information using a paper chart.**

---

[2]B. I. Blum, *Clinical Information Systems* (New York: Springer-Verlag, 1986).

Figure 2-1 shows the workflow of traditional charts:

1. Forms control is the first step. Committees meet to design and approve forms to be used in the facility. Forms are then distributed to various departments.
2. Caregivers record nurses' notes, doctor's orders, and other documents during the patient's stay.
3. Upon discharge, the patient's chart is collected, assembled, and analyzed by the health information management (HIM) department.
4. The chart is then abstracted and assigned codes for billing.
5. The chart is examined for completeness. If documents or signatures are missing, HIM personnel contact doctors or other departments to correct the chart deficiencies.
6. When the chart is complete, it is filed.

Regulatory reporting, billing, and accreditation requirements made it increasingly necessary to be able to abstract, aggregate, and report information collected from the charts of all patients treated by the facility. It became obvious that the task had evolved from managing health records to managing health information (which included managing the charts). Thus, in 1991 the American Medical Record Association became the American Health Information Management Association and the name for this profession was changed to health information management.

## HIM, HIT, and HIS

The renamed health information management (HIM) departments continued to compile, provide, and control access to patient records, as well as ensure the completeness and accuracy of those records. Other HIM functions include coding, abstracting, and aggregating health information for billing, reporting, and research purposes. However, two other changes significantly affected the field of health information management, as discussed next.

First, beginning in about 1970, hospitals began to install computer systems. At first these were large central computers called *mainframes,* which required special technicians to operate. Although mainframes did not contain much actual patient medical information, the department was called the health information system (HIS) department. By 1990, computer terminals and networked computers were prevalent in every department. By 1996 the majority of ambulatory facilities had computerized as well; 85 percent of physicians in private practices were using computers to run their offices.[3]

Facilities were becoming computerized but the HIS or information technology (IT) department was not usually a part of HIM. Furthermore, IT employees were not health information technicians (HITs), who report to the health information management administrator. This was a problem. If health information was going to be stored on and managed by computers, there needed to be coordination in defining content and maintaining security. One solution common at many facilities is to place both departments under the chief information officer (CIO).

The second major change for HIM occurred in 1996 when Congress passed the Health Insurance Portability and Accountability Act (HIPAA). HIPAA will be covered extensively in Chapter 3, but briefly its effect on HIM and HIS was threefold:

1. It mandated protection for the privacy of patient records.
2. It established specific standards for data codes and data sets.
3. It required security policies for patient information stored electronically.

---

[3]Medical Manager Research and Development, Alachua, FL.

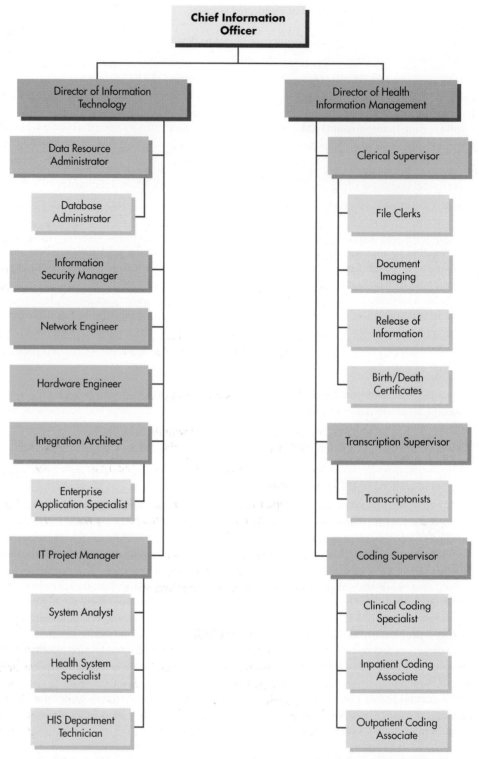

**FIGURE 2-2**    **Abridged organizational chart for IT and HIM departments under the CIO.**

## Increased Computerization

Hospitals and some ambulatory facilities are accredited by the Joint Commission (JCAHO) discussed in Chapter 3. The Joint Commission views health information as an important resource to be managed and states that "managing health information is an active, planned activity."[4] However, the increasing number of documents being produced per patient and the fact that information stored in thousands of paper charts is not easy to use to improve health brought about an interest in computerizing the records.

In the past century, medical records were primarily paper and, unfortunately, in most facilities they still are. In 1991 the Institute of Medicine (IOM) called for the creation of "an electronic patient record that resides in a system specifically designed to support users by providing accessibility to complete and accurate data, alerts, reminders, clinical decision support systems, links to medical knowledge, and other aids."[5]

Almost two decades later, ambulatory as well as acute care facilities are moving from paper to electronic medical record systems. As a result, health information managers must become well acquainted with information technology. Today, even paper forms are often designed to facilitate scanning into electronic health records.

As facilities have moved away from paper toward electronic records, the IT and HIM departments have become more intertwined. For that reason many healthcare facilities put both departments under the authority of the CIO as shown in the organizational chart in Figure 2-2.

Before proceeding to the next section, let us review some of the acronyms used for these departments and positions because they are so similar. Detailed job descriptions are provided later in the chapter.

- The chief information officer (CIO) is responsible for all of the hospital information systems, both HIM and IT departments.
- Health information management (HIM) is concerned with the security, accuracy and completeness of the health records and the information that can be reported from them.
  - A health information technician (HIT) is an HIM employee usually focused on a specific aspect of the HIM department.
- The information technology (IT) department operates the health information system (HIS) computers. The IT department may also be responsible for the phone systems and other computers as well.
  - IT technicians (also called network technicians, system analysts, database administrators, etc.) keep the computers operating. Although they may need to access patient information to do their job, they do not enter or use health information.

# Health Information Professionals

There are many nonclinical allied health professions available in the health information field. Some of these jobs are more prevalent in inpatient acute care facilities than outpatient settings. A large hospital may have a number of people who perform the same job, for example, coding specialists in the billing department. In smaller clinics, a single person may perform multiple jobs. For example, a small single-doctor practice may have only two office staff and they might each perform several HIM tasks.

Also some jobs are *outsourced* to a company that specializes in a particular HIM service. A typical example of this is medical transcription, which is often done by transcriptionists who work for a transcription service company, not the doctor. Another example might be computer security consultants or system trainers who may work for the HIS vendor, not the hospital or doctor.

---

[4]*Comprehensive Accreditation Manual for Hospitals* (Chicago: Joint Commission, 2005), IM-1.

[5]R. S. Dick and E. B. Steen, *The Computer-based Patient Record: An Essential Technology for Health Care* (Washington, DC: National Academy Press, 1991, revised 1997, 2000).

## Building an All-Digital Hospital

*By Tanya Townsend*

> *Tanya Townsend is the director of information technology at Saint Clare's Hospital in Schofield, Wisconsin. Tanya has a master's degree in medical informatics.*

When Ministry Health Care decided to construct Saint Clare's Hospital, one of the objectives was to try to use only digital records. Potentially, what was accomplished at our hospital could then be rolled out to the other 14 Ministry hospitals. I was fortunate to be involved in the development of this wonderful new facility.

I originally started out in health information management, but even as I was finishing school it was apparent that everything was going to change to electronic patient records. I wanted to get involved in the IT portion of making that happen, so I went on to get my master's in medical informatics.

Initially I worked as an analyst on a health information management system, which was perfect because of my HIM background. From there I continued to evolve in healthcare IT. I worked on starting a new hospital in Green Bay, Wisconsin. I was responsible for all of the application installation and coordination there. Saint Clare is actually the third new construction hospital I've had the opportunity to be a part of.

Our core objective at Saint Clare's was to come up with the highest level of operational efficiency that could be achieved using technology as well as patient safety, clinical excellence, and great customer service—all of that can be facilitated through technology.

Saint Clare's Hospital is partnered with an ambulatory setting, the Marshfield Clinic. We needed the hospital systems to integrate data with the ambulatory setting and any departmental applications that we had. Based on a detailed system selection process, we went with a best-of-breed approach and interfaced the systems by using HL7 and CCOW. *[Author's note: HL7 stands for Health Level Seven and CCOW stands for Clinical Context Object Workgroup.]*

We wanted to make sure we were supporting and optimizing the flow of information across the continuum of healthcare. So whether you are in the ambulatory clinic, in the hospital, in the emergency department, even in the OR [operating room], we have all of those systems tied together. Eliminating duplication and providing information anytime, anyplace is a win for the patient as well as the provider.

One of the key things that made us very successful was that [the process] was very collaborative. For this campus we used a project management office extensively on both IT as well as non-IT projects to pull everything together.

As we started developing and designing, we realized there were no maps to follow as we were pioneers in building this all-digital hospital. It was suggested we document each process. What steps were involved in performing a given task? We created a map of the procedure to ensure we were all on the same page, operating under the same assumptions. We called these *process maps* and developed 8,400 pages of them. That was integral for the rest of our success.

One of the challenges with a new facility is not having any patient population while designing it. A key piece of our implementation was taking those 8,400 process maps and working through simulations, just to make sure there were no errors and that it was going to flow the way we envisioned it. It was a good practice that we continue even today. If we are adding a new service line or adding a new order set, we do simulations of walking it through to make sure we didn't miss anything.

When it came to selecting systems, we didn't necessarily need to start completely from scratch. We could examine tools used within other hospitals in the organization and see what was working well for them. We also worked closely with Marshfield Clinic, which already had a home-grown EMR (electronic medical record) and had collaborated with St. Joseph's Hospital for many years. So we already had working relationships and interfaces across our organizations. Once we selected what would be used from existing systems, we then did a gap analysis.

One of the core gaps we found in our analysis was a need for scanning (to eliminate paper records). For example, a patient referral, a patient transfer, or anything that comes in on paper is scanned at the point of service. We immediately send the paper to HIM so they can do a quality check and make sure the scanning went through okay, and then they destroy the paper.

There are also some events that might be initially documented on paper. For example, a trauma event where we don't know who the patient is gets started on paper. However, as soon as we get the patient identified we scan that document in and it becomes a digital record.

Another solution developed because of that gap analysis is called *digital ink over forms*. This is a unique tool developed by Marshfield Clinic that allows us to bridge gaps knowing that we don't have a technological solution for every form we can imagine. We can create a digital form that looks like a PDF (Portable Document Format); then using a Tablet PC and the stylus we can document it online and save it in the patient's chart.

The hospital doors opened in October 2005. It has been a unique opportunity with a brand new building, new people, and new systems to start with an all-digital record. As we continue to evolve, we continue to use the techniques that worked initially and we now have a change control process rolling out enhancements to the system on a continuous basis. We do integration testing at different stages of development and use our process maps to make sure we understand how a change will flow in actual use.

## HIM Department Professionals

Figure 2-3 shows how some of the jobs listed in this chapter would be arranged on an organizational chart for the HIM department of an acute care hospital. The chart shows the chain of command, or responsibility, for various positions typically found in such a facility. Not all of the jobs discussed next are shown in the organizational chart. Also job titles may vary slightly by facility.

**HEALTH INFORMATION DIRECTOR or MANAGER**   The health information manager is responsible for the HIM department and services. This includes implementing and monitoring HIM systems, policies, and procedures; educating employees; and enforcing confidentiality, information security, information storage and retrieval, and record retention policies. The HIM manager or director also coordinates preparation for audits by accreditation groups and regulatory agencies. The health information director's qualifications nearly always include being a Registered Health Information Administrator (RHIA).

**REGISTERED HEALTH INFORMATION ADMINISTRATOR**   Health information administrators serve as managers or directors of the HIM department. They are responsible for other HIM workers who enter, store, retrieve, and protect medical records data. They are also involved in forms control and liaison with nearly every department concerning health information and strategic planning. A Registered Health Information Administrator (RHIA) has a bachelor or master's degree and has passed a certification exam offered by AHIMA.

**REGISTERED HEALTH INFORMATION TECHNICIAN**   Health information technicians enter medical records data into computer systems and validate their accuracy and completeness. Health information technicians may also perform coding for billing departments, work with the cancer registry, or generate reports from patient data to support administrative functions of the hospital. Health information technicians who pass certification exams can become Registered Health Information Technicians (RHITs), which is a step toward advancement into management and supervisory positions.

**CLINICAL DATA SPECIALIST**   The clinical data specialist is responsible for ensuring the accuracy and completeness of clinical coding, validating the data, and performing clinical research reports. A clinical data specialist audits the accuracy of clinical coding specialists, and validates data the facility uses for reporting to various disease registries. Research includes preparing outcomes management, utilization analyses, and patient and provider profile reports, as well as extracting information for special clinical research projects.

**CLINICAL CODING SPECIALIST**   Clinical coding specialists, also called coding and reimbursement specialists, review a patient's medical records for an inpatient stay or outpatient encounter to assign standard codes for the patient's diagnosis and the services the patient received. The codes are necessary for billing the patient's insurance plan and standardizing the data.

The coding specialist typically enters the codes into a computer system, which determines the amount to be billed from a *charge master*. If the codes have already been entered by someone else or sent over from another system, the coding specialist reviews the codes for correctness. In cases where the clinical documents are incomplete or inconsistent, the coding specialist communicates with the provider to clarify the record.

The codes used are national standards, such as the International Classification of Diseases, Ninth Revision, Clinical Modification (ICD-9-CM) and Healthcare Common Procedure Coding System (HCPCS) and procedure modifier codes. Every year the organizations that maintain the standard codes add new codes and delete old ones. Clinical coding specialists must keep up with the annual changes as well as changes in rules as to when certain codes may or may not be used.

If the coding specialist is employed at an inpatient facility, the diagnosis-related groups (DRGs) or ambulatory payment classification (APC) codes also need to be determined.

Coding specialists may be credentialed by two professional organizations, AHIMA and AAPC.

**CODING ASSOCIATE**   Coding associate is an entry-level position. They review patients' medical records and assign the correct ICD-9-CM and HCPCS codes for billing purposes. Their work is then reviewed by a coding specialist.

**Abridged organizational chart for an acute care HIM department.**

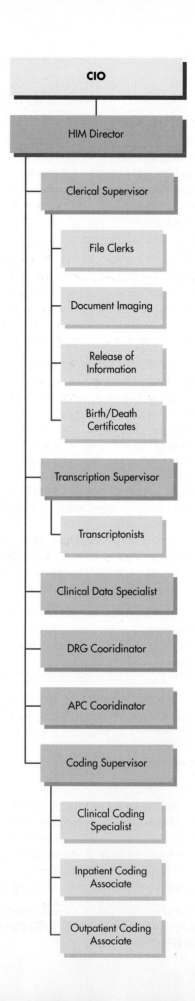

**DRG COORDINATOR**    The DRG coordinator works at inpatient hospitals where billing and reimbursement is tied to Medicare diagnosis-related groups (DRGs). The DRG coordinator reviews inpatient records to ensure the correct ICD-9-CM and DRG codes have been assigned. A DRG coordinator must be thoroughly familiar with all DRG rules and keep abreast of changes to the codes, guidelines, and billing rules.

The DRG coordinator's job is to optimize reimbursement through correct billing and documentation. This includes responding to DRG change and denial notices by supplying appropriate source documentation to the quality improvement organization (QIO) when appealing a QIO decision. (Note QIO was formerly called peer review organization or PRO.) DRG coordinators also study the inpatient case mix to monitor trends and determine is if changes are due to changing patient demographics or coding errors.

**APC COORDINATOR**    Medicare uses an ambulatory payment classification (APC) system to determine reimbursement for outpatient claims. The APC coordinator works for an inpatient facility that offers outpatient services to Medicare patients. The APC coordinator reviews encounter and claim data to verify that the correct ICD-9-CM, HCPCS codes, procedure modifiers, and APC groups have been used. The coordinator also checks to see if any secondary diagnoses or procedures have been missed. The coordinator's job also includes keeping up with any new APC mandates or outpatient reporting requirements to ensure continuing facility compliance.

**MEDICAL TRANSCRIPTIONIST**    A medical transcriptionist creates medical documents by listening to a recording and typing what is heard into a document. Most commonly these are history and physical reports, operative reports, discharge summaries, consultations, progress notes, and radiology reports. The finished document is reviewed and signed by the physician, then made part of the patient's chart. Transcriptionists also transcribe letters, referrals, and summary reports sent between physicians. In hospitals they may also transcribe minutes of committee meetings.

The Association for Healthcare Documentation Integrity (AHDI) (formerly American Association for Medical Transcription) offers a voluntary credentialing exam to individuals who wish to become Registered Medical Transcriptionists (RMTs). After two years of acute care experience, transcriptionists can become Certified Medical Transcriptionists (CMTs) by passing the AHDI certification exam.

Speech recognition software can replace medical transcription by converting the spoken word directly into text using a computer. However, computer speech recognition software is imperfect and medical transcriptionists are often employed to review, edit, and format the computer-generated text.

**CANCER REGISTRAR**    Cancer or tumor registrars collect and report cancer statistics to state cancer registries. The cancer registrar works with physicians, surgeons, and healthcare administrators to collect data, enter it into a cancer database, and generate reports, which are submitted to appropriate agencies. The cancer registrar is responsible for collecting and maintaining complete, accurate records. Cancer registrars can become certified through the ACS.

**HIM COMPLIANCE SPECIALIST**    An HIM compliance specialist provides training to hospital personnel including doctors, coding staff, billing staff, and ancillary departments about topics such as appropriate documentation and accurate coding to further the organization's HIM compliance program. The HIM compliance specialist may also be involved in monitoring and auditing the accuracy of coding and completeness of documentation and may serve on HIM compliance committees.

**OPTICAL IMAGING COORDINATOR**    An optical imaging coordinator implements and trains users on document imaging systems, monitors the workflow, and serves as a liaison between the HIM and IT departments. As more facilities have begun to store paper charts as images in computer records systems, employment in this profession has become more prevalent.

## IT Department Professionals

Figure 2-4 shows how some of the jobs listed below would be arranged on an organizational chart for the IT department of an acute care hospital. As with the previous chart, not all of the jobs listed below are shown in the organizational chart.

**FIGURE 2-4**

**Abridged organizational chart for a hospital IT department.**

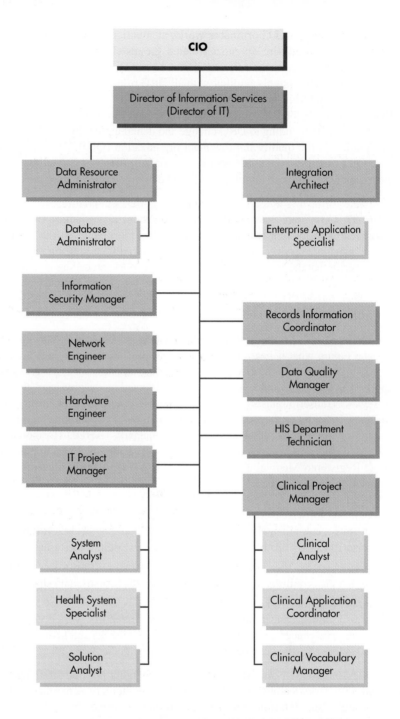

**INFORMATION SERVICES OR INFORMATION TECHNOLOGY DIRECTOR OR MANAGER**    The information services or IT director or manager oversees all aspects of the hospital computer systems and is responsible for the infrastructure of the health information system, technical staff, and budget. Responsibilities include supervising the computer network, databases, programming, applications, network security and administration, database administration, strategic planning, and development of new information services. In some facilities the telecom systems are also the responsibility of the director of IT. The information services director works closely with the HIM director.

**CLINICAL PROJECT MANAGER AND IT PROJECT MANAGER**    Project managers help organizations determine the scope of work, objectives, budget, schedule, and who is responsible for each component. Once the project is under way, the project manager tracks the progress of each component and advises management when projects are off budget or schedule. The job is very detail oriented and also requires good planning, risk analysis, and communication skills.

Clinical project managers and IT project managers do the same work, within their respective areas of the organization. When the two areas overlap, the project managers will communicate with each other frequently.

**CLINICAL ANALYST**    A clinical analyst studies the workflow of electronic health record (EHR) users, and then adds data or customizes the EHR to make it as efficient and as easy to use as possible. EHR systems may or may not come with a standardized nomenclature. The clinical content supplied with the system may not be organized in a way the provider can access quickly. The clinical analyst designs and builds forms, lists, order sets, and other clinical content into the EHR systems to help users quickly document patients' medical information.

Clinical analysts often meet with multidisciplinary teams to determine what is needed. They often are responsible for testing their designs and training users on modifications to the system. Clinical analysts develop a broad knowledge of their facilities' EHR systems and often test and troubleshoot problems with the applications.

**CLINICAL VOCABULARY MANAGER**    As you will learn in Chapter 7, most EHR systems use standardized codes and terms for recording symptoms, diseases, drugs, and many other medical components of the patient record. These are variously referred to as *clinical terminologies, vocabularies,* or *nomenclatures.* They are different from and more detailed than the codes used by coding specialists for billing.

Because there are many different aspects of the medical record, many different coding standards, and many different software systems in use, larger organizations may assign a person to coordinate it all. A clinical vocabulary manager has responsibility for recommending and maintaining the clinical vocabularies to be used.

Where multiple software applications use different codes, the clinical vocabulary manager supervises data tables that translate codes between different systems. Clinical vocabulary managers keep up with developments in standardized nomenclature and handle requests for new codes if users determine that the vocabulary is missing certain terms.

**CLINICAL APPLICATIONS COORDINATOR**    Clinical applications coordinators work for an inpatient facility that uses multiple software packages. They coordinate the issues of integrating different applications, follow up with vendors to correct deficiencies in the software, and manage the software parameters that affect the applications. They also coordinate implementation of new software and schedule training for users.

**DATA QUALITY MANAGER**    The data quality manager is responsible for ensuring that the healthcare data used for coding and reimbursement, health records, and documentation is accurate and consistent. The data quality manager does this by implementing and maintaining a data quality plan, by auditing the quality of the data, and by review of the data entry processes.

Where data is received from other hospitals or other healthcare partners, the data quality manager works to ensure that the data is accurate and meets the organization's standards.

**DATA RESOURCE ADMINISTRATOR**    The data resource administrator is responsible for data resource management policies and procedures to ensure that the organization's data are secure, accessible, accurate, and reliable. The data resource administrator works with HIM, IT, the data quality manager, database manager, and data analysts to manage the organization's data repository and data warehouse.

As the organization's information storage needs increase, the data resource administrator participates in forecasting growth, strategic planning, budgeting, and purchases of new IT systems.

**DECISION SUPPORT ANALYST**    The decision support analyst coordinates data and research for senior managers at the corporate level of the integrated system, providing ongoing data analysis relevant to the healthcare market and assisting in problem solving, solution development, decision making, and strategic planning. For example, the decision support analyst may extract statistical data from the hospital's database for comparison to similar measures extracted from a national database.

**HEALTH INFORMATION SERVICES DEPARTMENT TECHNICIAN**    HIS technicians provide technical and administrative assistance and implement HIS policies and procedures. They also assist in accreditation review preparation.

**ENTERPRISE APPLICATIONS SPECIALIST** In large organizations where many different software applications are interfaced, an enterprise application specialist provides expertise and guidance to ensure that data stored in different systems is available throughout the *enterprise* (organization). This includes communicating with those responsible for the various applications as well as the master patient index that ties them all together.

Because enterprise-wide sharing of information must conform to HIPAA and other privacy regulations, the enterprise application specialist works closely with the privacy and security officers and must be knowledgeable concerning privacy and security policies and procedures. The enterprise application specialist must understand the EHR, clinical data repository, any enterprise-wide software, and the systems with which they interact.

**INTEGRATION ARCHITECT** Healthcare facilities that use software applications from multiple vendors must connect the data from those applications to create a unified health information system. The integration architect develops and manages the HL7 interfaces between diverse systems to ensure the smooth and seamless flow of information and data across the organization. As upgrades for various systems are planned, the integration architect is involved in creating test scenarios, monitoring the upgrade process, and converting of any data tables affected by a new or upgraded application.

**HEALTH SYSTEMS SPECIALIST** A health systems specialist is knowledgeable in one or more applications used by the facility, its file or database structure, system requirements, and operational use. This person supports the users, trainers, and maintenance of the application software and data.

**SOLUTION ANALYST** A solution analyst works either for the healthcare organization or the software vendor to document workflow, functional design requirements, and test plans to create new or enhanced software.

**SOLUTION CONSULTANT** A solution consultant works either for the healthcare organization or the software vendor to recommend appropriate solutions that further the organization's goals of automation and process improvement. An effective consultant must possess in-depth knowledge of clinical information systems, healthcare organizations, and workflow processes.

**SYSTEMS ANALYST** A systems analyst works with system users and department heads in the organization to determine the needs and technical requirements for software applications and systems. Systems analysts also participate in implementation, training, support, and troubleshooting applications once they are installed. The systems analyst translates the technical workings of a system into something the user can understand and communicates users' requests in terms the technicians and programmers understand.

**INFORMATION SECURITY MANAGER** The information security manager reviews all information system security plans and is responsible for security activities related to the availability, integrity, and confidentiality of information within the healthcare organization.

**RECORDS AND INFORMATION COORDINATOR** The records and information coordinator processes incoming information by sorting, classifying, and verifying coded data for integration into the healthcare systems. The records and information coordinator maintains logs, computerized indexes, and databases and provides reference services to all departments.

## Officers and Other Positions

Two officers are found in every inpatient and ambulatory facility that were not shown in the previous organizational charts. These are the privacy officer and the security officer. There are also several IT and HIM positions that were not listed in the organizational charts. Descriptions of these officer and other positions are provided in the following subsections. Also discussed are two HIM positions not typically found in an inpatient setting, medical office manager and health insurance specialist (claims examiner).

**PRIVACY OFFICER** The privacy officer in a large healthcare organization reports directly to the chief executive office (CEO) or CIO. In a small ambulatory setting, the privacy officer may be simply an additional role taken on by the office manager, HIM director, or other office administrator. The privacy officer oversees all ongoing activities related to the development,

## A REAL-LIFE STORY

## Examples of Project Management

### By David Goldbaum

*David Goldbaum is a senior project manager at a 500+-bed hospital in the Midwest.*

Project management involves coordination between various people who might be focused on only their particular aspect of a project. Right now we are adding a new surgical building. I am working with the construction people, also with people who pull copper wire and the fiber optic cable through the structure, our telephony people, our HIS people, and those who provide the software and documentation.

Like every hospital we have systems that are tied to HIS or CIS (clinical information system), our organization-wide nursing software. Then we have some that are technically stand-alone systems that need to get tied into the unified structure. When the hospital builds on or adds a major department, there is an opportunity to improve how that department's data integrates into the patient's health record.

For example, our surgical department uses software that was purchased sometime ago from a different vendor than our main system. Heretofore, they used it in a very minimal way, so today the data from the surgical system comes into our EHR not as data but as scanned paper documentation. However, the new building will increase our cardiovascular services and there are newly evolving functions that would better serve our cardiovascular initiative if it were integrated into our clinical documentation system.

The hospital has a committee that deals with documentation that is looking at the needs of cardiovascular and another committee that looks at information technology, but the committees are not even connected. Project management's job is to connect them.

Another example is the nurse call system. Traditionally, this is the little light that goes on when patients push a button at their bedside. This system is usually the responsibility of the biomedical department but we have added new capability that incorporates RFID (radio-frequency identification). RFID allows us to track the location of equipment and personnel as they are moved from room to room. Applying that technology to the nurse call system improved patient care. We can detect when the call was made, when the nurse entered the room, and it is tied into our paging system so if someone hasn't come to the room after a reasonable interval it can generate a page.

This upgrade required a project manager because the biomedical equipment began using a topology that is maintained by IT, and the paging aspect is the responsibility of our telephony department. Project management coordinated the efforts of the biomedical, IT, telephony, and nursing departments to make the implementation a success.

Most projects in a hospital are of a clinical nature, but the project manager needs a good understanding of both the technical and clinical side to better facilitate communications between all parties involved.

---

implementation, maintenance of, and adherence to the organization's policies and procedures covering the privacy of, and access to, protected health information (PHI).

The position of privacy officer is required by HIPAA. This person is responsible for addressing patient complaints, recording and tracking incidents, and ensuring compliance with the organization's published privacy policy and relevant state and federal laws.

**INFORMATION PRIVACY COORDINATOR**   An information privacy coordinator works with the privacy officer to assess risks to health information security and privacy, train employees on the privacy policy, and address information privacy issues.

**SECURITY OFFICER**   The position of security officer is required by HIPAA. The security officer is responsible for the development, implementation of, and adherence to the organization's security policies and procedures, but may assign specific security duties to others with more technical expertise. The security officer must track and deal with security incidents and breaches.

In a large healthcare organization, the security officer reports directly to the CEO or CIO. In a small ambulatory setting, the security officer may be simply an additional role taken on by the office manager, IT director, or computer administrator.

**COMPLIANCE OFFICER**   Healthcare organizations are subject to regulation by numerous government agencies and voluntary organizations. They also have contractual obligations and must follow generally acceptable medical ethics. (This will be covered in Chapter 6.) The compliance officer keeps abreast of the rules, regulations, and contracts that affect the organization and develops policies and procedures to ensure compliance. The position of compliance officer is generally only be found in inpatient facilities or very large healthcare organizations. A compliance officer usually reports directly to the CEO or Board of Directors.

**UTILIZATION MANAGER**   Utilization management (formerly known as utilization review) is required by Medicare and other insurance programs to ensure that any services provided are medically necessary. The utilization manager (sometimes called a case manager) is responsible for managing prospective, concurrent, and retrospective cases, communicating with the QIO, obtaining preapproval or precertification from payers for procedures and continued patient stays, and preparing replies to QIO denials. The utilization manager collects and reports data on the utilization of medical services, clinical practice guidelines, care protocols, and quality care issues.

**QUALITY IMPROVEMENT DIRECTOR**   The quality improvement director (sometimes called the quality manager) is responsible for administering and managing the facility's quality improvement program. Quality improvement seeks to ensure quality care for the patients, improve outcomes, and comply with standards from accreditation bodies such as the Joint Commission. The quality improvement director collects, analyzes, and summarizes performance data, identifies opportunities for improvement, and advises internal quality improvement teams from various departments.

**SENIOR DOCUMENT COORDINATOR**   A senior document coordinator enters data concerning adverse events into a safety database, tracks them through completion, and generates reports.

**RISK MANAGEMENT SPECIALIST**   The risk management specialist improves patient safety through risk analysis, prevention, and employee education.

**HEALTH SERVICES MANAGER**   Health services managers plan and coordinate patients' healthcare. They are typically employed at inpatient facilities such as hospitals and nursing homes. Home healthcare organizations also employ health services managers to coordinate home visits and staffing needs according to physicians' plans of care for their patients.

**PATIENT INFORMATION COORDINATOR**   The patient information coordinator is responsible for ensuring that patients, their families, and healthcare providers receive appropriate, timely, and accurate health information about the services provided, financial services, social services, and other medical and legal issues. The goal of the patient information coordinator is continuing patient satisfaction with the facility and services.

**CLINICAL RESEARCH ASSOCIATE**   A clinical research associate works in a healthcare organization that participates in clinical studies. Each clinical study will have a protocol for the study and may have regulatory or participation requirements. The clinical research associate monitors clinical practices, procedures, and informed consent forms to ensure adherence to the study protocols. The clinical research associate may participate in the organization and reporting of study data as well as the development of protocols for follow-up studies.

**MEDICAL OFFICE MANAGER**   The office manager is typically the top supervisory position in an ambulatory medical practice. The medical office manager usually wears many hats, supervising scheduling, coding, billing, collections, patient relations, and acting as liaison between the providers and the clerical staff. In small practices the office manager may also have additional jobs such as the HIPAA privacy officer and security officer positions.

**MEDICAL ASSISTANT**   Medical assistants perform administrative and clinical tasks. In addition to the clinical duties described in Chapter 1, medical assistants perform administrative tasks. They answer telephones, greet patients, handle correspondence, schedule patient appointments, and have billing and bookkeeping duties. Administrative medical assistants also update and file patients' medical records, fill out insurance forms, arrange for hospital admissions and laboratory services, and make calls on behalf of the physician's office.

**HEALTH INSURANCE SPECIALIST**   A health insurance specialist, sometimes called a *claims examiner,* is normally employed by an insurance company, managed care plan, or third-party administrator. The health insurance specialist is knowledgeable about billing codes and payer guidelines and examines health claims to determine if the costs are within guidelines and if the procedures were medically necessary.

# Organizations of Importance to HIM or IT Professionals

Just as there are professional organizations for physicians, specialists, nurses and other healthcare providers, as discussed in Chapter 1, there are several organizations for allied healthcare professionals in health information management and health information systems. These organizations are dedicated to making improvements in their respective fields and providing credentialing and continuing education opportunities for their members. Several of these organizations develop and maintain the standards by which the entire healthcare industry must abide. Most of them offer membership to students at a reduced rate.

## American Health Information Management Association

The American Health Information Management Association (AHIMA) is the leading organization for HIM professionals. AHIMA's goals are to improve healthcare by advancing best practices and standards for health information management and to be a trusted source for education, research, and professional credentialing.

AHIMA traces its history back to the Association of Record Librarians of North America (ARLNA), which was formed by the American College of Surgeons to "elevate the standards of clinical records in hospitals and other medical institutions." Today AHIMA has more than 50,000 members.

In line with its mission, AHIMA offers certification examinations by which HIM professionals become credentialed. These include Certified Coding Associate, Certified Coding Specialist, Registered Health Information Technician, and Registered Health Information Administrator. AHIMA also offers credentials in healthcare privacy and security.

AHIMA has formulated a code of ethics by which all AHIMA members, credentialed nonmembers, and most HIM departments abide. The AHIMA Professional Ethics Committee investigates complaints of violations. A copy of the AHIMA Code of Ethics is provided at the end of Chapter 6.

If you are interested in becoming an HIM professional you will certainly want to join AHIMA. Special memberships are offered to students enrolled in accredited HIM programs or other approved programs in medical coding.[6]

## Healthcare Information and Management Systems Society

The Healthcare Information and Management Systems Society (HIMSS) is a global organization dedicated to providing leadership for the optimal use of healthcare IT and management systems. HIMSS frames and leads healthcare public policy and industry practices through its advocacy, educational, and professional development initiatives, which are designed to promote information and management systems' contributions to ensuring quality patient care.

HIMSS's 20,000 members lead change in the healthcare information and management systems field through knowledge sharing, advocacy, collaboration, innovation, and community affiliations. HIMSS members include executives such as CEOs, CIOs, chief operating officers (COOs), other senior executives, and industry specialists such as senior managers, IS technical staff, physicians, nurses, consultants, attorneys, financial advisers, technology vendors, academicians, management engineers, and students.

If you are interested in becoming an IT professional in healthcare, you may wish to join HIMSS. Membership in HIMSS is available to full-time students at a reduced rate.[7]

## American Medical Informatics Association

The American Medical Informatics Association (AMIA) is dedicated to the development and application of biomedical and health informatics in support of patient care, teaching, research, and healthcare administration. AMIA participates with HIMSS in its annual conference. Full-time students interested in a career in medical informatics can join AMIA at a reduced rate.[8]

---

[6]American Health Information Management Association, www.ahima.org.
[7]Healthcare Information and Management Systems Society, www.himss.org.
[8]American Medical Informatics Association, www.amia.org.

## Medical Group Management Association

The mission of the Medical Group Management Association (MGMA) is to continually improve the performance of medical group practice professionals and the organizations they represent. The 21,000 members of MGMA principally work in ambulatory settings such as physician group practices. MGMA has set up an affiliate program, ACMPE (see below), for development and certification of professional managers.

Students interested in a career in medical practice management can get a membership in both MGMA and ACMPE at a reduced rate.[9]

## American College of Medical Practice Executives

The American College of Medical Practice Executives (ACMPE), an affiliate of MGMA, was established to provide board certification, self-assessment, and leadership development for medical practice executives. ACMPE has a code of ethics and professional conduct committee similar to, but distinct from, that of the AHIMA.[10]

## American National Standards Institute

The American National Standards Institute (ANSI) oversees the creation, promulgation and use of thousands of standards and guidelines for nearly every sector of business.

In healthcare two of the ANSI standards developing organizations (SDOs) have great impact. The Data Interchange Standards Association (DISA) SDO committee X12i develops and maintains the electronic data interchange (EDI) formats required for most HIPAA transactions. The HL7 SDO (discussed next) develops and maintains the specifications health systems use to exchange data.

## Health Level Seven

Health Level Seven, known as HL7, is an organization of healthcare experts and information scientists collaborating to create standards for the exchange, management, and integration of electronic healthcare information. Using a consensus process, HL7 develops specifications for the most widely used messaging standard that enables disparate healthcare applications to exchange clinical and administrative data.

HL7 promotes the use of such standards within and among healthcare organizations to increase the effectiveness and efficiency of healthcare delivery for the benefit of all. HL7 joined ANSI, to become one of its SDOs for healthcare.[11]

Membership in either DISA X12i or HL7 is usually sponsored by your employer.

## Association for Healthcare Documentation Integrity

The Association for Healthcare Documentation Integrity (AHDI; formerly known as the American Association for Medical Transcription, or AAMT). If you are considering a career in medical transcription, AHDI offers certification of medical transcriptionists.

## National Cancer Registrars Association

The National Cancer Registrars Association (NCRA) is a not-for-profit association representing cancer registry professionals and Certified Tumor Registrars (CTRs). The primary focus of NCRA is education and certification with the goal of ensuring that all cancer registry professionals have the required knowledge to be superior in their field.[12]

## American Academy of Professional Coders

The American Academy of Professional Coders (AAPC) provides certified credentials to medical coders in physician's offices, hospital outpatient facilities, ambulatory surgical centers, and payer organizations. All members of AAPC agree to a code of ethics that ensures high levels of

---

[9]Medical Group Management Association, www.mgma.org.
[10]Ibid.
[11]Health Level Seven, www.hl7.org.
[12]National Cancer Registrars Association, www.ncra-usa.org.

professionalism, integrity, and ethical behavior.[13] Registered students can obtain a membership in AACP at a reduced rate.

### National Association for Healthcare Quality

The National Association for Healthcare Quality (NAHQ) promotes and provides leadership in the delivery of quality healthcare in the most efficient and cost-effective manner possible. NAHQ goals are to facilitate the communication, cooperation, and sharing of knowledge among individuals and entities within the field of healthcare and to support and advocate the interests of patients in receiving quality healthcare and in all other actions affecting their health and welfare.[14] NAHQ has about 5,000 members.

## Skills for Success

Healthcare information management is being transformed by technology. As HIM and IT merge, you need to understand both subjects to advance your career in either. Furthermore, you must understand the basic concepts and terminology of healthcare to converse with those who provide patient care. Finally, healthcare is also a business. Principles of accounting, management, and project management apply.

Figure 2-5 illustrates some of the overlapping skill sets a career in healthcare management or technology requires. If you already have a background in some aspect of healthcare, consider

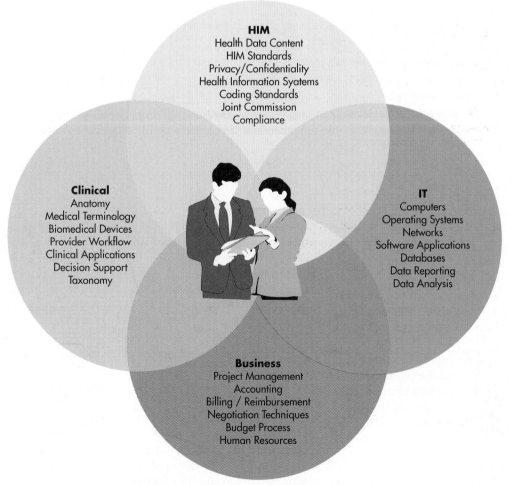

**FIGURE 2-5**

**Overlapping skill sets of the HIM or IT worker.**

---

[13]American Academy of Professional Coders, www.aapc.com.
[14]By-laws, Article I, National Association for Healthcare Quality, Chicago, IL.

developing yourself in areas that are not part of your current job. For example, many of the jobs described earlier involved managing an ongoing function or group of tasks. Although your first job might not be as a manager, the ability to accurately estimate the time required for a project and to deliver expected results in a timely fashion is bound to help you advance your career. Learn project management.

If your background is more clinical, you should learn computers. Each day another aspect of healthcare is being computerized. Whether you work in pharmacy, nursing, or medical records, you will be expected to use a computer. Understanding and being comfortable with computers frees you to focus on the patient.

Conversely, if your experience is completely technical, take a course in medical terminology. Although you may be able to troubleshoot a workstation or wire a network, the users in your work environment speak in a clinical vocabulary. If you can understand and converse with them you will be able to help them use your systems.

In preparing this text, real people who perform the jobs listed in this chapter were interviewed. Each of them was asked "What do students need to know?" Here is some of their advice:

- *Medical vocabulary.* Everyone queried recommended that students take a course in this subject.
- *Embrace technology.* Learn everything you can and don't be afraid of computers.
- *Learn about what physicians do.* They are at the core of the healthcare system. If you understand a little more of what they do and why they do it, you can better help them.
- *Think big picture.* It's not all about your particular job. How does your profession fit within all of the processes at your facility?
- *Understand workflow.* What is being done and how? What is the easiest way to accomplish a task? How do you make it efficient?
- *Learn a little project management.* How do you break down a project into tasks? How do you estimate a timeline? Which components are conditional on completion of other parts of the project?
- *Learn a little accounting.* This applies to jobs as varied as billing, database management, patient services, computer programming (health systems), or any managerial position.

# Chapter 2 Summary

### History of Health Information Management and Organizations

In 1918, the American College of Surgeons' (ACS') Hospital Standardization Program required hospitals to keep "accurate and complete medical records for all patients, filed in an accessible manner." This created the need for medical records clerks and is considered the forerunner of health information management.

In 1928 medical records clerks formed the Association of Record Librarians of North America, the precursor of the health information profession. Its name later changed to the American Association of Record Librarians (1941), then to the American Medical Record Association (1970), and finally to the American Health Information Management Association (1991).

### Health Information Professionals

Nonclinical allied health professions are those occupations in healthcare that do not involve medical or diagnostic services to the patient, but do handle and safeguard the medical information vital to those who provide direct services. This category includes all HIS, IT, HIM, and HIT professions. Some examples are medical office managers, registration and scheduling clerks, medical records clerks, transcriptionists, computer system analysts, IT managers, and billing and coding specialists.

Nonclinical allied health professionals impact the ability of the clinic to care for the patient by their attention to accuracy and detail. These professionals ensure successful operation of the healthcare delivery system. For example, HIM functions include compiling, storing, retrieving, and controlling access to the patient's records. Other HIM functions include coding, abstracting, and aggregating health information for billing, reporting, and research purposes. HIS/IT functions involve the computerization of those records and developing and maintaining the systems and infrastructure that deliver them.

Healthcare organizations large enough to have HIM and IT departments usually have an officer or CIO who is responsible for both departments.

## Organizations of Importance to HIM or IT Professionals

Associations whose members are healthcare professionals support their members and establish standards to improve patient care. Just as doctors have the American Medical Association and nurses have the American Nurses Association, in this chapter we listed many helpful organizations for workers in the HIM and IT fields. These associations set the standards for ethical conduct and provide education, certification, and credentials for many HIM positions. Most of the organizations listed offer memberships, often at a reduced rate, to students interested in a career in health information.

## Skills for Success

As computerized patient health records and delivery systems become more common in the various healthcare fields, the HIM and HIS or IT departments will continue to merge. Professionals already working in the field today recommend students become acquainted with multiple skill sets regardless of which career most interests them. These include medical terminology, computer technology, health information management, workflow, project management, and accounting principles. Familiarity with time management and budgeting principles will help you advance into management positions. Being conversant in both computer and medical vocabulary allows you to better communicate with others in healthcare facilities.

# Critical Thinking Exercises

1. Although you are just being introduced to the health information profession, think about the several different allied health professional occupations that were described in this chapter. Which of them piqued your interest the most and why?
2. Two important organizations for health information professionals, AHIMA (www.ahima.org) and HIMSS (www.himss.org), were discussed in this chapter. Visit each of their websites and learn more about them. Which of them interested you most and why?
3. On each of the websites mentioned in Exercise 2, locate the information about becoming a student member. (You do not have to join as part of this exercise.) Describe the benefits of a student membership. Describe the requirements to become a student member for each organization.

# Testing Your Knowledge of Chapter 2

1. What does the acronym HIM stand for?
2. What does the acronym HIT stand for?
3. Give an example of how the fields of HIM and IT are merging.
4. In what year did the American College of Surgeons establish standards for hospital records?
5. What is forms control?
6. How would understanding medical terminology help a billing clerk?

*For each of the following allied health professions, indicate if the job is clinical or nonclinical by circling the correct answer:*

7. Clinical applications coordinator

    *Clinical    Nonclinical*

8. Lab technician

    *Clinical    Nonclinical*

9. Coding specialist

    *Clinical    Nonclinical*

10. Cancer registrar

    *Clinical    Nonclinical*

11. In the HIM profession what is *abstracting*?
12. What are two requirements to become a Registered Health Information Administrator?

*For each of the following statements circle true if it is correct, or false if the statement is not true:*

13. Diagnosis-related groups are used for Medicare billing and reimbursement.

    *True    False*

14. A Registered Health Information Technician is required to implement and train users on imaging systems.

    *True    False*

15. A security officer is a position found exclusively at inpatient facilities or very large medical practices.

    *True    False*

# 3

# Accreditation, Regulation, and HIPAA

## LEARNING OUTCOMES

After completing this chapter, you should be able to:

- Discuss the importance of accreditation
- List HIPAA transactions and uniform identifiers
- Understand HIPAA privacy and security concepts
- Apply HIPAA privacy policy in a medical office
- Discuss HIPAA security requirements and safeguards
- Follow security policy guidelines in a medical facility

## ACRONYMS USED IN CHAPTER 3

Acronyms are used extensively in both medicine and computers. The following acronyms are used in this chapter.

| | | | |
|---|---|---|---|
| **ACS** | American College of Surgeons | **FDA** | Food and Drug Administration |
| **CAP** | College of American Pathologists | **HHS** | U.S. Department of Health and Human Services |
| **CARF** | Commission on Accreditation of Rehabilitation Facilities | **HCPCS** | Healthcare Common Procedure Coding System |
| **CDC** | Centers for Disease Control and Prevention | **HIPAA** | Health Insurance Portability and Accountability Act |
| **CMS** | Centers for Medicare and Medicaid Services (formerly known as Health Care Financing Administration) | **ICD-9-CM** | International Classification of Diseases, Ninth Revision, Clinical Modification |
| **COB** | Coordination of Benefits | **JCAHO** | Joint Commission on Accreditation of Healthcare Organizations (now referred to simply as the Joint Commission) |
| **COP** | Conditions of Participation (Medicare) | | |
| **CPT-4®** | Current Procedural Terminology, Fourth Edition | **MOU** | Memorandum of Understanding (between Government Entities) |
| **DEA** | Drug Enforcement Agency | **NPI** | National Provider Identifier |
| **DRG** | Diagnosis-Related Group | **OCR** | Office of Civil Rights |
| **EDI** | Electronic Data Interchange | | |
| **EHR** | Electronic Health Record | **PHI** | Protected Health Information |
| **EIN** | Employer Identification Number | **PIN** | Personal Identification Number |
| **EPHI** | Protected Health Information in Electronic Form | **PPS** | Prospective Payment System |
| **FBI** | Federal Bureau of Investigation | **PRO** | Peer Review Organization (now Quality Improvement Organization) |

| **PSRO** | Professional Standards Review Organization | **UM** | Utilization Management |
|---|---|---|---|
| **QIO** | Quality Improvement Organization (formerly Peer Review Organization) | **WAN** | Wide-Area Network |

# Accreditation and Regulation

Healthcare facilities and practitioners are licensed and regulated by federal, state, and local governments and laws. Additional self-regulation by following a set of recognized standards for healthcare organizations and voluntary participation in audits by accreditation organizations can assist in compliance with government requirements.

Government regulation influences healthcare delivery organizations in two ways. First, entities are directly controlled by agencies that issue permits and licenses to operate facilities and various departments within them. Second, healthcare organizations are influenced by the rules of government agencies that reimburse them for treating patients. The most prominent among these is the Centers for Medicare and Medicaid Services (CMS).

## Centers for Medicare and Medicaid Services

Medicare and Medicaid have been in existence since 1965. Medicare provides healthcare coverage for people ages 65 and older as well as people with disabilities and those with end-stage renal disease (kidney failure). Medicaid provides healthcare benefits (partially paid by the states) for people who are poor, blind, or have a disability, for pregnant women, and for some persons over age 65 (in addition to Medicare).

Medicare and Medicaid are both governed by a federal agency, the Centers for Medicare and Medicaid Services, which is under the U.S. Department of Health and Human Services (HHS). Both programs are administrated on a state level by *intermediaries,* companies that have a contract to handle claims processing, payments, authorizations, and provider inquiries for a region or a state. Often these intermediaries are health insurance plans such as the local Blue Cross/Blue Shield plan.

The influence of CMS on the healthcare delivery system cannot be underestimated. Here are just a few examples of its influence:

- Since its inception, Medicare has required utilization reviews to ensure that the services provided were medically necessary. Utilization review is now referred to as utilization management (UM). This led to the establishment of professional standards review organizations (PSROs) to perform concurrent review of the services provided during a patient's stay. Subsequently this evolved into peer review organizations (PROs) to review the necessity for inpatient admissions even before the patient was admitted. PROs are now referred to as quality improvement organizations (QIOs). The QIO process is also used by Blue Cross and private insurance plans and is the basis for the preadmission and preauthorization requirements common with many health plans today.

- In an effort to control healthcare costs, Medicare and Medicaid also established rates at which facilities and providers would be reimbursed for approved services. By law, providers could not collect more from a Medicare patient that the approved amount. This again became the model emulated by many health insurance plans, where participating providers enter into a contractual agreement ensuring that patients will not be charged more than the amount "approved" by the plan.

- In addition to payment systems that set the amount reimbursed for services delivered, Medicare led the way in establishing a prospective payment system (PPS), which paid for inpatient stays at a fixed amount based on the type of case, not the length of stay. The concept of diagnosis-related groups (DRGs) was created to establish the reasonable costs for care based on the patient's diagnosis at the time of discharge. The DRG concept was also embraced by Blue Cross and other plans. PPSs are now being applied to outpatient services.

- To ensure that patients receive quality care, Medicare established rules and standards of care and required facilities to comply with its conditions of participation (COP). Among other things, facilities are subject to audit and inspections to ensure the quality of the provider and compliance with standard policies and procedures. One of the ways a healthcare organization can comply is by voluntary participation in the accreditation process of the Joint Commission (discussed below). Medicare and other agencies recognize the rigorous standards of certain accreditation organizations that meet or exceed their own. Rather than submit to the time-consuming process of inspections by Medicare, Blue Cross, multiple agencies, and health plans, a facility can obtain a *deemed status*, whereby Medicare deems that if the facility has met the Joint Commission standards it would have also met the COP requirements.

- When the Health Insurance Portability and Accountability Act (HIPAA) became law, CMS was also instrumental in its implementation. HIPAA contained, among other things, a subsection on administrative simplification that required standardization of electronic transactions as well as the setting of standards for privacy and security of health records. CMS exerted pressure on Medicare intermediaries to adopt the required standards for their transactions or risk losing their contracts. CMS was also given the powers to enforce the HIPAA security standards. (HIPAA is discussed in more detail later in the chapter.)

These examples are only a few of the ways in which Medicare influences facilities, providers, and other insurance plans. HIPAA, DRG, accreditation, and many of the other concepts introduced here will be discussed in more detail later.

## Federal, State, and Local Laws

In addition to the laws concerning safety, employees, business practices, and zoning that apply to all types of businesses, healthcare entities are subject to further regulations. For instance, all states require healthcare facilities to be licensed. The caregivers (discussed in Chapter 1) who work in the facilities must be licensed by the state as well.

State laws provide detailed regulations concerning the operation of facilities, sanitation, medical and nursing staff requirements, and patient records. Even within the licensure of the hospital, the state may limit what services can be offered or require special licenses to operate certain departments within the facility.

In some cases licensing decisions can be very political. A state may restrict which facilities can perform certain cardiac procedures. For example, a hospital surgery department with surgeons qualified in the procedures may have difficulty getting licensed because of the political pressure exerted on the licensing board by larger competing hospitals in the region.

Licensing and state regulations differ by the facility type as well. For example, long-term care and rehabilitation facilities are subject to requirements that are different from those that must be followed by an acute care facility.

State agencies that regulate and license healthcare delivery conduct regular visits and inspections of healthcare facilities and their record keeping, operations, and compliance with state requirements. Local governments in many areas also require county or city licenses and may conduct inspections as well.

Earlier, we discussed CMS, an agency of the HHS, but there are additional federal agencies within HHS that also regulate or impact healthcare facilities. These include the Food and Drug Administration (FDA), Drug Enforcement Agency (DEA), Centers for Disease Control and Prevention (CDC), and the Office of Civil Rights (OCR). Licenses are required for providers who prescribe drugs, the pharmacists who prepare and dispense drugs, and the caregivers who administer them. A license is also required to operate a hospital pharmacy. Licenses and regulations also govern the use and handling of radioactive materials by radiology and nuclear medicine departments in healthcare facilities.

In addition to the licenses and inspections we just discussed, healthcare facilities are also required to report incidents that involve infectious diseases, child abuse, and certain injuries such as gunshots. State and federal governments also require facilities to report a substantial amount of statistical data concerning birth defects, cancer tumors, and the patients using the facility.

## The Joint Commission

As mentioned earlier, one way of meeting the requirements of operating a healthcare facility, and limiting a number of the time-consuming audits and inspections by numerous agencies and health insurance plans, is to voluntarily comply with the standards of a recognized accreditation organization. For acute care facilities, the most respected entity is the Joint Commission.

The name Joint Commission is derived from its history. Nearly a century ago, the American College of Surgeons (ACS) created a Hospital Standard Program describing how medical care should be documented and how hospitals should be operated. These standards continued to evolve. In 1952, the American Hospital Association and the Canadian Medical Association collaborated with the ACS to form a Joint Commission of Hospitals. Thirty-five years later, the word *Hospital* was dropped because the standards-setting body had expanded to include long-term, behavioral health, and ambulatory care settings as well as acute care hospitals. The new name was Joint Commission on Accreditation of Healthcare Organizations (JCAHO). Today the work of JCAHO is so widely recognized that the name has been shortened to the Joint Commission.

The Joint Commission establishes the optimum standards for patient care, medical documentation, and clinical data. Facilities adhering to these standards submit to accreditation surveys and audits by the Joint Commission to earn and maintain their accreditation. Here is the Joint Commission's list of benefits:

### Benefits of Joint Commission Accreditation and Certification

- Strengthens community confidence in the quality and safety of care, treatment and services
- Provides a competitive edge in the marketplace
- Improves risk management and risk reduction
- Provides education on good practices to improve business operations
- Provides professional advice and counsel, enhancing staff education
- Enhances staff recruitment and development
- Recognized by select insurers and other third parties
- May fulfill regulatory requirements in select states

Joint Commission standards address the organization's level of performance in key functional areas, such as patient rights, patient treatment, and infection control. The standards focus not simply on an organization's ability to provide safe, high-quality care, but on its actual performance as well. The standards set forth performance expectations for activities that affect the safety and quality of patient care.[1]

To help organizations measure outcomes and improve the quality of care, ongoing collection of performance measures was incorporated into the accreditation process. ORYX® is the name the Joint Commission gave to the initiative that integrates performance and outcome measures into the accreditation process.

Accredited hospitals now submit specific performance measurement data to the Joint Commission on a regular basis. The Joint Commission can then work with the facility to help it improve its quality of care. CMS has worked with the Joint Commission to ensure that the agency and the commission's performance measures are precisely aligned. Figure 3-1 shows the resulting improvements in hospital quality performance for selected illnesses reported by Joint Commission—accredited hospitals over a six-year period of time.[2]

In addition to the Joint Commission, several other organizations accredit some of the same facilities. Two important ones are discussed next.

---

[1]*Facts about the Joint Commission,* www.jointcommission.org.
[2]The Joint Commission 2008 Report.

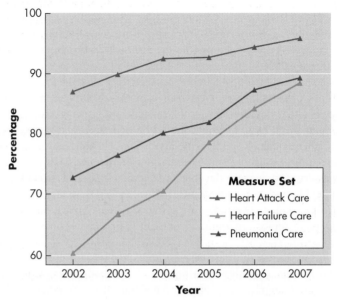

FIGURE 3-1   Measures of improvement in heart attack, heart failure, and pneumonia care.

## College of American Pathologists

The College of American Pathologists (CAP) is the principal professional organization for board-certified pathologists. Among the organization's diverse activities is the accreditation of medical laboratories. "The goal of the CAP Laboratory Accreditation Program is to improve patient safety by advancing the quality of pathology and laboratory services through education, standard setting, and ensuring laboratories meet or exceed regulatory requirements."[3]

Figure 3-2 shows a technician in a laboratory; however, CAP accreditation surveys go beyond the physical confines of the laboratory, ensuring that nurses and caregivers who use devices such as glucose meters to administer tests in patients' rooms have been thoroughly trained and are qualified to conduct those tests.

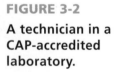

**FIGURE 3-2**

**A technician in a CAP-accredited laboratory.**

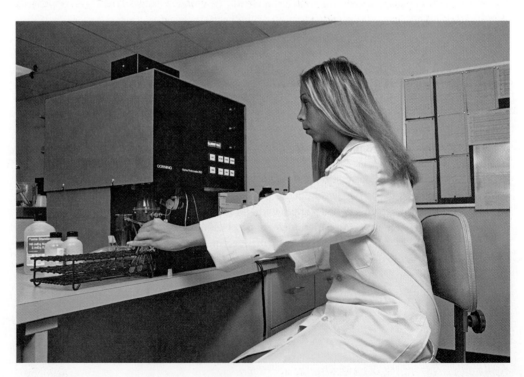

[3]*About the Laboratory Accreditation Program,* College of American Pathologists, www.cap.org.

Because the CAP accreditation process is so thorough, the Joint Commission accepts accreditation of a hospital laboratory by CAP as sufficient to meet the Joint Commission's standards in regard to that portion of their survey. CAP has also been designated by CMS as an authority, whereby a laboratory facility with a CAP accreditation is deemed to have complied with Medicare COP standards.

## Commission on Accreditation of Rehabilitation Facilities

The Commission on Accreditation of Rehabilitation Facilities (CARF) provides accreditation for organizations offering behavioral health, physical, and occupational rehabilitation services as well as assisted living, continuing care, community services, employment services, and others.

Although the Joint Commission also offers accreditation of rehabilitation facilities, CARF's approach is more consultative and less like an inspection. There are also some services for which CARF is the only accrediting body. Because the two commissions have somewhat different requirements, they have worked together to offer coordinated surveys in cases where facilities desire accreditation by both commissions.

CARF includes standards for adult day care, stroke specialty programs, person-centered long-term care communities, and dementia care specialty programs. CARF has developed accreditation for other human services that are not associated with rehabilitation, for example, the administration of one-stop career centers.[4]

# HIPAA

Let us return to our discussion of HIPAA, which has had a great impact on the field of health information and the health information management professional. Although you may not initially be positioned to make some of the policy and planning decisions discussed in this chapter, you will be required to understand and comply with them in a healthcare workplace. The remainder of this chapter will provide you with a thorough understanding of HIPAA and its impact on your job. The following sections make extensive use of documents prepared by the U.S. Department of Health and Human Services, the government authority on HIPAA.

## HIPAA's Administrative Simplification Subsection

In 1996 Congress passed legislation called the Health Insurance Portability and Accountability Act, or HIPAA. The law was intended to accomplish the following:

- Improve portability and continuity of health insurance coverage.
- Combat waste, fraud, and abuse in health insurance and healthcare delivery.
- Promote use of medical savings accounts.
- Improve access to long-term care.
- Simplify administration of health insurance.

HIPAA law regulates many things. However a portion known as the Administrative Simplification Subsection[5] of HIPAA covers entities such as health plans, clearinghouses, and healthcare providers. When you work in the healthcare field, these regulations govern your job and behavior. Therefore, it is not uncommon for healthcare workers to use the term *HIPAA* when they actually mean only the Administrative Simplification Subsection of HIPAA.

The Administrative Simplification Subsection has four distinct components:

1. Transactions and Code Sets
2. Uniform Identifiers
3. Privacy
4. Security

---

[4]*Answering Your Questions about CARF,* www.carf.org.
[5]HIPAA, Title 2, subsection f.

## HIPAA Transactions and Code Sets

The first section of the regulations to be implemented governs the electronic transfer of medical information for business purposes such as insurance claims, payments, and eligibility. We will discuss these and other electronic communications in more detail in a subsequent chapter.

When information is exchanged electronically both systems must use the same format in order to make the information intelligible to the receiving system. Here is an example to help you understand this concept: Perhaps a friend has e-mailed you a picture or video file you could not open with your computer. The most likely reason was that the file was in a format that your computer did not recognize. So while your friend's computer could display the image, your computer could not.

Before HIPAA, nearly every insurance plan used a format that contained variations which made it different from other plans' formats. This meant that plans could not easily exchange or forward claims to secondary payers and that most providers could only send claims electronically to a few plans. Too often the rest of the claims were sent on paper.

**EIGHT HIPAA TRANSACTIONS** HIPAA standardized formats by requiring specific transaction standards for eight types of electronic data interchange (EDI). Two additional EDI transactions are not yet finalized. The HIPAA transactions are:

1. Claims or equivalent encounters and coordination of benefits (COB)
2. Remittance and payment advice
3. Claims status
4. Eligibility and benefit inquiry and response
5. Referral certification and authorization
6. Premium payments
7. Enrollment and de-enrollment in a health plan
8. Health claims attachments (not final)
9. First report of injury (not final)
10. Retail drug claims, coordination of drug benefits, and eligibility inquiries.

In an EDI transaction, certain portions of the information are sent as codes. For the receiving entity to understand the content of the transaction, both the sender and the receiver must use the same codes.

For example, in an insurance claim, charges for patient visits are sent as procedure codes instead of their long descriptions. The medical reasons for the procedure are sent in the claim as diagnosis codes. HIPAA requires the use of standard sets of codes. Two of those standards are:

- ICD-9-CM codes for diagnoses (and some inpatient procedures)
- CPT-4 and HCPCS codes for outpatient procedures

Under HIPAA, any coded information within a transaction is also subject to standards. Just a few examples of the hundreds of other codes include codes for sex, race, type of provider, and relation of the policy holder to the patient.

Health information technicians are involved in coding claims, sending or managing electronic data transactions, and setting up or maintaining tables of standard codes used to ensure that claims are correctly coded.

## HIPAA Uniform Identifiers

You can see the importance of both the sending and receiving system using the same formats and code sets to report exactly what was done for the patient. Similarly, it is necessary for multiple systems to identify the doctors, nurses, and healthcare businesses sending the claim or receiving the payment. ID numbers are used in a computer processing instead of names because, for example, there could be many providers named John Smith.

However, prior to HIPAA, each provider had multiple ID numbers assigned to them for use on insurance claims, prescriptions, etc. A provider typically received a different ID from each plan and sometimes multiple numbers from the same plan. This created a problem for the billing office to get the right ID on the right claim and made electronic coordination of benefits all but impossible.

HIPAA established uniform identifier standards to be used on all claims and other data transmissions. These include:

■ *National Provider Identifier (NPI):* This type of identifier is assigned to doctors, nurses, and other healthcare providers.

■ *Employer Identifier:* This identifier is used to identify employer-sponsored health insurance. It is the same as the federal Employer Identification Number (EIN) employers are assigned for their taxes by the Internal Revenue Service.

■ *National Health Plan Identifier:* This identifier has not yet been implemented, but when it is it will be a unique identification number assigned to each insurance plan and to the organizations that administer insurance plans, such as payers and third-party administrators.

---

**COVERED ENTITY**

HIPAA documents refer to healthcare providers, insurance plans, and clearinghouses as *covered entities*. A clearinghouse is a business that converts nonstandard HIPAA transactions into the correct format required by HIPAA.

As a future HIM employee, think of a covered entity as a healthcare organization and all of its employees.

---

## Privacy and Security of Patient Records

The remaining two portions of HIPAA's Administrative Simplification Subsection are concerned with the protection and confidentiality of patient information. As someone who will work with patient's health records, it is especially important for you to understand the regulations regarding privacy and security.

### HIPAA Privacy Rule

The HIPAA privacy standards are designed to protect a patient's identifiable health information from unauthorized disclosure or use in any form, while permitting the practice to deliver the best healthcare possible. When the HIPAA legislation was passed, "Congress recognized that advances in electronic technology could erode the privacy of health information. Consequently, Congress incorporated into HIPAA provisions that mandated the adoption of Federal privacy protections for individually identifiable health information."[6]

---

**PROTECTED HEALTH INFORMATION**

HIPAA privacy rules frequently refer to PHI or protected health information. PHI is the patient's personally identifiable health information.

---

Healthcare providers have a strong tradition of safeguarding private health information and have established privacy practices already in effect for their offices. For instance:

■ By speaking quietly when discussing a patient's condition with family members in a waiting room or other public area;

■ By avoiding using patients' names in public hallways and elevators, and posting signs to remind employees to protect patient confidentiality;

---

[6]*Guidance on HIPAA Standards for Privacy of Individually Identifiable Health Information* (Washington, DC: U.S. Department of Health and Human Services Office for Civil Rights, December 3, 2002, and revised April 3, 2003).

- By isolating or locking file cabinets or records rooms; or
- By providing additional security, such as passwords, on computers maintaining personal information.

However, The Privacy Rule establishes, for the first time, a foundation of Federal protections for the privacy of protected health information. The Rule does not replace Federal, State, or other law that grants individuals even greater privacy protections, and covered entities are free to retain or adopt more protective policies or practices.[7]

To comply with the law, privacy activities in the average medical office might include the following:

- Providing a copy of the office privacy policy informing patients about their privacy rights and how their information can be used.
- Asking the patient to acknowledge receiving a copy of the policy and/or signing a consent form.
- Obtaining signed authorization forms and in some cases tracking the disclosures of patient health information when it is to be given to a person or organization outside the practice for purposes other than treatment, billing, or payment purposes.
- Adopting clear privacy procedures.
- Training employees so that they understand the privacy procedures.
- Designating an individual to be responsible for seeing that the privacy procedures are adopted and followed.
- Securing patient records containing individually identifiable health information so that they are not readily available to those who do not need them.

Let us examine some of these key points.

## PRIVACY POLICY

The HIPAA Privacy Rule gives individuals a fundamental new right to be informed of the privacy practices of their health plans and of most of their healthcare providers, as well as to be informed of their privacy rights with respect to their personal health information. Health plans and covered healthcare providers are required to develop and distribute a notice that provides a clear explanation of these rights and practices. The notice is intended to focus individuals on privacy issues and concerns, and to prompt them to have discussions with their health plans and healthcare providers and exercise their rights.
    Covered entities are required to provide a notice in *plain language* that describes:

- How the covered entity may use and disclose protected health information about an individual.
- The individual's rights with respect to the information and how the individual may exercise these rights, including how the individual may complain to the covered entity.
- The covered entity's legal duties with respect to the information, including a statement that the covered entity is required by law to maintain the privacy of protected health information.
- Whom individuals can contact for further information about the covered entity's privacy policies.[8]

The privacy policy must meet the requirements of HIPAA law and the use or disclosure of PHI must be consistent with the privacy notice provided to the patient.

---

[7]Ibid.
[8]Ibid.

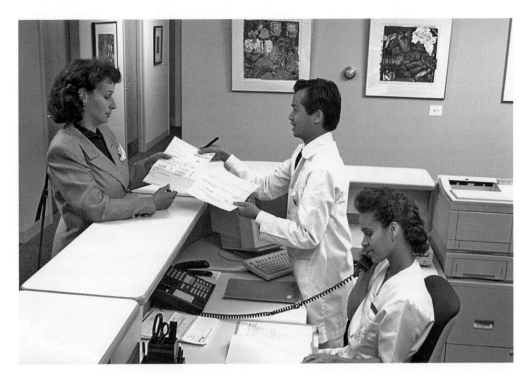

**FIGURE 3-3**

**A patient acknowledges receipt of a medical office's privacy policy.**

**CONSENT**   The term *consent* has multiple meanings in a medical setting. *Informed consent* refers to the patient's agreement to receive medical treatment having been provided sufficient information to make an informed decision. Consent for medical procedures must still be obtained by the practice.

Under the Privacy Rule the term *consent* is only concerned with use of the patient's information, and *should not be confused with consent for the treatment itself*. The Privacy Rule originally required providers to obtain patient "consent" to use and disclose PHI except in emergencies. The rule was almost immediately revised to make it easier to use PHI for purposes of treatment, payment, or operation of the healthcare practice.

Under the revised Privacy Rule, the patient gives consent to use their PHI by acknowledging that they have received a copy of the privacy policy. Figure 3-3 shows a patient receiving a copy of a medical office's privacy policy. The office has the patient sign a form acknowledging receipt of the privacy policy.

Although most healthcare providers who see patients obtain HIPAA "consent" as part of the routine demographic and insurance forms that patients sign, the rule permits some uses of PHI without the individual's authorization:

- A healthcare entity may use or disclose PHI for its own treatment, payment, and healthcare operations activities. For example, a hospital may use PHI to provide healthcare to the individual and may consult with other healthcare providers about the individual's treatment.

- A healthcare provider may disclose PHI about an individual as part of a claim for payment to a health plan.

- A healthcare provider may disclose PHI related to the treatment or payment activities of any healthcare provider (including providers not covered by the Privacy Rule). Consider these examples:

  A doctor may send a copy of an individual's medical record to a specialist who needs the information to treat the individual.

  A hospital may send a patient's healthcare instructions to a nursing home to which the patient is transferred.

  A physician may send an individual's health plan coverage information to a laboratory who needs the information to bill for tests ordered by the physician.

A hospital emergency department may give a patient's payment information to an ambulance service that transported the patient to the hospital in order for the ambulance provider to bill for its treatment

- A health plan may use protected health information to provide customer service to its enrollees.

Others within the office can use PHI also. For example, doctors and nurses can share the patient's chart to discuss what the best course of care might be. The doctor's administrative staff can access patient information to perform billing, transmit claims electronically, post payments, file the charts, type up the doctor's progress notes, and print and send out patient statements.

The office can also use PHI for operation of the medical practice, for example, to determine how many staff they will need on a certain day, whether they should invest in a particular piece of equipment, what types of patients they are seeing the most of, where most of their patients live, and any other uses that will help make the office operate more efficiently.

**Modifying HIPAA Consent** "Individuals have the right to request restrictions on how a covered entity will use and disclose protected health information about them for treatment, payment, and healthcare operations. A covered entity is not required to agree to an individual's request for a restriction, but is bound by any restrictions to which it agrees.

"Individuals also may request to receive confidential communications from the covered entity, either at alternative locations or by alternative means. For example, an individual may request that her healthcare provider call her at her office, rather than her home. A healthcare provider must accommodate an individual's reasonable request for such confidential communications."[9]

**AUTHORIZATION**   Authorization differs from consent in that it *does* require the patient's permission to disclose PHI. A signed "consent" document is not a valid permission to use or disclose protected health information for a purpose that requires an "authorization" under the Privacy Rule.

Some examples of instances that would require an authorization include sending the results of an employment physical to an employer and sending immunization records or the results of an athletic physical to the school.

The appearance of an authorization form is up to the practice, but the Privacy Rule requires that it contain specific information. Specific elements required by HIPAA are highlighted in yellow on the sample form shown in Figure 3-4. The required elements are:

- Date signed
- Expiration date
- To whom the information may be disclosed
- What is permitted to be disclosed
- For what purpose the information may be used.

Unlike the Privacy Rule concept of consent, authorizations are not global. A new authorization is signed each time there is a different purpose or need for the patient's information to be disclosed.

**Research**   Authorizations are usually required for researchers to use PHI. The only difference in a research authorization form is that it is not required to have an expiration date. The authorization may be combined with consent to participate in a clinical trial study for example.

**Research Exceptions**   To protect the patient's information while at the same time ensuring that researchers continue to have access to medical information necessary to conduct vital research, the Privacy Rule does allows some exceptions that permit researchers to access PHI without individual authorizations. Typically these are cases where the patients are deceased; where the researcher is using PHI only to prepare a research protocol; or where a waiver has been issued by an internal review board, specifying that none of the information will be removed or used for any other purpose.

---

[9]Ibid.

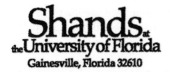

**Shands** at
the **University of Florida**
Gainesville, Florida 32610

**Medical Record Number**

**RI0001**

**Authorization for Use or Disclosure of
Protected Health Information**

**Health Information and Record Management Department**

Patient's Name: _____ Soc. Sec. #: _____
　　　　　　　　　Last　　　　　　First　　　　　Middle
Telephone #: _____ Date of Birth: _____

Check if the patient is a: ☐ Shands at UF employee　☐ University of Florida Physician

Send information to *(name of person, organization, or agency with full address):*

> Name: _____
>
> Attention: _____　Telephone #: _____
>
> Address: _____
>
> City: _____　State: _____　Zip: _____

Purpose of release *(For example: continued care, personal, etc.):* _____

Specific items or dates needed: _____
☐ Cardiovascular Reports　☐ EKG Report　☐ Laboratory Results　☐ Pathology Report　☐ Radiology (X-ray) Reports
☐ History & Physical　☐ Operative Report　☐ Discharge Summary　☐ Emergency Room　☐ Other: _____

Needed for doctor's appointment on: _____
　　　　　　　　　　　　　　　　　(Date)　　　　　　　　　　　(Time)

This authorization is for release of medical records and information including diagnosis, treatment, and/or examination related to mental health (psychiatry or psychology), drug and/or alcohol abuse, HIV testing/AIDS, and sexually transmissible diseases.

As required by state and federal law, Shands at the University of Florida may not use or disclose your health information, except as provided in our Notice of Privacy Practices, without your authorization. Your signature on this form indicates that you are giving permission for the uses and disclosures of the protected health information described on this form.

I understand that state law prohibits the re-disclosure of the information disclosed to the persons/entities listed above without my further authorization, but that Shands at the University of Florida cannot guarantee that the recipient of the information will not re-disclose this information contrary to such prohibition.

I understand that this authorization will remain in effect for one (1) year or until I revoke it in writing. I understand that I may revoke this authorization at any time. I understand that if I revoke this authorization, I must do so in writing to Health Information and Record Management, Shands at the University of Florida, PO Box 100345, Gainesville, FL 32610-0345. I further understand that any such revocation does not apply to information already released in response to this authorization.

I understand that I am under no obligation to sign this authorization. I further understand that my ability to obtain treatment will not depend in any way on whether I sign this authorization.

I understand that I have a right to inspect and to obtain a copy of any information disclosed.

I hereby release Shands at the University of Florida and its employees from any and all liability that may arise from the release of information as I have directed.

I understand that I may be charged a fee of up to $1.00 per page (plus applicable tax and handling) for every page copied. This fee is waived for copies provided to a health care provider for continuing medical care. I understand that this fee is within the limits allowable by Florida law.

I hereby authorize Shands at the University of Florida to release health information as described above.

Patient's Signature: _____ Date: _____

Signature of Parent or Guardian: _____ Date: _____

Relationship to Patient: _____

After completing this release, please return it to:
　　　　Medical Reports Section
　　　　Health Information and Record Management
　　　　Shands at the University of Florida
　　　　PO Box 100345
　　　　Gainesville, FL 32610-0345

Or fax it to: (352) 265-1098, telephone number: (352) 265-0131.

| For Department Use Only | | |
|---|---|---|
| # Copied: _____　Initials: _____ | | |
| Encounter: _____ | | |
| AN _____ | EM _____ | OT _____ |
| AU _____ | EN _____ | PF _____ |
| CC _____ | ER _____ | PN _____ |
| CH _____ | FS _____ | PO _____ |
| CL _____ | HP _____ | PR _____ |
| CO _____ | IM _____ | PS _____ |
| DS _____ | LA _____ | PT _____ |
| EC _____ | LD _____ | PX _____ |
| EE _____ | OP _____ | XX _____ |
| EK _____ | | |
| Other: _____ | | |
| Date: _____ | | |

Rev.12/21/06　　　　　　　　　　　　　　　　　　PS1985

**FIGURE 3-4**　Sample Authorization Form with elements required by HIPAA.

**Marketing** The Privacy Rule specifically defines marketing and *requires* individual authorization for all uses or disclosures of PHI for *marketing purposes* with limited exceptions. These exceptions are generally when information from the provider is sent to all patients in the practice about improvements or additions to the practice or when information is sent to the patient about his or her own treatments. For example, a reminder about an annual check-up is *not* considered marketing.

**Government Agencies** One area that permits the disclosure of PHI without a patient's authorization or consent is when it is requested by an authorized government agency. Generally such requests are for legal (law enforcement, subpoena, court orders, etc.) or public health purposes. A request by the FDA for information on patient's who are having adverse reactions to a particular drug might be an example. Another example might be an audit of medical records by CMS to determine if sufficient documentation exists to justify Medicare claims.

The Privacy Rule permits the disclosure of PHI, without authorization, to public health authorities for the purpose of preventing or controlling disease or injury and for maintaining records of births and deaths. Similarly, providers are also permitted to disclose PHI concerning on-the-job injuries to workers' compensation insurers, state administrators, and other entities to the extent required by state workers' compensation laws.

To ensure that covered entities protect patients' privacy as required, the Privacy Rule requires that health plans, hospitals, and other covered entities cooperate with efforts by the HHS Office for Civil Rights (OCR) to investigate complaints or otherwise ensure compliance.

**MINIMUM NECESSARY** The Privacy Rule *minimum necessary* standard is intended to limit unnecessary or inappropriate access to and disclosure of PHI beyond what is necessary. For example, if an insurance plan requests the value of a patient's hematocrit test to justify a claim for administering a drug, then the minimum necessary disclosure would be to send only the hematocrit result, not the patient's entire panel of tests.

> ### NO RESTRICTIONS ON PHI FOR TREATMENT OF THE PATIENT
>
> The minimum necessary standard does not apply to disclosures to or requests by a healthcare provider for PHI used for treatment purposes.

"The minimum necessary standard does not apply to the following:

- Disclosures to or requests by a healthcare provider for treatment purposes.
- Disclosures to the individual who is the subject of the information.
- Uses or disclosures made pursuant to an individual's authorization.
- Uses or disclosures required for compliance with the Health Insurance Portability and Accountability Act (HIPAA) Administrative Simplification Rules.
- Disclosures to the Department of Health and Human Services (HHS) when disclosure of information is required under the Privacy Rule for enforcement purposes.
- Uses or disclosures that are required by other law."[10]

**INCIDENTAL DISCLOSURES** "Many customary healthcare communications and practices play an important or even essential role in ensuring that individuals receive prompt and effective healthcare. Due to the nature of these communications, as well as the various environments in which individuals receive healthcare, the potential exists for an individual's health information to be disclosed incidentally.

---

[10]Ibid.

For example, a hospital visitor may overhear a provider's confidential conversation with another provider or a patient, or may glimpse a patient's information on a sign-in sheet or nursing station whiteboard.

The HIPAA Privacy Rule is not intended to impede customary and essential communications and practices and, thus, does not require that *all* risk of incidental use or disclosure be eliminated to satisfy its standards. In fact the Privacy Rule permits certain incidental uses and disclosures of protected health information to occur where there is in place reasonable safeguards and minimum necessary policies and procedures that normally protect an individual's privacy.[11]

**A PATIENT'S RIGHT TO KNOW ABOUT DISCLOSURES**  Whether the practice has disclosed PHI based on a signed authorization or to comply with a government agency, the patient is entitled to know about it. Therefore, in most cases the medical office must track the disclosure.

The Privacy Rule gives individuals the right to receive a report of all disclosures made for purposes *other than* treatment, payment, or operation of the healthcare facility. The report must include the date of the disclosure, whom the information was provided to, a description of the information, and the stated purpose for the disclosure. The patient can request the report at any time and the practice must keep the records for at least six years.

**PATIENT ACCESS TO MEDICAL RECORDS**  In addition to protecting privacy, the law generally allows patients to be able to see and obtain copies of their medical records and request corrections if they identify errors and mistakes. Health plans, doctors, hospitals, clinics, nursing homes, and other covered entities generally must provide access to these records within 30 days of a patient request, but may charge patients for the cost of copying and sending the records.

**HEALTH INFORMATION MANAGEMENT RESPONSIBILITIES**  Managing the portions of the HIPAA Privacy Rule discussed so far are almost always a function performed by the health information management professionals responsible for patient medical records. Duties often include ensuring that the appropriate forms for consent or authorization are on file, that requests for release of information are within the time frame of the authorization, that only the minimum necessary portion of the chart is sent as a result of a request, and that the disclosure is properly tracked. HIM professionals in the medical records office will also likely have responsibility for providing patients with copies of their records and disclosure reports.

**PERSONAL REPRESENTATIVES**  "There may be times when individuals are legally or otherwise incapable of exercising their rights, or simply choose to designate another to act on their behalf with respect to these rights. Under the Rule, a person authorized to act on behalf of the individual in making healthcare related decisions is the individual's *personal representative*.

"The Privacy Rule requires covered entities to treat an individual's personal representative as the individual with respect to uses and disclosures of the individual's protected health information, as well as the individual's rights under the Rule. . . . In addition to exercising the individual's rights under the Rule, a personal representative may also authorize disclosures of the individual's protected health information."[12]

In general, the personal representative's authority over privacy matters parallels their authority to act on other healthcare decisions.

As an HIM professional you may need to determine who may authorize access to a patient's records on the patient's behalf. When in doubt, consult with the privacy officer at your facility. Figure 3-5 provides a chart of people who, by virtue of their relationship to a patient, must be automatically recognized as the personal representative for certain categories of individuals.

---

[11]Ibid.
[12]Ibid.

**FIGURE 3-5**

**Persons automatically recognized as personal representatives for patients.**

| If the Individual Is: | The Personal Representative Is: | Examples: |
|---|---|---|
| An Adult or an Emancipated Minor | A person with legal authority to make health care decisions on behalf of the individual | Health care power of attorney Court appointed legal guardian General power of attorney |
| A Minor (not emancipated) | A parent, guardian, or other person acting in loco parentis with legal authority to make health care decisions on behalf of the minor child | Parent, guardian, or other person (with exceptions in state law) |
| Deceased | A person with legal authority to act on behalf of the decedent or the estate (not restricted to health care decisions) | Executor of the estate Next of kin or other family member Durable power of attorney |

**MINOR CHILDREN**    In most cases, the parent, guardian, or other person acting as parent is the personal representative and acts on behalf of the minor child with respect to PHI. Even if a parent is not the child's personal representative, the Privacy Rule permits a parent access to a minor child's PHI when and to the extent it is permitted or required by state or other laws.

Conversely, regardless of the parent's status as personal representative, the Privacy Rule prohibits providing access to or disclosing the child's PHI to the parent, when and to the extent it is expressly prohibited under state or other laws.

"However, the Privacy Rule specifies three circumstances in which the parent is not the personal representative with respect to certain health information about the minor child. The three exceptional circumstances when a parent is not the minor's personal representative are:

- When State or other law does not require the consent of a parent or other person before a minor can obtain a particular healthcare service, and the minor consents to the healthcare service;
- When a court determines or other law authorizes someone other than the parent to make treatment decisions for a minor;
- When a parent agrees to a confidential relationship between the minor and the physician.

**Example:**

A physician asks the parent of a 16-year-old if the physician can talk with the child confidentially about a medical condition and the parent agrees."[13]

If state or other laws are silent or unclear about parental access to the minor's PHI, the Privacy Rule grants healthcare professionals the discretion to allow or deny a parent access to a minor's PHI based on their professional judgment.

**BUSINESS ASSOCIATES**    "The HIPAA Privacy Rule applies only to covered entities—healthcare providers, plans, and clearinghouses. However, most healthcare providers and health plans do not carry out all of their healthcare activities and functions by themselves. Instead, they often use the services of a variety of other persons or businesses.

---

[13]Ibid.

"The Privacy Rule allows covered providers and health plans to disclose protected health information to these *business associates* if the providers or plans obtain written satisfactory assurances that the business associate will use the information only for the purposes for which it was engaged by the covered entity, will safeguard the information from misuse, and will help the covered entity comply with some of the covered entity's duties under the Privacy Rule.

"The covered entity's contract or other written arrangement with its business associate must contain the elements specified in the Privacy Rule. For example, the contract must:

■ Describe the permitted and required uses of protected health information by the business associate;

■ Provide that the business associate will not use or further disclose the protected health information other than as permitted or required by the contract or as required by law; and

■ Require the business associate to use appropriate safeguards to prevent a use or disclosure of the protected health information other than as provided for by the contract."[14]

It will generally fall to the privacy officer, or in larger healthcare organizations to the legal department, to ensure that business associate agreements are on file for clearinghouses, transcription services, and other businesses with whom you will exchange PHI as an HIT or HIM professional.

## A REAL-LIFE STORY

## The First HIPAA Privacy Case[15]

The first legal case under the privacy rule concerned the theft of patient demographic information (name, address, date of birth, Social Security number) by an employee in a medical office.

The former employee of a cancer care facility pled guilty in federal court in Seattle, Washington, to wrongful disclosure of individually identifiable health information for economic gain.

The ex-employee admitted that he obtained a cancer patient's name, date of birth, and Social Security number while employed at the medical facility, and that he disclosed that information to get four credit cards in the patient's name. He also admitted that he used several of those cards to rack up more than $9,000 in debt in the patient's name. He used the cards to purchase various items, including video games, home improvement supplies, apparel, jewelry, porcelain figurines, groceries, and gasoline for his personal use. He was fired shortly after the identity theft was discovered.

"Too many Americans have experienced identity theft and the nightmare of dealing with bills they never incurred. To be a vulnerable cancer patient, fighting for your life, and having to cope with identity theft is just unconscionable," stated U.S. Attorney John McKay. "This case should serve as a reminder that misuse of patient information may result in criminal prosecution."

The case was investigated by the Federal Bureau of Investigation (FBI) and prosecuted by the United States Attorney's Office. The man was sentenced to a term of 10 to 16 months. He has also agreed to pay restitution to the credit card companies and to the patient for expenses he incurred as a result of the misuse of his identity.

Though identity theft is serious, the consequences are much greater in a medical setting than if the same information had been stolen from an ordinary business. Why? Because even the patient's name and date of birth are part of the PHI. Additionally, the disclosure of medical information for financial gain could have resulted in a sentence of 10 years for each violation. The case serves as a reminder for everyone in the healthcare field of the personal responsibility for protecting PHI.

Although the patient privacy rule under HIPAA does not restrict the internal use of health information by the staff for treatment, payment, and operation of the healthcare facilities, you should make every effort to protect your patients' privacy and always follow the privacy policy of the practice.

---

[14]Ibid.

[15]Press release, United States Attorney's Office, Western District of Washington, August 19, 2004.

### CIVIL AND CRIMINAL PENALTIES

> The OCR within HHS oversees and enforces the Privacy Rule, while CMS oversees and enforces all other Administrative Simplification requirements, including the Security Rule.

"Congress provided civil and criminal penalties for covered entities that misuse personal health information. For civil violations of the standards, OCR may impose monetary penalties up to $100 per violation, up to $25,000 per year, for each requirement or prohibition violated. Criminal penalties apply for certain actions such as knowingly obtaining protected health information in violation of the law. Criminal penalties can range up to $50,000 and one year in prison for certain offenses; up to $100,000 and up to five years in prison if the offenses are committed under "false pretenses"; and up to $250,000 and up to 10 years in prison if the offenses are committed with the intent to sell, transfer or use protected health information for commercial advantage, personal gain or malicious harm."[16]

## HIPAA Security Rule

To fully comply with the Privacy Rule, it is necessary to understand and implement the requirements of the Security Rule. In this section you will learn about the Security Rule.

There are clearly areas in which the two rules supplement each other because both the HIPAA Privacy and Security Rules are designed to protect identifiable health information. However, the Privacy Rule covers PHI in all forms of communications, whereas the Security Rule covers only electronic information. Because of this difference, security discussions are assumed to be about the protection of electronic health records, but the Security Rule actually covers all PHI that is stored electronically. This is called EPHI.

### PHI—EPHI

> The Security Rule applies only to EPHI, whereas the Privacy Rule applies to PHI that may be in electronic, oral, and in paper form.

If you are interested in becoming an IT professional, especially if you will work in the computer network or operations aspects of an HIS department, you will be involved in or responsible for many of the aspects of security discussed here. However, whether you work in HIM or IT, it is important that you participate in the security training and follow the security policy and procedures of your healthcare organization.

### THE PRIVACY RULE AND SECURITY RULE COMPARED

The Privacy Rule sets the standards for, among other things, who may have access to PHI, while the Security Rule sets the standards for ensuring that only those who should have access to EPHI will actually have access. The primary distinctions between the two rules follow:

- Electronic versus oral and paper: The Privacy Rule applies to all forms of patients' protected health information, whether electronic, written, or oral. In contrast, the Security Rule covers only protected health information that is in electronic form. This includes EPHI that is created, received, maintained or transmitted.

---

[16]*Fact Sheet: Protecting the Privacy of Patients' Health Information* (Washington, DC: U.S. Department of Health and Human Services Press Office, April 14, 2003).

- "Safeguard" requirement in Privacy Rule: While the Privacy Rule contains provisions that currently require covered entities to adopt certain safeguards for PHI, the Security Rule provides for far more comprehensive security requirements and includes a level of detail not provided in the safeguard section of the Privacy Rule.

- HHS regulates and enforces HIPAA using two different divisions for enforcement. OCR or Office of Civil Rights enforces the Privacy Rule while CMS enforces the Security Rule.

## Security Standards

The security standards in HIPAA were developed for two primary purposes. First, and foremost, the implementation of appropriate security safeguards protects certain electronic healthcare information that may be at risk. Second, protecting an individual's health information, while permitting the appropriate access and use of that information, ultimately promotes the use of electronic health information in the industry—an important goal of HIPAA.

"The security standards are divided into the categories of administrative, physical, and technical safeguards. Each category of the safeguards is comprised of a number of standards, which generally contain of a number of implementation specifications.

- *Administrative safeguards:* In general, these are the administrative functions that should be implemented to meet the security standards. These include assignment or delegation of security responsibility to an individual and security training requirements.

- *Physical safeguards:* In general, these are the mechanisms required to protect electronic systems, equipment and the data they hold, from threats, environmental hazards and unauthorized intrusion. They include restricting access to EPHI and retaining off-site computer backups.

- *Technical safeguards:* In general, these are primarily the automated processes used to protect data and control access to data. They include using authentication controls to verify that the person signing onto a computer is authorized to access that EPHI, or encrypting and decrypting data as it is being stored and/or transmitted.

"In addition to the safeguards [listed above], the Security Rule also contains several standards and implementation specifications that address organizational requirements, as well as policies and procedures and documentation requirements."[17]

## Implementation Specifications

An implementation specification is an additional detailed instruction for implementing a particular standard. Implementation requirements and features within the categories were listed in the Security Rule by alphabetical order to convey that no one item was considered to be more important than another.

Implementation specifications in the Security Rule are either "required" or "addressable." *Addressable* does *not* mean optional.

To help you understand the organization of safeguards, security standards, and implementation specifications, a matrix of the HIPAA Security Rule is provided in Figure 3-6. The matrix is a part of the official rule and published as an appendix to the rule. You may wish to refer to Figure 3-6 as we discuss each of the following sections.

---

[17]Adapted from *Security 101 for Covered Entities*, HIPAA Security Series (Baltimore, MD: Centers for Medicare and Medicaid Services, November 2004 and revised March 2007).

## Security Standards Matrix

### Administrative Safeguards

| Standards | Section of Rule | Implementation Specifications | Required or Addressable |
|---|---|---|---|
| Security Management Process | § 164.308Addressable(1) | Risk Analysis | Required |
| | | Risk Management | Required |
| | | Sanction Policy | Required |
| | | Information System Activity Review | Required |
| Assigned Security Responsibility | § 164.308Addressable(2) | | Required |
| Workforce Security | § 164.308Addressable(3) | Authorization and/or Supervision | Addressable |
| | | Workforce Clearance Procedure | Addressable |
| | | Termination Procedures | Addressable |
| Information Access Management | § 164.308Addressable(4) | Isolating Health Care Clearinghouse Function | Required |
| | | Access Authorization | Addressable |
| | | Access Establishment and Modification | Addressable |
| Security Awareness and Training | § 164.308Addressable(5) | Security Reminders | Addressable |
| | | Protection from Malicious Software | Addressable |
| | | Log-In Monitoring | Addressable |
| | | Password Management | Addressable |
| Security Incident Procedures | § 164.308Addressable(6) | Response and Reporting | Required |
| Contingency Plan | § 164.308Addressable(7) | Data Backup Plan | Required |
| | | Disaster Recovery Plan | Required |
| | | Emergency Mode Operation Plan | Required |
| | | Testing and Revision Procedure | Addressable |
| | | Applications and Data Criticality Analysis | Addressable |
| Evaluation | § 164.308Addressable(8) | | Required |
| Business Associate Contracts and Other Arrangement | § 164.308(b)(1) | Written Contract or Other Arrangement | Required |

**FIGURE 3-6   HIPAA's Security Standards matrix.[18]**

### Administrative Safeguards[19]

The name *Security Rule* sounds like it would be mostly technical, but the largest category of the rule is administrative safeguards. The administrative safeguards comprise more than half of the HIPAA security requirements.

---

[18]*Security Standards: Administrative Safeguards,* HIPAA Security Series #2 (Baltimore, MD: Centers for Medicare and Medicaid Services, May 2005 and revised March 2007), 27–29.

[19]Adapted from *Security Standards: Administrative Safeguards,* HIPAA Security Series #2 (Baltimore, MD: Centers for Medicare and Medicaid Services, May 2005 and revised March 2007).

## Physical Safeguards

| Standards | Section of Rule | Implementation Specifications | Required or Addressable |
|---|---|---|---|
| Facility Access Controls | § 164.310Addressable(1)) | Contingency Operations | Addressable |
| | | Facility Security Plan | Addressable |
| | | Access Control and Validation Procedures | Addressable |
| | | Maintenance Records | Addressable |
| Workstation Use | § 164.310(b)Required | | Required |
| Workstation Security | § 164.310(c)Required | | Required |
| Device and Media Controls | § 164.310(d)(1) | Disposal | Required |
| | | Media Re-use | Required |
| | | Accountability | Addressable |
| | | Data Backup and Storage | Addressable |

## Technical Safeguards

| Standards | Section of Rule | Implementation Specifications | Required or Addressable |
|---|---|---|---|
| Access Control | § 164.312Addressable(1) | Unique User Identification | Required |
| | | Emergency Access Procedure | Required |
| | | Automatic Logoff | Addressable |
| | | Encryption and Decryption | Addressable |
| Audit Controls | § 164.312(b) | | Required |
| Integrity | § 164.312(c)(1) | Mechanism to Authenticate Electronic Protected Health Information | Addressable |
| Person or Entity Authentication | § 164.312(d) | | Required |
| Transmission Security | 164.312(e)(1) | Integrity Controls | Addressable |
| | | Encryption | Addressable |

**FIGURE 3-6    HIPAA's Security Standards matrix. (Continued)**

Administrative safeguards are the policies, procedures, and actions required to manage the implementation and maintenance of security measures to protect EPHI. We discuss each standard in the following sections.

**SECURITY MANAGEMENT PROCESS**    The Security Management Process standard is the first step. It is used to establish the administrative processes and procedures. There are four implementation specifications in the Security Management Process standard:

1. **Risk Analysis**
   Identify potential security risks and determine how likely they are to occur and how serious they would be.

**2. Risk Management**

Make decisions about how to address security risks and vulnerabilities. The risk analysis and risk management decisions are used to develop a strategy to protect the confidentiality, integrity, and availability of EPHI.

**3. Sanction Policy**

Define for employees what the consequences of failing to comply with security policies and procedures are.

**4. Information System Activity Review**

Regularly review records such as audit logs, access reports, and security incident tracking reports. The information system activity review helps to determine if any EPHI has been used or disclosed in an inappropriate manner.

**ASSIGNED SECURITY RESPONSIBILITY**    Similar to the Privacy Rule, which requires an individual be designated as the privacy official, the Security Rule requires one individual be designated the security official. The security official and privacy official can be the same person, but do not have to be. The security official has overall responsibility for security; however, specific security responsibilities may be assigned to other individuals. For example, the security official might designate the IT Director to be responsible for network security. Figure 3-7 shows a staff meeting at which security policy is being reviewed.

**WORKFORCE SECURITY**    Within the Workforce Security standard there are three addressable implementation specifications:

**1. Authorization and/or Supervision**

Authorization is the process of determining whether a particular user (or a computer system) has the right to carry out a certain activity, such as reading a file or running a program.

**2. Workforce Clearance Procedure**

Ensure that members of the workforce with authorized access to EPHI receive appropriate clearances.

**3. Termination Procedures**

Procedures must be in place to remove access privileges as soon as an employee, contractor, or other individual leaves the organization.

**FIGURE 3-7**

**Office staff review security policy and appoint a security official.**

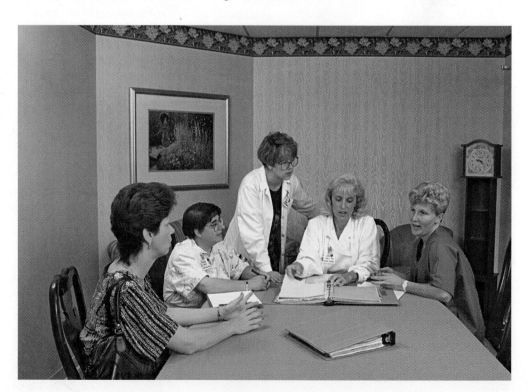

**INFORMATION ACCESS MANAGEMENT**    Restricting access to only those persons and entities with a need for access is a basic tenet of security. By managing information access, the risk of inappropriate disclosure, alteration, or destruction of EPHI is minimized. *Note:* This safeguard supports the "minimum necessary standard" of the HIPAA Privacy Rule.

The Information Access Management standard has three implementation specifications:

1. **Access Authorization**

   In the Workforce Security standard (see preceding section) the healthcare organization determined who has access. This section requires the organization to identify who has authority to grant that access and the process for doing so.

2. **Access Establishment and Modification**

   Once a covered entity has clearly defined who should be allowed access to what EPHI and under what circumstances, it must consider how access is established and modified.

3. **Isolating Healthcare Clearinghouse Functions**

   A clearinghouse is a unique HIPAA-covered entity whose function is to translate nonstandard transactions into HIPAA standards. In the very rare case that your healthcare organization also operates a clearinghouse, the rule requires the isolation of clearinghouse computers from other systems in the organization.

**SECURITY AWARENESS AND TRAINING**    Regardless of the administrative safeguards an organization implements, those safeguards will not protect the EPHI if the workforce is unaware them. Many security risks and vulnerabilities within an organization are internal. This is why the security awareness and training for all new and existing members of the workforce is required by this standard. In addition, periodic retraining should be given whenever changes at the facility could affect the security of EPHI. An employee is being trained in Figure 3-8.

The Security Awareness and Training standard has four implementation specifications:

1. **Security Reminders**

   Security reminders might include notices in printed or electronic form, agenda items and specific discussion topics at monthly meetings, and focused reminders posted in affected areas, as well as formal retraining on security policies and procedures.

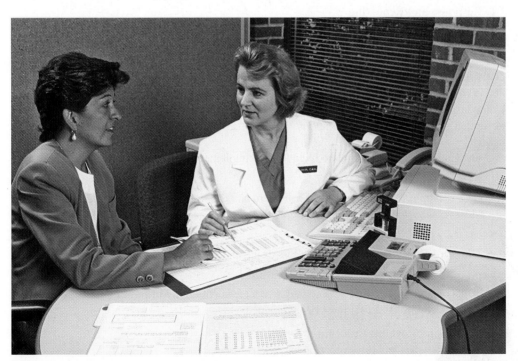

**FIGURE 3-8**

**Training a new employee on Security Policy and Procedures.**

## 2. Protection from Malicious Software

One important security measure that employees need to be reminded of is that malicious software is frequently brought into an organization through e-mail attachments and programs that are downloaded from the Internet. As a result of an unauthorized infiltration, EPHI and other data can be damaged or destroyed, or at a minimum, require expensive and time-consuming repairs.

## 3. Log-in Monitoring

Security awareness and training should also address how users log onto systems and how they are supposed to manage their passwords. Typically, an inappropriate or attempted log-in is when someone enters multiple combinations of user names and/or passwords to attempt to access an information system. Fortunately, many information systems can be set to identify multiple unsuccessful attempts to log in. Other systems might record the attempts in a log or audit trail. Still other systems might disable a password after a specified number of unsuccessful log-in attempts.

## 4. Password Management

In addition to providing a password for access, employees must be trained on how to safeguard it. Establish guidelines for creating passwords and changing them periodically.

**SECURITY INCIDENT PROCEDURES** Security incident procedures address how to identify security incidents and require that the incident be reported to the appropriate person or persons. Examples of possible incidents include:

- Stolen or otherwise inappropriately obtained passwords that are used to access EPHI
- Corrupted backup tapes that do not allow restoration of EPHI
- Virus attacks that interfere with the operations of computers containing EPHI
- Physical break-ins leading to the theft of media with EPHI on it
- Failure to terminate the account of a former employee that is then used by an unauthorized user to access information systems with EPHI
- Providing media with EPHI, such as a PC hard drive or laptop, to another user who is not authorized to access the EPHI.

There is one required implementation specification for this standard.

## 1. Response and Reporting

Establish adequate response and reporting procedures for these and other types of events.

**CONTINGENCY PLAN** What happens if your organization experiences a power outage, a natural disaster, or other emergency that disrupts normal access to healthcare information? A contingency plan consists of strategies for recovering access to EPHI should the organization experience a disruption of critical business operations. The goal is to ensure that EPHI is available when it is needed.

The Contingency Plan standard includes five implementation specifications:

## 1. Data Backup Plan

Data backup plans are an important safeguard and a required implementation specification. Most organizations already have backup procedures as part of current business practices.

## 2. Disaster Recovery Plan

These are procedures to restore any loss of data.

## 3. Emergency Mode Operation Plan

When operating in emergency mode due to a technical failure or power outage, security processes to protect EPHI must be maintained.

## 4. Testing and Revision Procedure

Periodically test and revise contingency plans.

## A REAL-LIFE STORY

### Contingency Plans Ensure Continued Ability to Deliver Care

*By Tanya Townsend*

*Tanya Townsend is the director of information technology at Saint Clare's Hospital in Schofield, Wisconsin.*

Saint Clare's is a new hospital that opened in 2005. We use all-digital health records; that is, there are no paper patient records, charts, or orders. As I talk to other hospitals and IT professionals about our accomplishments one question I am frequently asked is "What are your contingency plans in case of a power or system failure?"

Much of our plan is designed to avoid an outage in the first place. We have several redundancies in place to prevent that. For example, we have two WAN (wide-area network) connections; completely separate links going out different sides of the building to our core data center. The idea is that if one of those lines were to become disconnected for any reason, the other would seamlessly continue to function. In actual capacity they are balanced to make sure that can be accomplished. We also have redundancies on the local-area network with wireless access points. As mobile as we are, we are very dependent on wireless.

For data protection we have multiple data centers. On the hospital side we have two different data centers that are redundant. On the ambulatory side there are three. In addition to these data centers, we also back up all the data real-time to another off-site location in Madison, which is a couple of hours away.

Should we lose connectivity because both links are down we have a satellite antenna on the roof that can access the backup data in Madison. So as long as you can still power up your computer, you can get to the historical information. Electrical power can be supplied by an emergency generator that is designed to come online automatically in the event of a power loss.

Should the systems ever be completely down, we still need to take care of patients. In that event we have downtime procedures for utilizing paper forms that would allow us to continue to function. The necessary forms can be printed on demand but we have some preprinted copies on hand in case a power loss prevented us from printing. Once the system again becomes available, we have a policy and process for incorporating that paper documentation back into the system so we are not forced to carry that paper record forward.

The other area where we have built redundancy is our voice communications. We are using Voice-over-IP technology for our telecommunications, so a power or network outage would mean our phones wouldn't work either. We plan for that by having cell phones and radios available. We also have certain phones that use traditional phone lines so we can continue to communicate.

We do a practice run, a mock downtime situation twice a year. One time is just simulated, but for the second one we actually take the systems down to make sure that we know how we are going to function. We also have planned outages, where we need to take the system down because we are upgrading it or doing maintenance on it. We continue to strive to keep those outages as brief as possible, but in those events we go to our downtime procedures and we continuously learn and improve on these.

5. **Application and Data Criticality Analysis**

Analyze software applications that store, maintain, or transmit EPHI and determine how important each is to patient care or business needs. A prioritized list of specific applications and data will help determine which applications or information systems get restored first and/or which must be available at all times.

**EVALUATION**  Ongoing evaluation of security measures is the best way to ensure that all EPHI is adequately protected. Periodically evaluate strategy and systems to ensure that the security requirements continue to meet the organization's operating environments.

**BUSINESS ASSOCIATE CONTRACTS AND OTHER ARRANGEMENTS**  The Business Associate Contracts and Other Arrangements standard is comparable to the Business Associate Contract standard in the Privacy Rule, but is specific to business associates that create, receive, maintain, or transmit EPHI. The standard has one implementation specification:

1. **Written Contract or Other Arrangement**

Covered entities should have a written agreement with business associates ensuring the security of EPHI. Government agencies that exchange EPHI should have a memorandum of understanding in place.

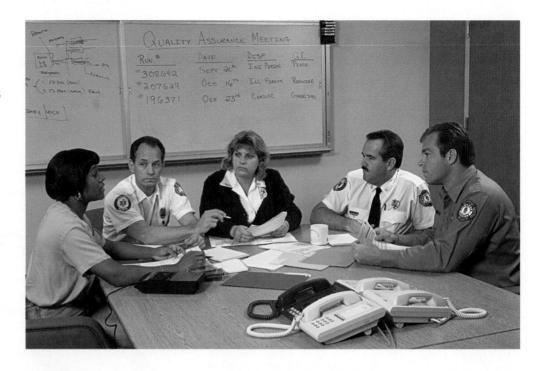

## Physical Safeguards[20]

The Security Rule defines physical safeguards as "physical measures, policies, and procedures to protect a covered entity's electronic information systems and related buildings and equipment, from natural and environmental hazards, and unauthorized intrusion."

**FACILITY ACCESS CONTROLS**   The Facility Access Controls standard deals with policies and procedures that limit physical access to electronic information systems and the facility or facilities in which they are housed. Facility access controls, like all security measures, should be reviewed periodically (Figure 3-9). There are four implementation specifications:

1. **Access Control and Validation Procedures**
   Access control and validation procedures determine which persons should have access to certain locations within the facility based on their roles or functions.

2. **Contingency Operations**
   Contingency operations refer to physical security measures to be used in the event of the activation of contingency plans.

3. **Facility Security Plan**
   The facility security plan defines and documents the safeguards used to protect the facility or facilities. In addition, all staff or employees must know their roles in facility security. Some examples of facility safeguards include:

   • Locked doors, signs warning of restricted areas, surveillance cameras, alarms

   • Property controls such as property control tags and engravings on equipment

   • Personnel controls such as identification badges, visitor badges, and/or escorts for large offices

   • Private security service or patrol for the facility.

---

[20]Adapted from *Security Standards: Physical Safeguards,* HIPAA Security Series #3 (Baltimore, MD: Centers for Medicare and Medicaid Services, February 2005 and revised March 2007).

### 4. Maintenance Records

Document facility security repairs and modifications such as changing locks, making routine maintenance checks, or installing new security devices.

**WORKSTATION USE**    Inappropriate use of computer workstations can expose your organization to risks, such as virus attacks, compromise of information systems, and breaches of confidentiality. The organization should specify the functions that are proper on HIS workstations. The workstation use policies also apply to workforce members who work off-site using workstations that can access EPHI. This includes employees who work from home, in satellite offices, or in another facility.

**WORKSTATION SECURITY**    While the Workstation Use standard addresses the policies and procedures for how workstations should be used and protected, the Workstation Security standard addresses how workstations are to be physically protected from unauthorized users.

**DEVICE AND MEDIA CONTROLS**    The Device and Media Controls standard provides policies and procedures that govern the receipt and removal of hardware and electronic media that contain EPHI into and out of a facility, and the movement of these items within the facility.

The Device and Media Controls standard has four implementation specifications:

### 1. Disposal

When disposing of any electronic media that contains EPHI, make sure it is unusable and/or inaccessible.

### 2. Media Re-use

Instead of disposing of electronic media, the IT department may want to reuse it. The EPHI must be removed before the media can be reused.

### 3. Accountability

When hardware and media containing EPHI are moved from one location to another, a record should be maintained of the move. Portable computers and media present a special challenge. Portable technology is getting smaller, less expensive, and has an increased capacity to store large quantities of data, making accountability even more important and challenging.

### 4. Data Backup and Storage

This specification protects the availability of EPHI and is similar to the data backup plan detailed in the Contingency Plan administrative standard.

## Technical Safeguards[21]

The Security Rule defines technical safeguards as "the technology and the policy and procedures for its use that protect electronic protected health information and control access to it."

Because security technologies are likely to evolve faster than legislative rules, specific technologies are not designated by the Security Rule. Where the CMS guidance documents provide examples of security measures and technical solutions to illustrate the standards and implementation specifications, these are just examples. The Security Rule is *technology neutral*; healthcare organizations have the flexibility to use any solutions that help them meet the requirements of the rule.

**ACCESS CONTROL**    The Access Control standard outlines the procedures for limiting access to only those persons or software programs that have been granted access rights by the Information Access Management administrative standard (discussed earlier). Figure 3-10 shows one of the most common methods of access control.

---

[21] Adapted from *Security Standards: Technical Safeguards,* HIPAA Security Series #4 (Baltimore, MD: Centers for Medicare and Medicaid Services, May 2005 and revised March 2007).

**FIGURE 3-10**

**A clinician logs on to Allscripts Enterprise using a Unique User ID and Secure Password.**

(Courtesy of Allscripts, LLC.)

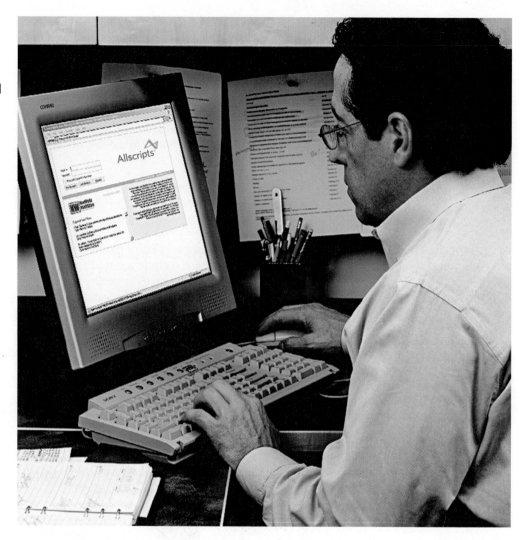

Four implementation specifications are associated with the Access Controls standard:

1. **Unique User Identification**
   The Unique User Identification specification provides a way to identify a specific user, typically by name and/or number. This allows the organization to track specific user activity and to hold users accountable for functions performed when logged into those systems.

2. **Emergency Access Procedure**
   Emergency access procedures are documented instructions and operational practices for obtaining access to necessary EPHI during an emergency situation. Under emergency conditions access controls may be very different from those used in normal operational circumstances.

3. **Automatic Logoff**
   As a general practice, users should log off the system they are working on when their workstation is unattended. However, there will be times when workers may not have the time, or will not remember, to log off of a workstation. Automatic logoff is an effective way to prevent unauthorized users from accessing EPHI on a workstation when it is left unattended for a period of time.

   Many applications have configuration settings for automatic logoff. After a predetermined period of inactivity, the application will automatically log off the user. As an example, your own computer may set up to go back to its log-in screen when you leave it unattended for too long. Though the operating system is not actually closing your applications, the concept is similar in that no one can see what was previously on your screen until you log in again.

### 4. Encryption and Decryption

Encryption is a method of converting regular text into code. The original message is encrypted by means of a mathematical formula called an *algorithm*. The receiving party uses a *key* to convert (decrypt) the coded message back into plain text. Encryption is part of access control because it prevents someone without the key from viewing or using the information.

**AUDIT CONTROLS**   Audit controls are "hardware, software, and/or procedural mechanisms that record and examine activity in information systems." Most information systems provide some level of audit controls and audit reports. These are useful, especially when determining if a security violation occurred. This standard has no implementation specifications.

**INTEGRITY**   Protecting the integrity of EPHI is a primary goal of the Security Rule. EPHI that is improperly altered or destroyed can result in clinical quality problems, including patient safety issues. The integrity of data can be compromised by both technical and nontechnical sources.

There is one addressable implementation specification in the Integrity standard.

### 1. Mechanism to Authenticate Electronic Protected Health Information

Once risks to the integrity of EPHI data have been identified during the risk analysis, security measures are put in place to reduce the risks.

**PERSON OR ENTITY AUTHENTICATION**   This standard requires "procedures to verify that a person or entity seeking access to electronic protected health information is the one claimed." It has no implementation specifications.

Some examples of ways to provide proof of identity for authentication include the following:

- Require something known only to that individual, such as a password or PIN.

- Require something that individuals possess, such as a smart card, a token, or a key. An example of a smart card is shown in Figure 3-11.

- Require something unique to the individual such as a biometric. Examples of biometrics include fingerprints, voice patterns, facial patterns, or iris patterns.

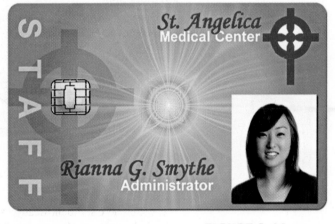

**FIGURE 3-11**

**A staff ID card that uses Smart Card Technology.**

(Courtesy of Digital Identification Solutions, LLC.)

Most covered entities use one of the first two methods of authentication. Many small provider offices rely on a password or PIN to authenticate the user.

**TRANSMISSION SECURITY**   Transmission Security is the "measures used to guard against unauthorized access to electronic protected health information that is being transmitted." The Security Rule allows for EPHI to be sent over an electronic open network as long as it is adequately protected. This standard has two implementation specifications:

### 1. Integrity Controls

Protecting the integrity of EPHI in this context is focused on making sure that the EPHI is not improperly modified during transmission. A primary method for protecting the integrity of EPHI being transmitted is through the use of network communications protocols. Using, these protocols, the computer verifies that the data sent is the same as the data received.

### 2. Encryption

As previously described in the Access Control standard, encryption is a method of converting an original message of regular text into encoded or unreadable text that is eventually decrypted into plain comprehensible text.

Encryption is necessary for transmitting EPHI over the Internet. Various types of encryption technology are available, but for encryption technologies to work properly, both the sender and receiver must be using the same or compatible technology. Currently no single interoperable encryption solution for communicating over open networks exists.

### Organizational, Policies and Procedures, and Documentation Requirements[22]

In addition to the administrative, physical, and technical safeguards, the Security Rule also has four other standards that must be implemented. These are not listed in the Security Standards matrix (Figure 3-6), but must not be overlooked.

**ORGANIZATIONAL REQUIREMENTS**    The two implementation specifications of this standard are:

1. **Business Associate Contracts**
   If business associates create, receive, maintain, or transmit EPHI, they must be contractually required to meet the Security Rule requirements.

2. **Other Arrangements**
   When both parties are government entities, there are two alternative arrangements:

   a. A memorandum of understanding (MOU) can be developed that accomplishes the objectives of the Business Associate Contracts section of the Security Rule.

   b. A law or regulation applicable to the business associate can be applied that accomplishes the objectives of the Business Associate Contracts section of the Security Rule.

**POLICIES AND PROCEDURES**    This standard requires covered entities to implement security policies and procedures, but does not define either "policy" or "procedure." Generally, policies define an organization's approach. Procedures describe how the organization carries out that approach, setting forth explicit, step-by-step instructions that implement the organization's policies.

**DOCUMENTATION**    The Documentation standard has three implementation specifications:

1. **Time Limit**
   Retain the documentation required by the rule for six years from the date of its creation or the date when it last was in effect, whichever is later.

2. **Availability**
   Make documentation available to those persons responsible for implementing the procedures to which the documentation pertains.

3. **Updates**
   Review documentation periodically, and update as needed, in response to environmental or operational changes affecting the security of the electronic protected health information.

The Security Rule also requires that a covered entity document the rationale for all security decisions.

## Chapter 3 Summary

### Accreditation and Regulation

Healthcare facilities and practitioners are licensed and regulated by federal, state, and local governments. In addition, voluntary compliance with standards set by recognized accreditation organizations can assist in meeting government requirements.

Government regulation influences healthcare delivery first by requiring licensure of both the facilities and their providers and, second, by requiring them to meet certain conditions to participate in programs such as Medicare that reimburse them for treating patients.

The Centers for Medicare and Medicaid Services (CMS) is an agency of the U.S. Department of Health and Human Services (HHS).

- Medicare provides healthcare coverage for people ages 65 and older as well as people with disabilities and those with end-stage renal disease (kidney failure).

---

[22]Adapted from *Security Standards: Organizational, Policies and Procedures and Documentation Requirements*, HIPAA Security Series #5 (Baltimore, MD: Centers for Medicare and Medicaid Services, May 2005 and revised March 2007).

- Medicaid provides healthcare benefits (partially paid by the states) for people who are poor, blind, or have a disability, for pregnant women, and for some persons over age 65 (in addition to Medicare).

Both programs are administered on a state level by *intermediaries,* companies that contract to handle claims processing, payments, authorizations, and provider inquiries for a region or a state.

In many cases, Blue Cross/Blue Shield, and commercial health insurance plans make rules similar to those set by CMS regarding preauthorization, payments, and coverage of medical services.

State laws provide detailed regulations concerning the operation of facilities, sanitation, medical and nursing staff requirements, and patient records. Even within the licensure of the hospital, the state may limit what services can be offered or require special licenses to operate certain departments within the facility. Local city and county governments may also regulate or license healthcare facilities.

In addition the licenses and inspections, healthcare facilities are also required to report incidents of infectious diseases, child abuse, and certain injuries such as gunshots. State and federal governments also require the facilities to report a substantial amount of statistical data concerning birth defects, cancer tumors, and the patients using the facility.

Participating providers and facilities are subject to inspection and audit by CMS as well as other insurance programs. Compliance with standards set by the Joint Commission, CAP, CARF, and other approved organizations can earn the facilities *deemed status,* meaning the accredited facility is deemed to have complied with CMS's conditions of participation (COP).

The Joint Commission, formerly known by the acronym JCAHO, is the leading accreditation organization for acute care facilities. In addition, the Joint Commission also accredits long-term, behavioral health, and ambulatory care settings. Acute care hospitals submit statistical data quarterly to the Joint Commission as part of a quality improvement initiative.

The College of American Pathologists (CAP) provides accreditation of medical laboratories as part of the organization's commitment to excellence in medical testing.

The Commission on Accreditation of Rehabilitation Facilities (CARF) provides accreditation for organizations offering behavioral health, physical, and occupational rehabilitation services as well as assisted living, continuing care, community services, employment services, and others.

## HIPAA

The Health Insurance Portability and Accountability Act, or HIPAA, was passed in 1996. The Administrative Simplification Subsection (Title 2, subsection f) (hereafter just called HIPAA) has four distinct components:

1. Transactions and Code Sets
2. Uniform Identifiers

3. Privacy
4. Security.

HIPAA regulates health plans, clearinghouses, and healthcare providers as "covered entities" with regard to these four areas.

HIPAA standardized EDI (electronic data interchange) formats by requiring specific transaction standards. These are currently used for eight types of transactions between covered entities. This section also requires the use of standardized code sets such as HCPCS, CPT-4, and ICD-9-CM.

HIPAA also established uniform identifier standards, which will be used on all claims and other data transmissions. These standards include:

- A national provider identifier (NPI) for doctors, nurses, and other healthcare providers
- A federal employer identification number that is used to identify employer-sponsored health insurance
- A National Health Plan Identifier, which is a unique identification number that will be assigned to each insurance plan and to the organizations that administer insurance plans, such as payers and third-party administrators.

### Privacy and Security of Patient Records

HIPAA's Privacy and Security Rules use two acronyms:

- PHI, which stands for protected health information
- EPHI, which stands for protected health information in an electronic format.

The HIPAA privacy standards are designed to protect a patient's identifiable health information from unauthorized disclosure or use in any form, while permitting the practice to deliver the best healthcare possible. Privacy activities in the average medical office might include:

- Providing a copy of the office privacy policy informing patients about their privacy rights and how their information can be used.
- Asking the patient to acknowledge receiving a copy of the policy and/or signing a consent form.
- Obtaining signed authorization forms and in some cases tracking the disclosures of patient health information when it is to be given to a person or organization outside the practice for purposes other than treatment, billing, or payment purposes.
- Adopting clear privacy procedures.
- Training employees so that they understand the privacy procedures.
- Designating an individual to be responsible for seeing that the privacy procedures are adopted and followed.
- Securing patient records containing individually identifiable health information so that they are not readily available to those who do not need them.

Providing the patient with a copy of the privacy policy implies consent for the practice to use PHI for almost anything related to treating the patient, running the medical practice, and getting paid for services. However, HIPAA consent is not the same as medical consent for treatment.

HIPAA authorization differs from HIPAA consent in that it *does* require the patient's permission to disclose PHI. Some examples of instances that would require an authorization would include sending the results of an employment physical to an employer and sending immunization records or the results of an athletic physical to the school.

The authorization form must include the date signed, an expiration date, to whom the information may be disclosed, what is permitted to be disclosed, and for what purpose the information may be used. The authorization must be signed by the patient or a representative appointed by the patient. Unlike the open concept of consent, authorizations are not global. A new authorization is signed each time there is a different purpose or need for the patient's information to be disclosed.

Practices are permitted to disclose PHI without a patient's authorization or consent when it is requested by an authorized government agency. Generally such requests are for legal (law enforcement, subpoena, court orders, etc.) public health purposes or for enforcement of the Privacy Rule itself. Providers are also permitted to disclose PHI concerning on-the-job injuries to workers' compensation insurers, state administrators, and other entities to the extent required by state law.

Whether the practice has disclosed PHI based on a signed authorization or to comply with a government agency, the patient is entitled to know about it. The Privacy Rule gives the individuals the right to receive a report of all disclosures made for purposes *other than treatment, payment, or operation of the healthcare facility*. Therefore, in most cases the medical office must track the disclosure and keep the records for at least six years.

Most healthcare providers and health plans use the services of a variety of other persons or businesses. The Privacy Rule allows disclosure of protected health information to these *business associates* if they obtain a written agreement that the business associate will appropriately safeguard the protected health information it receives or creates on behalf of the covered entity.

Congress has provided civil and criminal penalties for covered entities that misuse personal health information. The privacy rule is enforced by the HHS Office for Civil Rights (OCR).

The Privacy Rule sets the standards for, among other things, who may have access to PHI, whereas the Security Rule sets the standards for ensuring that only those who should have access to EPHI will actually have access. The Privacy Rule applies to all forms of patients' protected health information, whether electronic, written, or oral. In contrast, the Security Rule covers only protected health information that is in electronic form.

## Security Standards

Security standards were designed to provide guidelines to all types of covered entities, while affording them flexibility regarding how to implement the standards.

Security standards were designed to be "technology neutral." The rule does not prescribe the use of specific technologies, so that the healthcare community will not be bound by specific systems and/or software that may become obsolete.

The security standards are divided into the categories of administrative, physical, and technical safeguards:

- *Administrative safeguards:* These are the administrative functions that should be implemented to meet the security standards. These include assignment or delegation of security responsibility to an individual and security training requirements.
- *Physical safeguards:* These are the mechanisms required to protect electronic systems, equipment and the data they hold, from threats, environmental hazards and unauthorized intrusion. They include restricting access to EPHI and retaining off-site computer backups.
- *Technical safeguards:* These are primarily the automated processes used to protect data and control access to data. They include using authentication controls to verify that the person signing onto a computer is authorized, or encrypting and decrypting data as it is being stored and/or transmitted.

## Critical Thinking Exercises

1. You have a job in the HIM department. A friend of yours works for a lawyer. She comes to your facility to pick up copies of records for one of her boss's clients. She has forgotten to bring the client's authorization form. She is in a hurry and doesn't have time to go back to her office. You have known her for many years and are good friends. Do you give her the records without the authorization form?
2. If you decide to give your friend the records, what are the implications for your employer?
3. Is there a way to help your friend get the records without requiring her to drive back to her office?

# Testing Your Knowledge of Chapter 3

1. What is the advantage of Joint Commission accreditation?
2. Name the organization that accredits laboratory and testing personnel.
3. What does the CMS term *deemed status* refer to?
4. What do the acronyms PHI and EPHI stand for?
5. Compare the difference between consent and authorization in the context of HIPAA.
6. Does a provider need the patient's consent to share PHI with an authorized government agency?
7. List the four components of the HIPAA Administrative Simplification Subsection
8. Business associate agreements apply to which components of the Administrative Simplification Subsection?
9. What department of the U.S. government enforces HIPAA?
10. List the three categories of the security rule.
11. Name the *covered entities* under HIPAA.
12. Which components of the Administrative Simplification Subsection require employee training?
13. List the requirements for the medical office privacy policy.
14. Name three of HIPAA's technical safeguards.
15. Who may sign an authorization to release PHI?

# 4 Fundamentals of Information Systems

After completing this chapter, you should be able to:
- Understand fundamental concepts of computers
- Discriminate between hardware and software
- Define computer input and output
- Discuss components of a database
- Compare different types of computer data and explain relational data
- Describe different types of computer networks
- Understand how a wireless network functions
- Understand how interoperability standards help disparate systems exchange data

## ACRONYMS USED IN CHAPTER 4

Acronyms are used extensively in both medicine and computers. The following acronyms are used in this chapter.

| | | | |
|---|---|---|---|
| **ASCII** | American Standard Code for Information Interchange | **LAN** | Local-Area Network |
| **BLOB** | Binary Large Object | **LED** | Light Emitting Diode |
| **CAT** | Computerized Axial Tomography | **MDS** | Minimum Data Set |
| **CCOW** | Clinical Context Object Workgroup | **MRI** | Magnetic Resonance Imaging |
| **CD** | Compact Disk | **PACS OR PAC SYSTEM** | Picture Archiving and Communication System |
| **COLD** | Computer Output to Laser Disk | **PDA** | Personal Digital Assistant |
| **CPU** | Central Processing Unit | **PDF** | Portable Document Format |
| **DICOM** | Digital Imaging and Communication in Medicine | **PET** | Positron Emission Tomography |
| **DVD** | Digital Video Disk | **POP3** | Post Office Protocol, Version 3 |
| **HIM** | Health Information Management | **RAID** | Redundant Array of Independent Disks |
| **HIS** | Health Information System | **RAM** | Random Access Memory |
| **HL7** | Health Level 7 | **RIS** | Radiology Information System |
| **HTTP** | Hypertext Transfer Protocol | **SAN** | Storage Area Network |
| **IMAP** | Internet Message Access Protocol | **SMTP** | Simple Mail Transfer Protocol |
| **I/O** | Input/Output | **SSL** | Secured Socket Layer |
| **ISP** | Internet Service Provider | **TCP/IP** | Transmission Control Protocol/Internet Protocol |
| **JPEG** | Joint Photographic Experts Group | **TIFF** | Tagged Image File Format |

| **VPN** | Virtual Private Network | **WAN** | Wide-Area Network |
|---------|------------------------|---------|-------------------|
| **VOIP** | Voice-Over-Internet Protocol | **WI-FI** | Wireless Fidelity |

# The Technology behind Health Systems

As a student of this course you probably already use computers, but depending on your previous computer experience and previous courses you have taken, you may or may not understand them. The purpose of this chapter is to familiarize you with some of the terminology and concepts that make a computer work and that make dozens of computers work together as a health information system (HIS).

Computer systems are generally discussed in terms of two components: *hardware* and *software.*

## Hardware

*Hardware* refers to the components you can physically see and touch: the computer, circuit boards, computer chips, monitor screen, keyboard, mouse, cables, wires, printers, and so forth. When multiple computers are connected in a *network* (discussed later), the switches, routers, network cards, and cabling that connect them are also referred to as the hardware. Let's look at some specific types of hardware.

**CPU** The central processing unit (CPU) is sometimes referred to as the computer's brain. It is usually a single chip, which controls the flow of information to and from other parts of the computer. It often adds, subtracts, modifies, and otherwise "processes" the information passing through it according to instructions from the software.

**MEMORY AND STORAGE** Computers can hold vast quantities of information, but only a little of it is in the CPU at any one time. Information not currently being processed is stored elsewhere. Some of the places where it is stored include optical disks (CD or DVD), the hard drive, and computer memory chips. In most cases, the computer can both *read* the information stored on the device and *write* (save) information back to the device.

*Random access memory (RAM)* chips keep information in electronic circuits, which operate at or near the same speed as the CPU. This provides the CPU with the ability to access the information it needs very quickly such that the CPU can read and write information to RAM almost continuously. However, RAM information is only in memory while the computer is turned on. When the computer is turned off, the memory is cleared. Also, memory chips hold only a certain quantity of information; anything more than the chip can hold must be stored elsewhere.

*Hard drives* store information magnetically on disks that spin at high speeds inside a sealed unit. Unless the disk becomes damaged or exposed to a strong magnet, the information stored there is stable, and is retained even when the power is turned off. Hard drives can store vast quantities of information and are the computer's principal storage device. The CPU can both save and retrieve information from the hard drive. Though modern hard drives are very fast, they are considerably slower than the purely electronic circuits of RAM memory.

Figure 4-1 allows you to identify many of the hardware components discussed in this section. Because it generates intense amounts of heat, the CPU is covered by metal fins (heat sink) and a fan. The actual CPU is not visible in the picture.

*Optical disks,* such as CD-ROMs or DVDs, use lasers to burn information for long-term storage. The CPU can read and write optical disks just as it can hard drives, although an optical disk transfers information slower than does a hard drive. The advantage of an optical disk is that the storage is permanent. The disk is not affected by magnetism, has an extremely long life span, and can be removed from the computer when not needed. Although each disk has a fixed capacity, an unlimited number of disks can be used, making optical disks ideal for archiving records that are not frequently accessed.

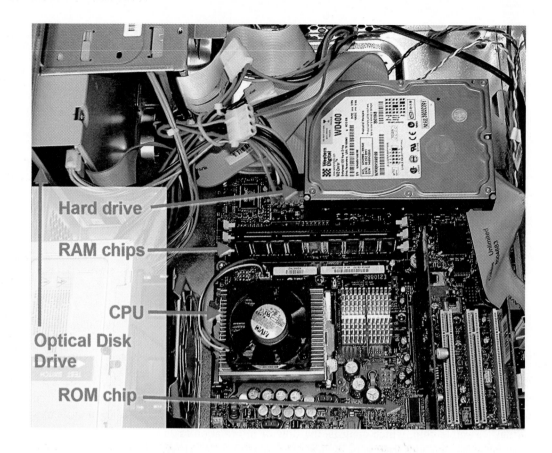

Although certain types of optical disks are reusable, optical disks cannot be written over accidentally. Optical disks are often used for the transfer and storage of large radiology images. They are a reliable media for permanent record archives.

*Read-only memory (ROM)* chips are computer chips with electronic circuits that retain information when the power is off. The CPU or other parts of the computer can read a ROM chip as quickly as a RAM chip, but cannot accidentally write over the information stored on the ROM. This type of memory is usually used to store instructions the computer needs to start up; also devices within the computer such as the hard drive may store information about its configuration on a ROM chip.

*Magnetic tape* was used in the early days of computing to actively store and retrieve data. Today it is used only to back up data stored on hard drives.

**INPUT AND OUTPUT DEVICES**   How does information get into the computer? Then once the information is in the computer, how do you see it? The computer terms for these concepts are *input* (putting information in) and *output* (information coming out of the computer). Sometimes the abbreviation I/O is used, which simply stands for input/output.

The main devices for inputting information into the computer are the keyboard and mouse. Likewise the most popular output device is the monitor or screen. Newer technology such as the Tablet PC (shown later in Figure 4-3) and touch screens, which are often used in kiosks, combine these functions, allowing the screen to act as both an input and an output device.

Printers are also output devices. The only output device for early computers was a teletype printer. Even after monitors came into use as the predominant display technology, business processes were so oriented toward paper records that most computer information was also printed, wasting tons of paper that also had to be stored.

In the 21st century businesses and healthcare organizations are increasingly using *scanners* to store images of documents instead of storing the paper documents. A scanner is an input device that looks and works much like a modern office copier, except where a copier prints a copy, a scanner sends it to a computer as a digital image. The image of the document can be retrieved and displayed on the computer screen or even reprinted whenever it is needed. A small scanner is shown in Figure 4-2.

However, if a document that an organization needs to keep, such as financial and other reports, was originally generated by a computer, then there is no need to waste time and paper printing the computer report, then scanning it back in as a document image. Some systems can directly create the report as an image file. This process, sometimes referred to by the acronym COLD (computer output to laser disk), will be discussed later in this chapter.

Other input devices include microphones and cameras, which can capture sound, digital pictures, and video to be saved directly in the computer. The monitor screen and computer speakers are the output devices for these types of files. Voice files and document image files can be converted to computer data using special computer programs (voice recognition and optical character recognition software, respectively).

Tablet PCs (Figure 4-3) and PDAs (personal digital assistants) can receive handwritten input. Using an inkless pen, called a stylus, that will not damage the screen, the user writes on the screen. Handwriting recognition software interprets the handwritten characters and changes them into typed letters and numbers, which can then be saved as computer data.

Medical images such as x-rays, CAT scans, MRIs, and PET scans are major input sources for health information systems. These diagnostic devices are able to save images directly from the medical device that captures them. Other medical devices that can output their information to an electronic patient chart include ultrasound and electrocardiogram devices and even those that measure vital signs.

So far the input and output methods we have discussed are those by which humans and computers interact, but for sheer quantity of data input and output, the greatest volume is the electronic exchange between computers. A small portion of this type of input and output is conducted using the memory storage devices we discussed earlier: CD-ROM, DVD, and portable RAM devices. However, most of the data exchanged between of computers is via *networks*, which are discussed later in this chapter.

**ERGONOMICS**   Because our primary method of inputting information into the computer is keyboarding, and our primary method of using that information is looking at a screen, workers who use a computer all day can develop various ailments from repeating the same motions, sitting at the same angle to the monitor, screen glare, and other factors. Computer *ergonomics* is the study of the physical effect of human/computer interaction on workers with the goal of minimizing or eliminating problems.

Ergonomics in the healthcare workplace goes beyond the computers. It is applied to the height and shape of desks, nurses' stations, wall units, portable carts, and the height at which monitors are mounted. Another consideration unique to healthcare is the ability to protect the keyboard, mouse, and the screens of portable devices so they can be sanitized without damaging the electronics.

Figure 4-4 shows a workstation mounted at a nurses' station using a bracket that allows the user to adjust the height and angle of both the monitor and keyboard for maximum ergonomics.

## Software

The second major component of our discussion is *software*. It consists of the logic, programs, and routines that make the

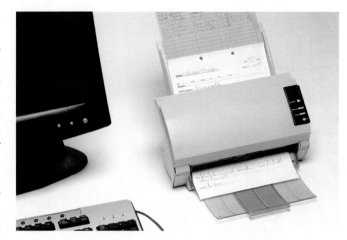

**FIGURE 4-2**

**A scanner captures an image of a document.**

(Courtesy of Allscripts, LLC.)

**FIGURE 4-3**

**Clinician using a tablet PC.**

(Courtesy of GE Healthcare.)

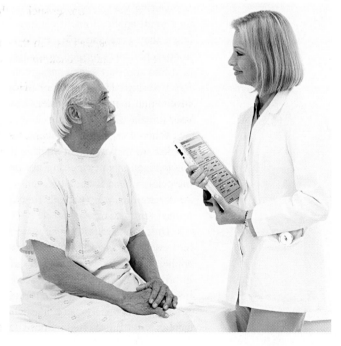

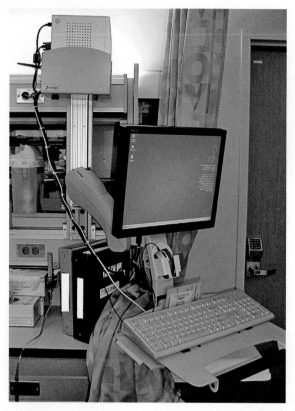

**FIGURE 4-4**

**Ergonomically mounted workstation in a nursing unit.**

hardware useful and provide instructions to the computer for processing the information it receives. It is referred to as "soft" because it is intangible. Unlike hardware, you cannot physically touch it. When you turn on your computer and when you start a desired program, those programs are temporarily loaded in the CPU and RAM. When you close a program those functions disappear.

Our discussion of software will be broadly grouped into two types: *operating system software* and *application software.*

**OPERATING SYSTEMS**   Operating system software consists of programs that enable us to work with a computer's hardware. This type of software includes functions that allow the CPU and other control chips to operate the monitor display, memory storage devices, and input/output devices, including the keyboard and mouse. You are probably most familiar with the Windows® or Macintosh operating systems; however, in HIS environments you may also find UNIX®, AIX®, HP-UX®, and LINUX®, which are also operating systems.

An operating system is not simply a single program, but rather thousands of little functions and programs that perform different operations. Generations of computer science advances have evolved into today's operating systems, making it possible for you to click the mouse, start a program, and see the characters you type appear on the screen. A few of the layers of this underlying technology are explained in the later section titled *Bits and Bytes—How Computers "Think."*

In a healthcare facility most of the computers are linked together into a *network.* The networking software is part of the operating systems just discussed, but we will learn more about networks later in this chapter.

**APPLICATION SOFTWARE**   Applications are the software that you use every day. They make the computer "apply" to the task we need done. A word processor is a good example of application software. To understand the differences between an operating system and application software, consider this simple example: Let us say you want to write a paper for class. You click on the word processor icon on your computer screen and the operating system loads the software into the CPU. You type your paper, spell check it, save it, and print it out.

During your word processing session, the operating system handled the many things common to all applications. It captured the signals from the keyboard and mouse, interpreted what letters they were, and provided those to the application. In contrast, the word processor kept track of how characters formed words, if they were spelled correctly, and when it was time to go to the next line and start a new paragraph or a new page. The application allowed you to decide what font was used and whether or not to center the title of your paper. Meanwhile, with each keystroke, the operating system communicated with your monitor so the characters appeared on your screen.

When you saved your work, the application called on the operating system, which stored it on the hard disk and kept track of its location for future retrieval. When you printed your paper, the application software sent not only the text but information about the margins, font changes, ink color, and so forth. However, it was the operating system that located the printer device, set up communications with it, regulated how fast the text was sent to it, and kept track of the printer's progress.

Unless you choose to become a computer or network technician, almost everything you do on a computer in an HIM profession will be focused on application software. Examples of HIS applications include patient registration and scheduling software, electronic health records, clinical information systems, computerized order entry systems, billing and coding software, document imaging systems, radiology information systems, and laboratory information systems, as well as generalized applications such as word processing, spreadsheets, and e-mail. Some of these applications will be discussed in more depth in later chapters.

## Bits and Bytes—How Computers "Think"

Computer processor and memory chips contain millions of transistors, each of which act like an on/off switch. These represent the smallest unit of information in the computer called a *bit*. Bits represent the values zero and one. If the transistor switch is off, the bit is zero; if the transistor switch is on, the bit is one. Imagine that the eight LED lights in Figure 4-5 represent a group of eight *bits*. Where the LED is green, the bit is on; where it is off, the LED is not lit.

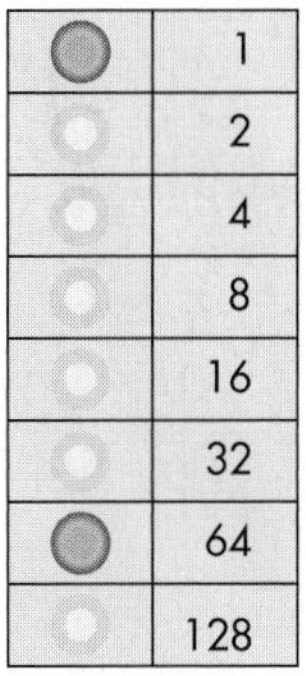

Look at the number next to each LED in Figure 4-5; notice that each successive number is twice as large as the one above it. When bits are grouped together, each succeeding bit in the group represents a number twice as large as the previous bit. From this humble beginning, the computer forms a binary number system. *Binary* means made up of two parts, in this case zero and a designated number.

Eight bits, grouped together, form the basic unit of computing called a *byte*. Figure 4-5 has eight bits, therefore it also illustrates one byte. The value of a byte is the cumulative total of its bits which are "on." For instance, in Figure 4-5 the LEDs next to bits 1 and 64 are on; the other LEDs represent bits that are "off" or zero. The sum of bits that are "on" represents the value of the byte, which in this figure is 65.

Logically, you can see how a computer could use this system to do math. For example, to add four to this number, turn on the third bit. The sum of the byte would then be (1 + 4 + 64 = 69). However, most of the data we see in the computer consists of letters, words, names, so how do bits become alphabetical?

In 1963 the American Standard Code for Information Interchange (ASCII) standardized text bytes by assigning a meaning to each possible combination of bits.[1] Bytes with values of 1 through 31 are used to control the flow of information in the computer. Bytes with values of 32 through 126 represent printable characters of the alphabet, punctuation, and numerals. Bytes with values of 128 through 255 are used as for extended characters. As an example, the table shown later in Figure 4-7 lists the values assigned to the alphabet characters in ASCII. For example, the value 65 shown in Figure 4-5 equates to the letter "A" in the ASCII standard.

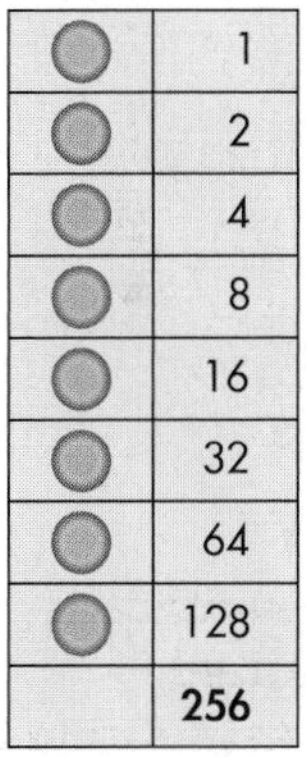

Although everything in computer memory is a function of bits being on or off, not everything is limited to 8-bit bytes. If all of the bits in Figure 4-6 are turned on, the highest number the computer could calculate would be 256. To go beyond this limit, *data types* are defined that use a larger number of bits. For example, a numeric *integer* is 16 bits. Integers can be used for whole numbers from −32,767 to 32,767. *Long integers* use 32 bits to handle larger whole numbers. Numeric data that has decimal fractions is a data type called *double,* which has 64 bits.

**EXTENDING FUNCTIONALITY**   So it's all math, right? Well, actually that is true. The genius of modern computer science has been the ability to take the basic arithmetic function derived from turning bits on and off and extend it into all of the possible data types we use today. Take color for example.

The smallest dot on a computer screen, called a *pixel,* can be displayed in millions of colors by using a large number of bits. If the pixel data were one bit, the only colors would be white (bit on) or black (bit off)—but define that pixel as eight bits and it can display 256 colors. When image data is defined as *true color,* it uses 32 bits and suddenly the computer can render all the nuances of a CAT scan or an MRI.

When images are scanned into a medical record, electronic circuits in the scanner capture the reflection of each pixel on the page and express it as a numerical value. The computer stores these digits in a file that it recognizes as image data.

Similarly, with sound files, a microphone captures the voice of a doctor dictating a note. A sound card converts the electrical signal into numbers representing the frequency of the sound wave at each instant. Computer software stores these in a file it recognizes as a sound file.

Even the computer software is really just ones and zeros stored in a type of file that the computer recognizes as program instructions. Virtually, everything in computer processing is a function of handling bits in specific size groups, defined as specific data types.

**FIGURE 4-5**

**LED lights illustrate 8 bits.**

| | |
|---|---|
| ● | 1 |
| ○ | 2 |
| ○ | 4 |
| ○ | 8 |
| ○ | 16 |
| ○ | 32 |
| ● | 64 |
| ○ | 128 |

**FIGURE 4-6**

**Maximum value of a byte is 256.**

| | |
|---|---|
| ● | 1 |
| ● | 2 |
| ● | 4 |
| ● | 8 |
| ● | 16 |
| ● | 32 |
| ● | 64 |
| ● | 128 |
| | 256 |

---

[1] ASCII characters use only seven bits. The eighth bit, called the parity bit, was originally reserved for error checking.

All that we see and hear from the computer is really just a marvelous expression derived from binary math. Computer science has built layer upon layer of functionality over these fundamental concepts, so that the user and even the programmer seldom need to think of bits and bytes.

Although an operating system's "data type" refers to how bits are grouped into logical units, in application software "data type" refers to how data is used: as a text character, a date, a mathematical value, and so forth. Hereafter, when we refer to a data type, we will be referring to the application-level definition.

# Databases

Thus far we have discussed the operating system and application software in terms of its ability to store, retrieve, and process information. In computer systems, information that is input is called *data*. Data is stored in an arrangement defined by the software to make it easy to identify and retrieve the data later. The structure defined by the application to hold the data is called a *database*. Healthcare systems typically have numerous databases.

A database can be structured in any of many different ways, but before exploring different types of databases, let us first discuss some of the key concepts of data.

## Characters

A *character* is the smallest unit of text data. Text characters (sometimes called *alphanumeric* characters) are limited to letters, numbers, a space, and punctuation marks as defined in the ASCII table shown in Figure 4-7. Some application software disallows certain punctuation marks; other software permits special symbols such as © to be used as data.

## Fields

*Fields* separate data into defined units that can be recognized later. For example, when you look at an envelope, your brain recognizes the street, city, state, and zip code by the way they are separated and the order in which they appear. Similarly, a database may have separate *fields* for the street address, the city, state, and zip code.

Storing data in defined fields not only allows the application software to retrieve and redisplay the data in the correct form, but it also allows the software to find and process pieces of data quickly. For example, having the zip code in its own field would make it possible for the application to sort and print addresses in zip code order.

**FIGURE 4-7**
**Decimal values for alphabet characters in the ASCII table.**

| Alphabet Portion of the ASCII Table (abridged) | | | | | | | | | |
|---|---|---|---|---|---|---|---|---|---|
| Value | Char. | Value | Char. | Value | Char. | Value | Char. | Value | Char. |
| Uppercase | | 75 | K | 86 | V | 95 | e | 106 | p |
| 65 | A | 76 | L | 87 | W | 96 | f | 107 | q |
| 66 | B | 77 | M | 88 | X | 97 | g | 108 | r |
| 67 | C | 78 | N | 89 | Y | 98 | h | 109 | s |
| 68 | D | 79 | O | 90 | Z | 99 | i | 110 | t |
| 69 | E | 80 | P | | | 100 | j | 111 | u |
| 70 | F | 81 | Q | Lowercase | | 101 | k | 112 | v |
| 71 | G | 82 | R | 91 | a | 102 | l | 113 | w |
| 72 | H | 83 | S | 92 | b | 103 | m | 114 | x |
| 73 | I | 84 | T | 93 | c | 104 | n | 115 | y |
| 74 | J | 85 | U | 94 | d | 105 | o | 116 | z |

Fields not only separate data into logical groups, but define the type of data in the field as well. Some basic *field types* are alphanumeric (text), numeric, and dates. Numeric fields are further defined as integers (whole numbers) or decimal numbers such as money.

Field types help the computer display and process the data correctly. For example, to print a report in chronological order, the computer needs to know that the number in a *date* field represents year, month, and day. When printing the amount field on the patient bill, the computer needs to know that the value in the *numeric* field is monetary and should be printed with two decimal places.

## Records

The next level of a database is a *record*. Records are made up of a group fields about a specific thing. For example, an address record may contain the fields for street address, city, state, and zip code. One record would hold the address data for patient Gloria Green; a separate address record would hold the address data for Rosa Garcia. The database could have thousands of address records for thousands of patients, but each record would have the same group of fields, arranged in the same order.

A database will have many different types of records. Each type of record can be made up of different fields, arranged in a different order, for a different purpose. We have discussed a record type for a patient's address, but the database also has a record type for the patient's insurance information, and yet another record type for the patient's visit.

Although spreadsheet programs are far simpler than the databases in healthcare, if you are familiar with Excel® you may be able to visualize the concepts of fields, records, tables, and files. For example, Figure 4-8 shows an Excel file containing patient information. Think of rows 2, 3, and 4 as records of data—one for each patient. Think of the columns as fields. Notice how each record has the same number of fields, even if there is no data. For example, Mr. Baker has no middle name, but the place for the middle name is reserved.

## Files and Tables

How are records stored? Some databases are a collection of many separate files, each holding a certain type of record. Other databases store all types of records in one or more large files and then define *tables* to group records of the same type together. Several data tables are shown later in Figure 4-10.

**DATA DICTIONARY**　Figure 4-8 was intended merely to provide a visual concept. A database would not usually have the field names in the data table. Fields and tables are defined elsewhere in the database or application and are referred to as the *data dictionary*.

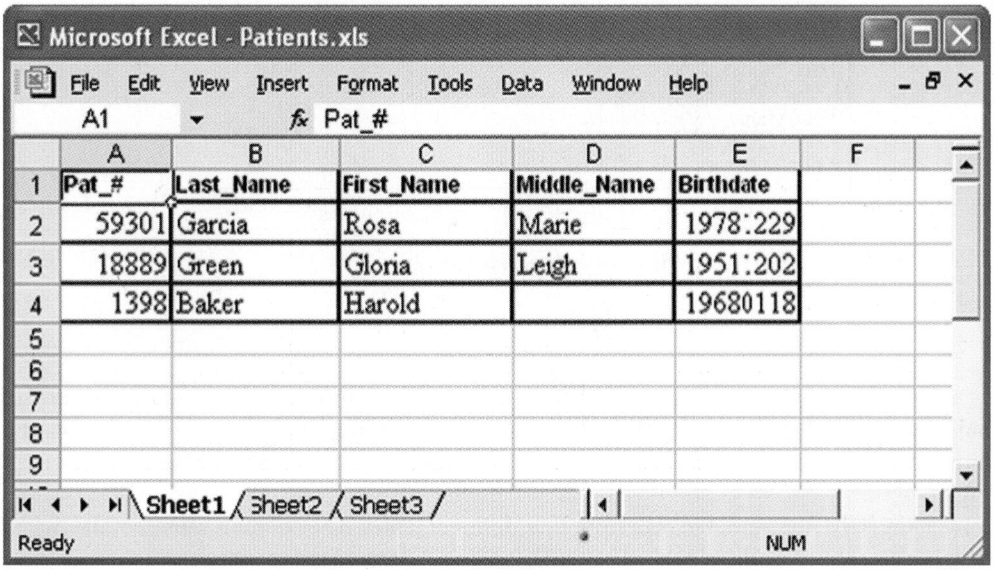

**FIGURE 4-8**

**Excel spreadsheet of patient information.**

| Patient Info Table | | |
|---|---|---|
| **Field Name** | **Len.** | **Data Type** |
| Pat_# | 12 | Integer |
| Last_Name | 22 | Alpha |
| First_Name | 15 | Alpha |
| Middle_Name | 15 | Alpha |
| Birthdate | 10 | Date |

| Patient Address | | |
|---|---|---|
| **Field Name** | **Len.** | **Data Type** |
| Pat_# | 12 | Long Integer |
| Address | 25 | Alpha |
| City | 25 | Alpha |
| State | 2 | Alpha |
| Zip | 10 | Alpha |

| Patient Visits | | |
|---|---|---|
| **Field Name** | **Len.** | **Data Type** |
| Pat_# | 12 | Long Integer |
| Encounter_# | 15 | Double |
| Date | 10 | Date |
| Time | 5 | Alpha |
| Provider_# | 4 | Integer |

| Provider Info Table | | |
|---|---|---|
| **Field Name** | **Len.** | **Data Type** |
| Provider_# | 12 | Integer |
| Last_Name | 22 | Alpha |
| First_Name | 15 | Alpha |
| Middle_Name | 15 | Alpha |
| Credentials | 10 | Alpha |

**FIGURE 4-9** **Data dictionary tables.**

The data dictionary defines the field name, the maximum length of data the field can hold, and the type of data the field will contain. It also defines the record layout; that is, the order of the fields in the record. Figure 4-9 illustrates a data dictionary for the tables used in Figure 4-10.

Figure 4-10 illustrates the data from four different tables. The columns represent the fields, and the rows represent the records. Each table holds a different kind of data.

| Patient Info Table | | | | |
|---|---|---|---|---|
| **Pat_#** | **Last_Name** | **First_Name** | **Middle_Name** | **Birthdate** |
| 59301 | Garcia | Rosa | Marie | 19781229 |
| 18889 | Green | Gloria | Leigh | 19511202 |
| 1398 | Baker | Harold | | 19680118 |

| Patient Address Table | | | | |
|---|---|---|---|---|
| **Pat_#** | **Address** | **City** | **State** | **Zip** |
| 59301 | 1301 Paces Ferry Rd | Atlanta | GA | 30339-1301 |
| 18889 | 3529 Cobb Dr | Smyrna | GA | 30080-3529 |
| 1398 | 9856 Peachtree Rd | Atlanta | GA | 30305-9856 |

| Patient Visits Table | | | | |
|---|---|---|---|---|
| **Pat_#** | **Encounter_#** | **Date** | **Time** | **Provider_#** |
| 59301 | 100875 | 20071220 | 09:00 | 1 |
| 59301 | 111219 | 20080211 | 11:15 | 2 |
| 59301 | 120547 | 20080601 | 16:30 | 1 |

| Provider Info Table | | | | |
|---|---|---|---|---|
| **Provider_#** | **Last_Name** | **First_Name** | **Middle_Name** | **Credentials** |
| 1 | Jones | Clive | Carl | MD |
| 2 | Smith | Marsha | Ann | ARNP |
| 3 | Lopez | Roseanne | | MD |

**FIGURE 4-10**   **Data tables for patients, addresses, encounters and providers.**

**RELATIONAL DATA**   The data dictionary may also indicate the relationship between records in one table to related records in another. Databases are designed to be very efficient. Long pieces of information that will be used many times can be stored once, and referenced only by an ID field that takes less space to store. Two examples of this can be found in Figure 4-10:

■ The HIS registration system has assigned each patient a unique ID number (stored in the first field). The Patient Address and Patient Visits records do not need the entire name, only the patient ID. Each time the application reads an address or visit record, it can automatically retrieve the patient's name from the *related* Patient Info record.

■ A second example, similar in concept, is that the Patient Visits records do not need to repeatedly store the full name of the doctor in every encounter record. It is only necessary to use an ID field that *relates* to a table of providers in the practice.

Virtually all healthcare information systems use *relational databases*. Well-designed relational databases store information efficiently, retrieve data very quickly, and expand easily as the organization's data grows.

Figure 4-11 illustrates how data from the different database tables in Figure 4-10 is used when printing a patient statement.

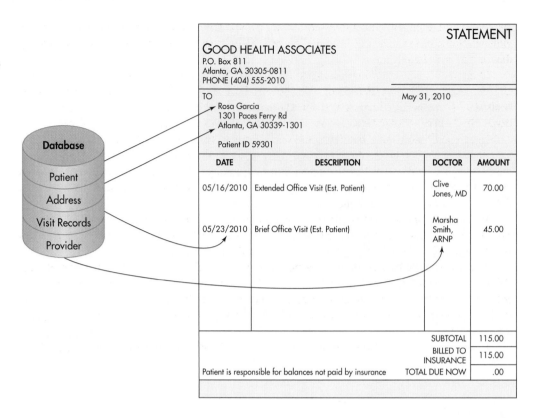

STATEMENT

GOOD HEALTH ASSOCIATES
P.O. Box 811
Atlanta, GA 30305-0811
PHONE (404) 555-2010

TO                                           May 31, 2010

Rosa Garcia
1301 Paces Ferry Rd
Atlanta, GA 30339-1301

Patient ID 59301

| DATE | DESCRIPTION | DOCTOR | AMOUNT |
|------|-------------|--------|--------|
| 05/16/2010 | Extended Office Visit (Est. Patient) | Clive Jones, MD | 70.00 |
| 05/23/2010 | Brief Office Visit (Est. Patient) | Marsha Smith, ARNP | 45.00 |
| | | SUBTOTAL | 115.00 |
| | | BILLED TO INSURANCE | 115.00 |
| Patient is responsible for balances not paid by insurance | | TOTAL DUE NOW | .00 |

## Images

Information stored in a healthcare system is not limited to the ASCII data we have discussed so far. Images that are used to diagnose the patient such as x-rays, MRIs, and CAT scans as well as scanned images of paper documents are also part of the patient's record. Images are captured and stored using different sets of standards. The DICOM (Digital Imaging and Communication in Medicine) standard is used for diagnostic images. Typical standards for photographs and scanned documents include these three:

- JPEG (Joint Photographic Experts Group)
- TIFF (Tagged Image File Format)
- PDF (Portable Document Format).

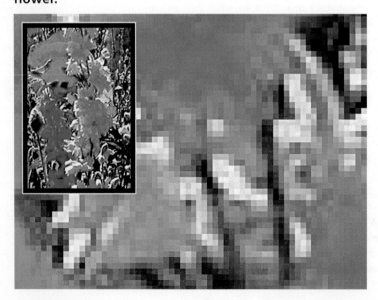

Conceptually, medical image files are made up of data similar to the photographs you take with your digital camera, except they are higher quality. A digital image consists of millions of dots, too small to see. In Figure 4-12 a portion of a digital photo is magnified to show the dots.

Whereas the smallest unit of ASCII data is a character (one byte), the smallest unit of an image is a *pixel*. A pixel represents the color, brightness, and contrast of a single dot in the image as a number. The amount of detail that can be seen in a digital image is a factor of the number of pixels (dots) per inch, and the number of *bits* used for each pixel. (Pixel size was discussed in more detail earlier in the *Bits and Bytes—How Computers "Think"* section.)

**IMAGE STORAGE: FILE OR BLOB**  Images can contain millions of pixels, making the amount of data enormous. Some of the image standards listed above permit the data to be compressed for storage and then restored to near original quality for viewing. Some of the standards keep the image in its original size and do not compress it, making the file size very large.

Diagnostic and radiology images are typically stored in a Picture Archiving and Communication System (PACS) or a Radiology Information System (RIS) computer. Some healthcare systems store images of scanned documents in the same system as the patient's electronic chart, whereas other systems use a separate computer for document image storage.

Images are *binary data,* but not ASCII data. Images vary in size, can be very large, and therefore do not fit well in the records and fields of the types of databases we have studied so far. There are two popular techniques for storing and retrieving images. Both methods use the database to catalog information about the image such as the patient, date, type of image, and a description. A field in the catalog record also indicates where the image is located.

In the first method, systems keep images as individual files on a hard drive, CD, or DVD. The database catalog records include a field containing the *path* (location) to the image files stored on the disk drive so the image can be accessed when desired.

The second method is to set up a portion of the database to hold binary large objects (BLOBs). Image data can then be stored directly in the database (though separate from the data stored in fields). When an application requests the image, the database retrieves the BLOB. The database recognizes that it is not data from a field and passes it on to the requesting application.

Image systems can also store many other types of digital information including audio or video files.

# Networks

In the early days, hospitals had a single giant computer called a mainframe. Users had screens and keyboards called terminals, but all of the computer processing was done by the mainframe. Today healthcare organizations of all sizes have hundreds of computers connected together as a *network*.

Networks allow computers to seamlessly pass information to one another and to share resources such as printers, scanners, application software, and central disk storage. Networks require special hardware and software, some of which is included in the operating system. There are several types of networks and many types of network software. Here we discuss but a few that are found in healthcare.

### Network Hardware

Networks require a network card for each computer (some newer computers have this built in). A network *router* is also required. The router is also sometimes called a *hub* or *switch*. It identifies each computer on the network and manages the flow of information throughout. Network cables, wires specially manufactured to handle data at high speeds, are run from the router to each computer. (Wireless networking is also used, as discussed in a later section.)

### Clients and Servers

Most healthcare organizations set up networks to allow many computers to share the information stored in one or more large databases. This is called a client/server configuration. The desktop computers throughout the facility need only a portion of the software (called the client) and rely on a main computer (called a server or host) to store, process, and retrieve the data.

Generally, the server is a larger, more powerful computer than the client computers, but its function is passive. That is, it waits for requests from the client, and then serves the requested data to the client. The client can be a typical desktop computer, a laptop, or a Tablet PC or other portable device. The client sends requests and waits for replies from the server.

A familiar example of this is e-mail. The application software you use to retrieve, write, and send e-mail messages is the *client*. Each time you receive or send a message, your computer is communicating with an e-mail *server*.

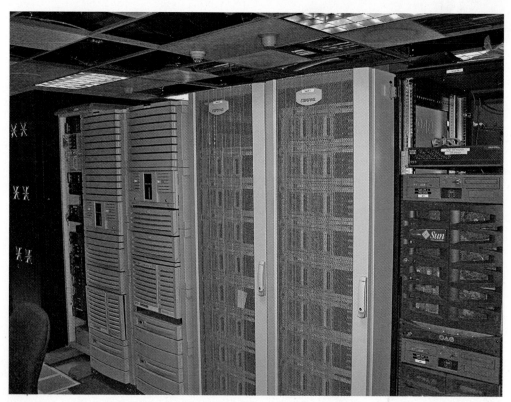

**FIGURE 4-13**  **Multiple servers at a large inpatient facility.**

Each client workstation in a healthcare facility typically communicates with multiple servers. Some examples might include a registration server, a clinical information system server (for medical records), image servers, e-mail servers, application servers, and print servers. Figure 4-13 shows a number of servers at a large inpatient facility.

### Local-Area Networks

Local-area networks (LANs) are computers that are connected by a network serving just the organization or facility in which they are located. Each computer on the network is called a *node*. A LAN allows computers to share printers, files, and other resources in common. The cables and switches used in a LAN allow for high-speed transfer of information within the network. A LAN can be managed locally and can be designed to keep the data very secure.

### Wide-Area Networks

Wide-area networks (WANs) function similar to a LAN except that they cover larger geographic areas. To do so, the WAN typically uses telecommunication lines to connect two or more LANs into one large private network. The phone company provides a secure connection that prevents computers not on the WAN from accessing it.

For example, a WAN might be used where a hospital owns several healthcare facilities that are miles apart. It would be too expensive for the hospital to run its own wires that distance, so the hospital would lease high-speed telephone lines to connect the LAN at each facility into one large network. Given permission to do so, any node on the network could communicate with computers at all of the other facilities as seamlessly as if they were in the same LAN.

A WAN may not transfer data as quickly as a LAN because the portion of the network using the phone lines may limit its speed. This is partially because the point at which the LAN connects to the phone lines can act as a bottleneck when large amounts of data are being sent over the WAN, and also because the cost of the phone lines will be based on their quality and capacity. Businesses have to balance the expected normal usage of the WAN with their budget.

Several types of telecommunications are available for a WAN. The two most prevalent are *leased line, point-to-point connections*, or *frame relay*. Frame relay uses a computer node at the phone company to securely send the data transparently through the phone circuits to a node near the other end of the WAN. Frame relay is cheaper for a geographically large WAN because the business leases a point-to-point connection only as far as the phone company node.

## Internet

LANs and WANs are private networks that can be accessed only by the users in that network. In contrast, the Internet is a worldwide public network that can be accessed by any computer anywhere. Most people know about the Internet because of the services they use on it such as e-mail, research, games, and web pages; however, it is also used to exchange data.

The Internet was created by interconnecting millions of smaller business, academic, and government networks. It is a very large network of networks, functionally similar to the other types of networks we have discussed.

**PROTOCOLS**    Different types of networks have certain things in common. Networks use a *protocol* or set of rules for how they are to communicate on the network. Networks also assign a unique ID or number to each computer on the network.

Although several standard protocols are in use for various LANs, the entire worldwide Internet uses one specific protocol: TCP/IP, which stands for Transmission Control Protocol/Internet Protocol. The TCP/IP protocol is now also commonly used for LANs and WANs.

The difference between the Internet and other networks is seen in how the Internet works. When a LAN or WAN is represented in a schematic design, lines connect each node of the network to the hub/switch or router. In contrast, the Internet is represented in the schematic as a cloud (as shown in Figure 4-14) because information goes into one side and out to its destination without relying on any predefined circuit.

To help you understand how this works, let us compare the post office and the phone company. When you make a phone call, the wires and circuits must establish an electrical connection

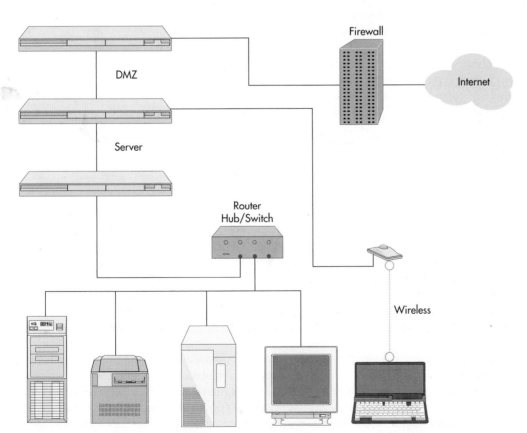

**FIGURE 4-14**

**Drawing of a network configuration.**

with the phone of the person you are calling *before* their phone rings and the call can go through. When you write a letter, you address the envelope and deposit it in the mailbox. You don't know how the post office will transport it or what roads the trucks will take, but in the end it is delivered to the address on the envelope.

The Internet Protocol encloses data in packets that have an address on them. The packets are sent through the various networks making up the Internet until they arrive at their address.

Figure 4-14 is a drawing of a LAN configuration. Each workstation is connected to the router, which is sometimes also called a hub or switch. The black connecting lines represent cables or wires that are run throughout the facility. Each server is also connected to the router.

Figure 4-14 also shows that the network is connected to the Internet. The Internet is shown as a cloud. Two components shown at the top of the figure are used to secure the network. The first is the firewall. This may be a special device, a component of the router, or a dedicated computer. The firewall screens packets coming in from the Internet. The firewall can be set up to limit connections to only certain networks, computers, or TCP/IP ports.

The second level of protection is the server at the top labeled DMZ. This is a computer that can provide information to the public or be used to send messages out of the network but which cannot be used to access the hospital's internal network from outside.

**SECURE REMOTE ACCESS**    The flexibility of the Internet protocol and its ability to get information to and from almost any point in a worldwide network obviously has a lot of potential for healthcare. Providers can access their patients' charts, communicate with patients, transmit medical images, and work from anywhere. However, the Internet is not very secure. The packets of data pass through many computers and networks on their way to their destination. They can be copied, opened, and read by anyone with enough technical savvy.

How do we secure the information so we can use the accessibility of the Internet, but protect the information? Two ways of doing this are to use a secured socket layer (SSL) or a virtual private network (VPN). Both of these rely on *encrypting* the transmission. There are other secure transmission schemes not covered here.

SSL adds security to HTTP (Hypertext Transfer Protocol) web pages, sending only encoded data within the packets, and then decrypting it when it is received to display the web page. This prevents anyone intercepting the transmitted packets from making sense of them. SSL, however, is limited to the type of things you can do on a web page.

Some providers and organizations want to run software that is on their network computers from home or elsewhere. As we discussed earlier, the most secure method would be a point-to-point connection to the hospital's network. However, if that is not possible or if the provider is not always accessing the network from the same location, a VPN may be used.

The VPN uses the Internet to transport packets of data, but it has its own software that encrypts and decrypts the packets between the sending and receiving systems. The VPN also verifies the identity of the person signing on, ensuring access only to those who are permitted to use the system. A VPN is not limited to web pages and may be used to secure the data being transmitted for other application software, such as an electronic health record system.

## Wireless Networks

Remote access today both in and out of the office includes wireless devices that access the network while the user is mobile. Wireless networks are connected to the LAN through a radio transceiver called an access point, which is actually wired to the router like other network nodes.

The portable device has a built-in radio transceiver and a unique ID. When it is near an access point, it sends packets of data using Wi-Fi, a high radio-frequency. The access point receives the packets and sends them along on the network. Where there are multiple access points, the closest point automatically takes over transmissions, as the user walks from one location to another.

Figure 4-15 illustrates the coverage area of an office with multiple access points. The red lines indicate the wired LAN cables connecting the computers and access points. The overlapping teal and lavender circles represent the range of radio signals from each access point. The laptop computer in the exam room is communicating with access point 1 due to its proximity. If the laptop were moved to one of the other exam rooms, access point 2 would automatically take over the connection.

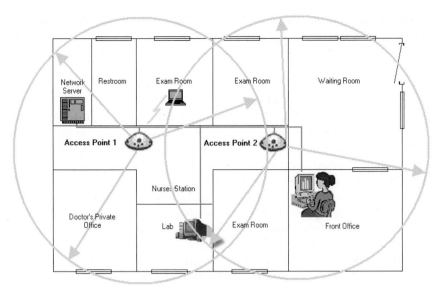

**FIGURE 4-15    Access points of a wireless network in a medical office.**

# Printers and Reports

In addition to sharing files and data, one of the main resources shared on a network are printers. Despite the move toward electronic records, healthcare organizations are anything but paperless. There is a frequent need to print orders, reports, and forms throughout the facility. The ability for a networked computer to send output to a printer that is not directly attached to it has many advantages, including these:

- Saves the cost of attaching a printer to every computer.
- Saves the desk space attached printers would occupy.
- Allows the use of faster printers with more features that would be too expensive to buy for individual workstations.
- Saves time because, rather than printing a report in one department and carrying it to another, it is possible to sent the output to a printer located right in the other department.

Many larger printers have their own network card, allowing them to be connected directly to the LAN without being connected to a workstation. However, printers that are connected to workstations may also be used as network printers if the workstation is configured for this.

### Report Server

Because reports make up a large portion of what is printed, we will discuss a related topic: the report server. The advantage of the large relational databases we discussed earlier in this chapter is that they contain a great deal of data that is useful for reporting purposes. For example, patient records contain information such as the dates the patient was seen, the procedures that were billed, the amount paid by insurance, and the amount outstanding. This data, gathered from all of the accounts, is then used to produce monthly financial reports, length of stay reports, and billing and productivity reports, to name just a few.

The report does not exist as organized data. To generate the report, the application software queries the database and begins collating and sorting data from fields within relevant records returned from the server. Finally, the organized data is formatted with headings and columns and sent to the printer as the finished product you see when you look at a report.

When an organization runs a lot of large or complicated reports, the gathering, sorting, and printing of the reports can impact the performance of the database server. To minimize this, some applications make use of a report server, a computer that is used only for the generation of reports. The database server is still queried for the relevant data records, but that information is copied temporarily to the report server, which handles the sorting, organizing, and printing of the report. Because the data in the report server is only a temporary copy, it is deleted when the report is finished.

### Cold

Businesses are required to keep copies of a large number of financial and compliance reports generated every month. Over time these records require a lot of storage space, so many organizations choose to keep those reports in a computer document imaging system of the type discussed earlier for use with patient records.

Organizations that intend to store reports in a document image system can do so without printing and then scanning them by using some type of COLD (computer output to laser disk) software. Rather than printing a paper copy, COLD software captures the printer output and converts it into an image file, exactly as it would appear on the piece of paper. The file is archived onto an optical disk (CD or DVD) for permanent storage.

Computer systems can also achieve similar results using software other than COLD. One example you may be familiar with is the PDF or Portable Document Format. If you participate in online banking services, you may be able to download your bank or credit card statement as a PDF file. In these examples, the bank may not be printing the statement you download, but rather their computers output an image of your statement directly into a PDF file.

## Interoperability Standards

The ability of various software systems to communicate with each other and to share data saves the time and effort of reentering the same information in multiple systems. Where group medical practices often use software from only one or two vendors the ability to share data within the application is assured. However, it is not uncommon for larger organizations such as hospitals to have from 60 to 600 software applications by various vendors.

Whereas the network protocols we have discussed so far enable the workstations and servers to exchange packets of data, nothing in the protocol has defined the content of those packets. Similarly, the databases we discussed defined the data in fields and records and data types, but nothing assured that the data in one database could be understood by another application or database.

To solve this problem, the health information industry has created *standards* that define the exchange of patient and medical data between applications. To facilitate the *interoperability* of diverse systems, vendors who create application software must support and adhere to the standards. Two concepts important to interoperability of healthcare systems are data elements and HL7.

### Data Elements

One might confuse the term *data elements* with fields or records that hold data, but the concept is broader. The term *data element* applies to paper records as well as computer records. Data elements do not define the layout of the database, but rather are a broad set of standards that establish what types of information health systems ought to keep. For example the patient's address is one of the standard data elements. However, we see in Figure 4-10 that the address is divided into four fields. A different database might use six fields for the address, but it would still be considered one data element.

Including standard data elements in a database design makes it likely that the application will have data similar to other systems. This not only improves interoperability but provides common elements for system-wide reports.

### Data Sets

A *data set* is a list of data elements collected for a particular purpose. For example, an admission record would need all the data elements of the patient demographics, insurance information, next of kin, and so forth. In a paper system, this would be done by making sure the paper form contained all of the appropriate boxes and that they were filled in correctly.

In an electronic system, many elements of the data are entered only once, and then assembled into the data set as needed. For example, the patient demographics, insurance information, and next-of-kin information would be retrieved from the patient registration system without reentering the data.

Usually a healthcare data set represents the minimum list of data elements that must be collected. Examples of standard data sets in healthcare will be discussed in Chapter 5.

## HL7

As you learned in Chapter 2, HL7 stands for Health Level Seven, a nonprofit organization that developed and maintains the leading messaging standard used to exchange clinical and administrative data between different healthcare computer systems. The acronym is also used as the name of the standard itself.

HL7 specifications are independent of any application or vendor; therefore, applications that can send and receive HL7 messages can potentially exchange information. If a hospital has one vendor's system for registration and another vendor's radiology system, the simple act of transferring patient information from the admissions office to the radiology department would not be easy without HL7.

Of course, HL7 goes much further than specifying the communication of patient admission, registration, and discharge information. It includes a wide range of clinical information messages. As such it is the primary standard for the communication of orders, lab results, radiology reports, clinical observations such as vital signs, and many other types of clinical data maintained in the patient's record.

HL7 has been successful because it is very flexible both in its structure as well as its support for multiple coding standards. Healthcare systems use codes in place of text in many database fields. Procedure codes, diagnosis codes, lab test codes, and many other types of codes not only save space but ensure accurate interpretation of the data later. Although there are uniform standard codes for some types of data, multiple code standards are being used for other types of data. Therefore, when a message is received, the codes and terms used by the other system may not match those used by the receiver. To overcome this problem, segments of the HL7 message that contain coded data also identify what coding standard is being used. A special computer program called an *HL7 translator* is used to match the codes in the message with the codes used by the other application. The translator can also reconcile differences between two systems using different versions of HL7.

## Maintaining Interoperability

One of the main challenges in a large HIS department is to maintain the interoperability between multiple systems. For example, cross-reference tables are used to reconcile differences in the way various systems codify data. One database might assign a unique code to each provider; another might use the doctor's Social Security number. As data is exchanged, a table of providers would help each application correctly match the ID for a patient's doctor to provider record in that system. When a new provider joins the practice, not only must that person be added to every database, but to the cross-reference table as well.

This seems complex enough, but application venders also regularly update their software to new versions. Often the update involves changes to that application's database. Every new version must be tested to ensure that it will not fail. The HIS department must then analyze any proposed database changes to ensure continued compatibility with the 60 or so other applications already running on the network. Healthcare organizations that use multiple vendors typically have a separate set of computers used to test software changes without risk to daily operations.

## CCOW

CCOW stands for the Clinical Context Object Workgroup, a subset of HL7. Like HL7 its acronym is used for the name of the group and the standard that the group developed. The purpose of the standard was to develop a means by which a facility that used applications from several different vendors for their electronic health record could make it easier for the users. For example, if one brand of software is used for the chart, but a different one for prescriptions and yet a third for writing lab orders, clinicians would have to log into three different applications and search for the same patient in each application before they could record the encounter and orders.

When CCOW is implemented, the user logs in once. When the user changes applications, the user is automatically logged into the new application and the patient, provider, and clinical encounter are automatically selected. This is called *context management*.

Although CCOW makes things simpler for the end user, implementation is very difficult. Each vendor's application software must be specifically written to enable CCOW, and the HIS department must set up special servers to handle the CCOW functions. CCOW is usually only found in inpatient settings, particularly teaching hospitals.

## Communication Systems

Thus far we have discussed systems used for the patient and business records of a healthcare organization. Equally important, however, are the communication systems used by the staff in the healthcare facility.

## A REAL-LIFE STORY

### A Look Behind the Hospital Network
*By Craig A. Gillespie*

*Craig Gillespie is a network specialist at a large hospital connected to multiple remote facilities.*

Our hospital has a variety of computer systems and operating systems linked not only by our internal LAN but also by a high-speed WAN, which connects the main hospital to our downtown business office and a couple of our other medical facilities.

Our network uses a Cisco backbone and multiple Cisco routers. Our servers include IBM AS 400s running IBM's proprietary O/S 400 operating system; IBM P series running AIX; and a number of Intel-based servers running Red Hat Linux. Our PACS (Picture Archiving and Communication System) runs on a Sun system (Unix). The dietary department is using an application that runs on a Novell network and a few other applications that run Citrix.

Oracle is the principal database our applications use. As the amount of data increases, the database grows in size. We usually have to manually increase the extent of the database about every five months. This is usually just because of the indexes. Because I don't like taking our system down to rebuild indexes, I would rather grow it a little bit and wait until the system is down for something else to rebuild them.

From a pure IT point of view, as a system administrator and database administrator, it doesn't matter to me what the application is. What matters is how important is it; what are the response time requirements; and what can I do to make sure those happen?

There are several things we do. First, a few of our systems are mirrored. That means the data is constantly written twice to two different systems, so if one goes down the other has the same up-to-the-minute data. In addition, the most important are stored on a SAN (storage area network) with a RAID 5 (redundant array of independent disks) with redundant connections all the way through. Should a hard disk become damaged, this type of configuration would allow us to swap out a disk drive without even bringing the system down.

Finally, of course, we regularly back up the systems. Our backup system uses a Robot tape library with eight drives in it.

With so many different applications in our facility, there are things we can do to help the teams that support those applications as well. For example, the database, operating system, network, and many of our applications create log records of certain events, such as user logon, connections, error messages, and so forth. When an application team identifies certain errors or conditions they need to be alerted to, I use script languages to write little programs to scan the logs checking for certain things outside of the standard application area. When the scripts find something, the team can be alerted.

When I talk to people who are interested in what I do I say, "Why don't you try a little project at home to see if this kind of work is for you?" Take an old computer, purchase a copy of Red Hat Linux (a low–cost, Unix-type operating system), and build a proxy server or a mail server. This exercise will get you involved enough to have an understanding of what is going on.

If you're still interested, then try a little web development and some degree of programming. You don't have to write a program, but learn enough to understand what is happening behind the scenes. These are suggestions to help you find out if the technology side of IT interests you.

### E-Mail Systems

E-mail has become a primary communication tool in all types of businesses. The IT department has responsibility for the hospital's e-mail system. These responsibilities include managing a mail server, assigning user e-mail addresses, managing e-mail record storage, and protecting the system from viruses and malicious software that can affect workstations, other servers, and the entire network.

E-mail was used earlier in this chapter as an example of a client/server architecture. The e-mail program on the workstation is the client, sending and receiving messages to the e-mail server. The e-mail server is typically set up to communicate through a larger server outside the network, called a *mail host*.

Like other components of networks, e-mail systems use a protocol. Several different protocols are available for e-mail. SMTP (Simple Mail Transfer Protocol) is the standard for sending messages; however, it cannot be used to retrieve messages.

E-mail is retrieved from the mail host using either IMAP (Internet Message Access Protocol) or POP3 (Post Office Protocol, version 3).

- IMAP holds messages on the host server until they are specifically deleted by the user.
- POP3 holds messages on the mail host server, deleting them from the host server once they are downloaded.

Most healthcare facilities use POP3 to retrieve e-mail from a host server operated by an Internet service provider (ISP). The downloaded e-mail is stored in the hospital's e-mail server. The typical hospital user's e-mail client communicates only with the hospital's e-mail server, not the mail host at the ISP. This arrangement helps shield the hospital's e-mail system from the public Internet.

### Telecommunications

Historically, responsibility for a facility's phone systems was assigned to engineering, physical plant, or another department. Increasingly, however, telecommunications systems are becoming the responsibility of IT departments. This makes sense for several reasons:

- The phone switching systems are now computer based, requiring IT expertise to manage them.
- As organizations upgrade the wiring in their facilities, many are eliminating phone wires and opting to use VoIP (Voice-over-Internet Protocol). VoIP uses special phones that provide phone service by sharing the computer network.
- The increase in wireless devices, including pagers, cordless intercoms, and medical telemetry devices, is more easily managed by one department than by several.

---

# Chapter 4 Summary

### The Technology behind Health Systems

Computer systems are generally discussed in terms of two components: *hardware* and *software*. Hardware refers to the components you can physically see and touch: the computer, circuit boards, computer chips, monitor screen, keyboard, mouse, cables, wires, printers, and so forth.

Software refers to the operating system and application programs, which provide instructions to the hardware to process the information the computer receives and stores; that is, computer software gives functionality to the computer hardware, making it useful. Software consists of program instructions that enable us to work. Operating systems and network software control computer hardware, input/output devices, and communications with other computers. Application software allows us to perform specific tasks on a computer such as write a letter, enter a medical record, view an x-ray, send an e-mail, or order a medication.

The fundamental unit of modern computing is called a *bit*. Bits are grouped together in logical units, the most common of which is called a *byte*. There are eight bits in one byte. Bits have a value of 0 or 1. When they are grouped together as a byte, the value of the byte can range from 0 to 256. Computers create alphabet characters by using the numbers 32 through 128 to represent letters, numerals, and punctuation marks. This is called the ASCII table.

The smallest unit of text data is a *character*. Text characters (sometimes called *alphanumeric* characters) are limited to letters, numbers, a space, and punctuation marks.

Bits are also grouped into larger units to represent large numbers, digital images, or other types of data. The smallest unit of a digital image is called a pixel. Pixels are typically comprised of 8 to 32 bits, depending on how many colors are represented by the pixel.

Computer *data* is information that can be stored and retrieved. Data and programs are stored on the hard disk, optical disks, or temporarily in RAM memory chips. Programs and data are retrieved and processed by a computer chip called the CPU or central processing unit.

## Databases

Data is stored on disk drives in files and databases. Databases store data in defined structures called tables. Tables have records. The records are made up of fields, which have a defined field type and format. Examples of field types include numeric and alphanumeric or text fields. Numeric fields can be further defined to hold specific types of data such as money or dates.

## Networks

Multiple computers can be linked together into a network. This allows them to communicate with each other to share files and information. A computer network consists of hardware such as cables, network cards, routers or switches, and networking software, which is sometimes included in the operating system. Wireless networks allow portable devices to communicate with the network using a radio signal called Wi-Fi. Antennas called access points are connected to the computer network. As a user moves throughout the facility, the portable computer automatically switches to the access point with the strongest signal, dynamically maintaining the connection to the network.

## Printers and Reports

Computer output devices include printers, screens or monitors, and COLD (computer output to laser disk) software. COLD software converts printer output directly into an image file, thus bypassing the steps of printing and then scanning the paper report.

## Interoperability Standards

Data is input into the computer using a keyboard, mouse, touch screen, microphone, camera, or scanner. Data can also be directly transferred from another computer or medical device. For computers to exchange data, it is necessary for the data to be in a format that both systems understand. In healthcare HL7 is the most prominent interoperability standard used today. (This is different from the HIPAA transactions discussed in Chapter 3 that are used for claims billing, reimbursement, and insurance eligibility.)

When a facility uses application software from many different vendors for their electronic health records it is necessary to use HL7 to maintain interoperability between the various applications. Even with HL7 in place the users may find that they have to sign into several applications to record the information about one patient. One solution to the problem is to allow the user to sign in and select the patient once, then to use CCOW to maintain the context while switching between applications.

## Communication Systems

The communication systems used by the staff in the healthcare facility include e-mail systems and telecommunications, which are now often placed in the IT department. One important advancement in application software is a networking application that allows the computer network to replace the hospital telephone system. The application is called VoIP and eliminates the need for the facility to maintain two different sets of wiring.

# Critical Thinking Exercises

1. Look at your personal or home computer (or a school computer if you do not have one of your own). What operating system is on your computer? Name at least three application programs on the computer.
2. See if you can determine how much RAM is installed in your computer or the school's computer. What are the steps you used to determine this?

# Testing Your Knowledge of Chapter 4

1. What does the acronym COLD stand for?

2. What part of the computer hardware only retains data while the computer is on?

3. How many bits are in a byte?

4. Describe the difference between computer hardware and computer software.

5. What type of data is stored in a PACS?

6. Is a document scanner an input or output device?

7. A character is the smallest unit of text data. What is the smallest unit of image data?

8. A database record can have different types of fields. Name three different field types.

9. What is the difference between a LAN and a WAN?

10. What is the acronym for the Internet protocol?

11. Name two ways discussed in this chapter for sending information securely over the Internet.

12. What is the name of the standard by which computers define alphabetical, numerical, and punctuation characters?

13. What is the acronym for the software that allows computer networks to be used for telephone systems?

14. What is a BLOB used for?

15. What computer chip is sometimes called the "brains" of the computer?

# Comprehensive Evaluation of Chapters 1-4

This comprehensive evaluation will enable you and your instructor to determine your understanding of the material covered so far.

1. The hospital emergency department is what kind of facility?
   a. acute
   b. subacute
   c. inpatient
   d. outpatient

2. What type of nurse can diagnose patients and write orders?
   a. triage nurse
   b. licensed nurse practitioner
   c. licensed vocational nurse
   d. doctor's nurse assistant

3. An inpatient was admitted June 10 and discharged June 14. What was the LOS?
   a. 3 days
   b. 4 days
   c. 10 days
   d. 14 days

4. What does the acronym CIO stand for?
   a. computer input/output
   b. computer interpreted observation
   c. chief information officer
   d. chief complaint

5. Which group first established standards for hospital records?
   a. American College of Surgeons
   b. American College of Pathologists
   c. American Medical Association
   d. American Hospital Association

6. A user authorized to view records on a document image system must be a:
   a. Registered Health Information Technician
   b. Registered Health Information Administrator
   c. registered health nurse
   d. none of the above

*For each of the following allied health professions, indicate whether the job is clinical or nonclinical:*

7. Clinical application specialist
   a. clinical
   b. nonclinical

8. Lab technician
   a. clinical
   b. nonclinical

9. Coding specialist
   a. clinical
   b. nonclinical

10. Cancer registrar
    a. clinical
    b. nonclinical

11. Diagnosis-related groups are used for:
    a. point of care documentation
    b. Medicare billing and reimbursement
    c. patient assessment
    d. decision support

12. Which of the following is **not** one of the four components of the HIPAA Administrative Simplification Subsection?
    a. Privacy
    b. Security
    c. Transactions and Code Sets
    d. Conditions of Participation

13. HIPAA security standards are divided into three categories. Which of the following is **not** one of those categories?
    a. Physical Safeguards
    b. Ambulatory Safeguards
    c. Administrative Safeguards
    d. Technical Safeguards

14. Which of the following is a covered entity under HIPAA?
    a. pharmaceutical manufacturers
    b. government agencies
    c. healthcare providers
    d. medical device manufacturers

15. HIPAA requires which of the following to disclose health records for TPO?
    a. signed informed consent form
    b. signed patient authorization form
    c. patient receipt of privacy policy
    d. U.S. government authorization

16. HIPAA requires an authorization to release PHI to be signed by:
    a. the patient or personal representative
    b. a physician or nurse
    c. the medical administrator or office manager
    d. a notary public

*Write the full name represented by each of the following acronyms:*

17. PHI _____

18. EDI _____

19. HIM _____

20. EHR _____

21. What type of the computer memory only retains data while the computer is on?
    a. ROM
    b. RAM
    c. CPU
    d. CRT

22. How many bits are in a byte?
    a. Two
    b. Four
    c. Seven
    d. Eight

23. A data dictionary defines:
    a. medical terminology
    b. field names and position
    c. communication standards
    d. clinical vocabulary

24. Which of the following is not an image file type?
    a. ASCII
    b. DICOM
    c. JPEG
    d. TIFF

25. CMS "deemed status" means that Joint Commission accreditation is deemed to have met CMS condition of participation requirements.
    T. true
    F. false

26. The position of security officer is exclusively found only in very large healthcare facilities.
    T. true
    F. false

27. A pixel is the smallest unit of text data.
    T. true
    F. false

28. A single database record can have more than one type of field.
    T. true
    F. false

29. Group medical practices are considered ambulatory facilities.
    T. true
    F. false

30. A physical exam must be performed on a patient within 72 hours of a hospital admission.
    T. true
    F. false

31. The hospital CEO is in charge of all medical staff.
    T. true
    F. false

32. Hospitals start a new chart each time a patient is admitted.
    T. true
    F. false

# 5 Healthcare Records

## LEARNING OUTCOMES

After completing this chapter, you should be able to:
- Discuss the functions that healthcare records serve
- Explain the difference between primary and secondary health records
- Identify different forms used to record patient information
- Discuss standard data elements and standard data sets
- Explain how health records assist in the continuity of care
- Define a RHIO
- Describe the various forms of telemedicine
- Explain an E-visit

## ACRONYMS USED IN CHAPTER 5

Acronyms are used extensively in both medicine and computers. The following acronyms are used in this chapter.

| | | | |
|---|---|---|---|
| **ALOS** | Average Length of Stay | **NCVHS** | National Committee on Vital Health Statistics |
| **CDC** | Centers for Disease Control and Prevention | **NHIN** | National Health Information Network |
| **CMS** | Centers for Medicare and Medicaid Services | **OASIS** | Outcome and Assessment Information Set |
| **CPR** | Cardiopulmonary Resuscitation | **PACS OR PAC SYSTEM** | Picture Archiving and Communication System |
| **CT** | Computed Tomography (also CAT, Computerized Axial Tomography) | **PET** | Positron Emission Tomography |
| **DEEDS** | Data Elements for Emergency Department Systems | **PHI** | Protected Health Information |
| | | **PHR** | Personal Health Record |
| **DNR** | Do Not Resuscitate | **RAI** | Resident Assessment Instrument |
| **ECG** | Electrocardiogram (also EKG) | | |
| **EEG** | Electroencephalogram | **RHIO** | Regional Health Information Organization |
| **EHR** | Electronic Health Record | | |
| **EKG** | Electrocardiogram (also ECG) | **SNF** | Skilled Nursing Facility |
| **HEDIS** | Health Plan Employer Data and Information System | **SOAP** | Subjective, Objective, Assessment, Plan |
| **HPI** | History of Present Illness | **UACDS** | Uniform Ambulatory Care Data Set |
| **IDN** | Integrated Delivery Network | | |
| **LOS** | Length of Stay | **UAMCMDS** | Uniform Ambulatory Medical Care Minimum Data Set |
| **MDS** | Minimum Data Set | | |
| **MPI** | Master Patient Index | **UCDS** | Uniform Clinical Data Set |
| **MRI** | Magnetic Resonance Imaging | **UHDDS** | Uniform Hospital Discharge Data Set |
| **NCDB** | National Cancer Data Base | | |

# Understanding Healthcare Records

Healthcare records have many purposes, the most important of which is to help healthcare providers with patient care. The patient health record is the repository of data and information about the patient, the condition of the patient's health, the care and treatments the patient received, and the outcome of that care. This chapter will familiarize you with some of the contents of health records and how they are used.

The term *patient health record* has replaced the term *patient medical record* because it encompasses a holistic view of patient care. Though the terms are used almost interchangeably, an acute care patient record is usually concerned with one stay or episode, whereas an outpatient medical record is usually limited to one group or clinic. Later in this chapter we will discuss efforts to overcome these limitations by regional providers sharing records electronically and the growing interest by patients in maintaining lifelong personal health records.

In Chapter 4 the term *data* was used to differentiate the information the computer processes from the software application. In this and future chapters the word *data* does not just mean computer information, but rather the information in a health record. Additionally, the term *health data* is sometimes used herein for what is technically *health information*. In a more precise definition, data and information are not the same thing. *Data* are records of facts. *Information* is data in a useful form that conveys meaning. For example, the numeric values 68, 70, 72 are data.

- If the data represent height in inches, they may be used to plot an adolescent's growth rate.
- If the data represent a patient's pulse, they are used to provide information about the patient's heart rate measured at different intervals.

Health information, therefore, is not just the patient data but the presentation of this data in a useful form and the association of other relevant details with it. Figure 5-1 shows a standard form used in pediatric practices. When patient height is recorded on this form, the doctor can easily see the rate of growth over time. Curved lines on the form compare a boy's height to the general population at the same age. In this chapter we will examine some typical health information forms and further explore the concepts of *data elements* and *data sets* introduced in the previous chapter.

# Functions of Healthcare Records

A patient's health record provides accurate information not only about the patient's treatment, but also about the patient's health history and previous treatments. As such, it serves as the primary communication document among various providers who might care for the patient at different times in different departments.

The patient record also provides the basis for all billing and reimbursement. Coding professionals review the record of the patient visit and determine what codes to put on the insurance claim. CMS and other health insurance auditors follow the dictum that "if it isn't documented, it wasn't done," meaning that medical claims will not be paid if the patient record does not have enough detail about the encounter or treatment to support the claim.

The health record is a legal document. Should a question arise as to the cause of a disease or injury, or to determine if a medical error was made, relevant portions of the patient's record may become evidence in a court of law.

Healthcare records provide the basis for improvements in health. Individually, a patient's record is evaluated and used to develop care plans for the patient. Collectively, health records can be used by the healthcare facility to improve the quality and processes of healthcare delivery.

Public health departments, Homeland Security, and law enforcement officials use information from health records to track births, deaths, communicable diseases, effects of exposure to hazardous materials, bioterrorism threats, gunshot wounds, child abuse, and other crimes.

Researchers use patient records from *clinical trials* to monitor the effectiveness and safety of new drugs.

De-identified health records are analyzed by researchers to find health trends in our society and measure which treatments seem to have the best outcomes.

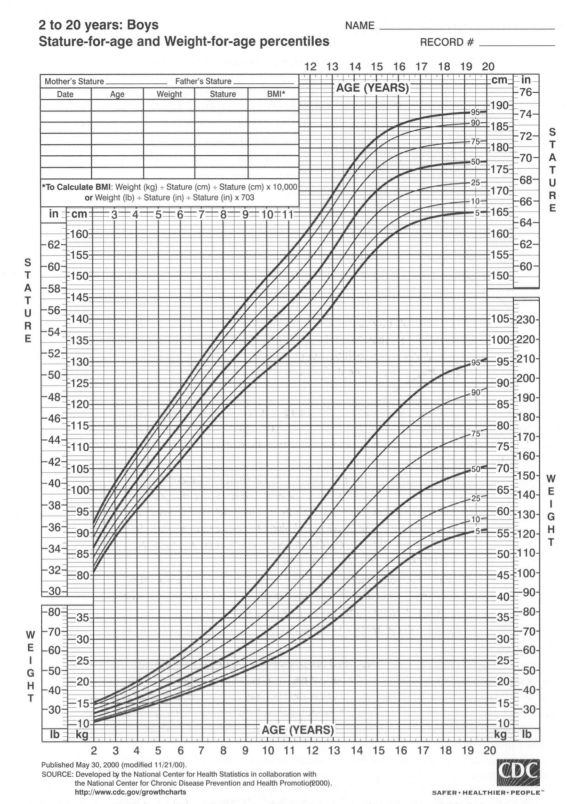

**FIGURE 5-1**   **Pediatric Growth Chart of Boys' Stature for Age and Weight for Age.**

# Primary and Secondary Records

Health information professionals classify health records as primary or secondary records:

- *Primary records* are those that are gathered directly from the patient and his or her providers, as well as records obtained from devices and diagnostic tests performed on the patient. Primary records are used for patient care and as legal documents.

- *Secondary records* are those that are created later, by analyzing, summarizing, or abstracting from the primary records. Secondary records are used in billing, research, and quality improvement.

## Types of Primary Health Records

Primary records may be electronic medical records or paper forms, but what they have in common is that they document the patient's history and state of health, the clinician's observations and actions, and all tests, treatments, and outcomes. As such, the patient's health record at a given facility is actually a collection of documents or computer records, descriptions of which are provided later in this chapter.

As you have learned in previous chapters, there are differences between inpatient and outpatient facilities. The type and quantity of information they keep also varies by the type of facility. For example, primary health records are generated and maintained by patients, doctors, nurses, home health providers, hospitals, rehabilitation facilities, dentists, chiropractors, and others.

The following examples illustrate some of the differences between health records at different providers' locations:

- *Acute care hospital* charts contain admission and discharge reports, nursing notes, physician examination notes, all orders, test results, operative reports, pathology and radiology reports, and administrative and demographic forms. However, in nearly all cases these are concerned with the current stay.

- *Ambulatory care facilities* (physician offices) tend to keep a single chart per patient, combining documents from all previous visits, medical history, consults, lab results, and reports from other providers. The principal document is the physician's note, which details the observation and findings, but often includes the physician's orders and plan of treatment. In addition to demographic and social history information, many offices keep records of communications with the patient and their insurance plans in the chart as well.

- *Home care agency* records are uniquely centered on a physician's orders for treatment at home. CMS has standardized the details that are required about a patient's home care. The nurses or therapists visiting the patient at home keep notes from each visit concerning the services performed and the patient's progress. These are updated in records maintained by the home care agency.

- *Dental records* generally contain *very* abbreviated notes about the treatments and procedures performed, but usually cover all visits the patient has ever had with the practice including dental hygienists and other dentists. Also, because dental x-rays are small, most offices store them in the patient's chart. This is different from medical facilities where x-rays and other diagnostic images are typically stored in a separate location or computer system.

## Types of Secondary Health Records

Secondary health records are those that are created by abstracting relevant details from the primary records. These secondary records are used for reimbursement (insurance claims), quality improvement at the facility, reporting to accreditation and government agencies, and research.

The following are some examples of secondary health records:

- *Health insurance claims* are created by selecting information from the patient record, such as procedures and diagnoses, assigning codes to them, and assembling them with information from the patient's demographic and insurance information. These are then submitted to the insurance plan for payment.

- The *master patient index* (MPI) is typically a computerized system intended to prevent duplicate registrations for the same patient. By taking key identifying facts from patient demographic information such as full name, date of birth, gender, and sometimes Social Security number, a list is created of all the patients registered anywhere in the healthcare facility. By checking the MPI first, registration clerks can see if the patient is already registered and thereby avoid creating duplicate records in the system.

- *Aggregate data* is collected by gathering selected items of information from many patients' charts and then analyzing it. For example, in Chapter 1 we discussed ALOS or average length of stay. By extracting the LOS of all of the patients in the hospital last month, the hospital can calculate the average. Similarly, aggregate data can be analyzed to determine the case mix or for quality improvement purposes. Case mix will be described further in Chapter 9.

### Transition from Paper to Electronic Records

Many social forces and practical reasons are causing healthcare providers to change from paper health records to electronic health records (EHRs). Social reasons include an increasingly mobile society where patients move and change doctors more frequently. Additionally, many patients today see multiple specialists for their care. This means their medical record no longer resides with a single general practitioner who provides their total care. Thus, the ability to share examination records and test results is increasingly important to the patient's continuity of care (discussed later in this chapter).

Practical reasons for the move to EHRs include the fact that paper records cannot be easily accessed or shared, the charts must be copied and faxed or transported from one office to another, and handwritten portions of the record are often abbreviated, cryptic, or illegible. Finally, searching the contents of paper charts requires manually opening every chart and reading it.

Chapter 7 will cover ways EHR systems can be used to help improve patient health, the quality of care, and patient safety by providing access to complete, up-to-date records of past and present conditions. Though many facilities are moving toward electronic health records, the transition will take several years.

## Contents of Health Records

Although the types of documents or data contained in medical records differ between inpatient and outpatient facilities, many of them serve a similar purpose. However, clinical records are not the only items stored in a patient's chart. For example, many ambulatory offices store nearly any document concerning a patient in the patient's chart. Figure 5-2 compares a list of some typical records in an inpatient and outpatient chart. Additional information and samples of many of the forms are provided later in this chapter.

### Administrative and Demographic Data

Whether health records are paper or electronic, certain administrative documents tend to originate as paper forms. Generally this is the registration information provided by the patient or relative and certain legal documents that the patient must sign. In an all-digital facility these paper documents are subsequently scanned as images and stored in the electronic record.

When a patient is first registered, demographic data such as name, address, phone numbers, next of kin, and emergency contact information is recorded. Registration will also record information used for billing such as account guarantor and insurance plans. Though some facilities allow the patient to enter this information directly using a web page, most facilities employ a registrar to enter the data into a computer.

In a paper-based facility the patient demographics form is called the *face sheet*. In facilities that are still transitioning from paper to electronic records, the information may be entered into the computer then printed out to create a face sheet for the paper chart.

Demographic and billing information is verified and updated if necessary for each return visit. Patients' insurance cards may also be photocopied or scanned into the computer during registration.

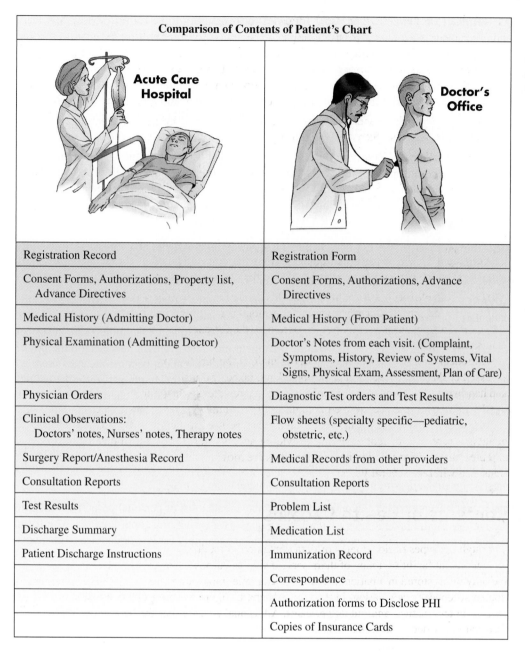

**Comparison of Contents of Patient's Chart**

| Acute Care Hospital | Doctor's Office |
| --- | --- |
| Registration Record | Registration Form |
| Consent Forms, Authorizations, Property list, Advance Directives | Consent Forms, Authorizations, Advance Directives |
| Medical History (Admitting Doctor) | Medical History (From Patient) |
| Physical Examination (Admitting Doctor) | Doctor's Notes from each visit. (Complaint, Symptoms, History, Review of Systems, Vital Signs, Physical Exam, Assessment, Plan of Care) |
| Physician Orders | Diagnostic Test orders and Test Results |
| Clinical Observations: Doctors' notes, Nurses' notes, Therapy notes | Flow sheets (specialty specific—pediatric, obstetric, etc.) |
| Surgery Report/Anesthesia Record | Medical Records from other providers |
| Consultation Reports | Consultation Reports |
| Test Results | Problem List |
| Discharge Summary | Medication List |
| Patient Discharge Instructions | Immunization Record |
|  | Correspondence |
|  | Authorization forms to Disclose PHI |
|  | Copies of Insurance Cards |

**FIGURE 5-2**

**Contents typical of acute care versus ambulatory patient charts.**

## Consent and Directives

A number of legal documents signed by the patient are included in the medical record. In some cases these are simple permission statements included on the patient information form; in other facilities the patient signs many individual forms, which are then filed in the chart or scanned into the computer. Some typical examples include the following.

**HIPAA CONSENT TO USE AND DISCLOSE PHI**   The patient acknowledges receipt of the Notice of Privacy Practices discussed in Chapter 3. This consent or acknowledgment may be included on the registration form or combined with another consent form.

**CONSENT TO TREATMENT**   A general consent to be treated by the healthcare practice or facility is usually included in the registration form. Additional *informed* consent forms are required for each operation or special procedure (discussed below).

**MEDICARE PATIENT RIGHTS STATEMENT**   CMS requires that patients be given a statement of their rights under Medicare. Patients will sign an acknowledgment that they have received the statement and their rights have been explained.

**ASSIGNMENT OF BENEFITS**    In order for a healthcare facility to be reimbursed by Medicare and other insurance plans, the policy holder must sign a form permitting the plan to pay the provider directly. This is called the *assignment of benefits*, and may be part of the insurance portion of the registration form or may be a blank insurance claim form signed by the policy holder. Note that a CMS-1500 paper insurance form has two signature blocks; one authorizes the patient's medical information to be sent to the plan and the other authorizes the assignment of benefits to the provider. (Refer to Chapter 10, Figure 10-4, to view an example of this form.)

**INFORMED CONSENT**    Written consent forms are signed by the patient or patient's legal representative before any operation or special procedure. The informed consent describes what is going to be done, the expected outcome, any risks associated with it, and possible alternatives to the procedure. This is done to ensure the patient has a complete understanding before going forward. Figure 5-3 shows a two-sided informed consent form.

**REFUSAL OF TREATMENT**    A patient may elect not to have a medically necessary procedure done. In such a case, a form documenting that the consequences of the decision are fully understood by the patient is signed and added to the chart.

**ADVANCE DIRECTIVES**    An advance directive is sometimes called a living will and permits patients to provide instructions regarding resuscitation and life-prolonging procedures in the event the patient should become terminally ill or injured and unable to communicate his or her wishes. The advance directive or separate document may also grant another person the power to make medical decisions on the patient's behalf should the patient become incapacitated.

The advance directive may include instructions not to resuscitate the patient in the case of death. When this is the case, inpatient facilities create a special order in the chart and clearly mark it DNR (do not resuscitate). If a DNR order is *not* present, consent to perform cardiopulmonary resuscitation (CPR) is presumed.

**ORGAN DONOR**    If a patient has agreed to donate organs or other tissues upon death, this is also noted in the record. If a patient dies without specifying an organ donor status, the patient's family must be given the opportunity to authorize organ donation.

**PERSONAL PROPERTY LIST**    Inpatient facilities may create a list of personal property brought to the facility by the patient such as jewelry, eyeglasses, hearing aids, and dentures. The form, signed by the patient, may release the facility from responsibility for loss or damage to the items. A similar disclaimer may absolve the facility of responsibility for a patient's vehicle parked on the premises while staying there.

**DISCLOSURE RECORDS**    As discussed in Chapter 3, HIPAA requires any disclosure of PHI for purposes *other than treatment, payment, or operations* of the facility to be tracked and recorded. In addition, copies of signed authorizations permitting release of partial or complete medical records are kept by the HIM department, sometimes with the health record itself.

## Clinical Documents

As you would expect, most of the information in the patient's medical record will be of a clinical nature. In both paper and electronic systems, diagnostic images are stored separately from the chart documents or data; however, some EHR systems may provide seamless access to images, giving the appearance that they are located within one system. In paper systems x-rays films are stored separately, usually in another part of the hospital.

The following are clinical documents typically found in the health record.

**MEDICAL HISTORY**    The primary source of a patient's medical history is the patient or a relative.

A medical history at an acute care facility will be obtained through an interview of the patient by the admitting doctor or a nurse.

At an ambulatory facility the history typically originates as a paper form that is filled out by the patient in the waiting room, though some modern medical practices allow patients to enter this data themselves on a computer using medical history software. A sample paper history form is shown in Figure 5-4.

## Informed Consent for Operative / Invasive Procedure CP2.10

Date _____ Time _____

I, the undersigned, consent to the following operation(s) and / or procedure(s); **Lumbar fusion with** **interbody allograft and pedicle screw fixation and iliac crest bone graft and/or allograft**

to be performed by Dr. _____ and his / her associates and assistants (including resident physicians), with knowledge that the attending physician will have primary responsibility for my care specific to the stated procedure. Dr. _____ has explained to me the nature and purpose of each operation(s) and / or procedure(s) as well as the substantial risks and possible complications involved, the benefits and the medically reasonable alternative methods of treatment.

The **SUBSTANTIAL RISKS** include but are not limited to: (check if applicable and add additional risks as indicated):
- ☑ perforation and / or injury to adjacent blood vessels, nerves and / or organs
- ☑ bleeding
- ☑ infection

Hemorrhage; infection; anesthetic reaction; neurological deficit including bowel, bladder or sexual dysfunction; CSF leak; recurrent disk rupture; no relief of symptoms; non-union; instrumentation failure; graft migration; visual loss; weakness; numbness; paralysis; off-label use of implant; degenerative change at adjacent segments; need for additional surgery

The **POTENTIAL BENEFIT(S)** include but are not limited to: Possible relief of symptoms; possible improved neurologic function.

The **MEDICALLY REASONABLE ALTERNATIVE(S)** options are: 1. Continued conservative treatment with physical therapy, rest, non-narcotic medications; 2. No treatment.

- I understand and consent to Shands' disposing of any tissue, parts or organs that are removed during the operation(s) and / or procedure(s), in accordance with its usual practice.
- I understand that the information I have received, about risks is not exhaustive and there may be other, more remote risks.
- I have had the opportunity to ask questions regarding the proposed procedure(s) and all my questions have been answered to my satisfaction.
- I have read or have had read to me, this Operative / Invasive Procedure Informed Consent form.
- I have had explained to me, and I understand the potential benefits and drawbacks, potential problems related to recuperation, the likelihood of success, the possible results of non-treatment, and any medically reasonable alternatives.
- I have received no guarantees from anyone regarding the results that may be obtained.
- I know the relationship, if any, of my physician or other practitioner, to any teaching facility involved in my care.

**Shands HealthCare**

‖‖‖‖‖‖‖‖‖‖‖‖‖ AC0001

Patient Name:

Patient Identification #:

*FACILITY* ___ **Shands at UF** ___
*please print facility name*

This form provided by Shands at UF as a courtesy to patients and their physicians
**Operative / Invasive Procedure Informed Consent** *(page 1 of 2)*
*If printed electronically, pages 1 & 2 must be stapled.*

Rev. 3/23/07                    PS55435

**FIGURE 5-3a** Informed Consent (front side).

My initials below indicate whether or not I consent to additional operations and / or procedures as are considered diagnostically or therapeutically necessary.

_____ I consent OR
_____ I do not consent

to additional operations and / or procedures as are considered diagnostically or therapeutically necessary on the basis of findings during the course of the operation(s) and / or procedure(s) described above and I accept the risks that may be associated with such additional operation(s) and / or procedure(s).

My initials below indicate whether observers may be present during my procedure, in accordance with my physicians' approval and hospital policy.

_____ I give permission to allow observers in the room during my procedure.
_____ I do not give permission to allow observers in the room during my procedure.

## CONSENT

I do hereby consent to the above described operation(s) and / or procedure(s).
Date _____

Patient Signature _____ Patient Printed Name _____

Witness Signature _____ Witness Printed Name _____

## SIGNATURES FOR CONSENT WHEN GIVEN BY REPRESENTATIVE OF PATIENT

**If patient is unable to consent, complete the following:**
☐ Patient is a minor, or
☐ Patient is unable to consent because: _____

Date _____

Patient's Name _____

Representative's Signature _____

Representative's Printed Name _____ Relationship to Patient _____

Witness Signature _____ Witness Printed Name _____

## SIGNATURES OF PHYSICIAN WHO OBTAINED CONSENT

I certify that the procedure(s) described above, including the substantial risks, benefits, possible complications, anticipated results, alternative treatment options, including non-treatment, the likelihood of success and the possible problems related to recuperation, were explained by me to the patient or his / her legal representative.

Date _____ Signature of Physician Who Obtained Consent _____

Physician Identification Number _____

| Patient Name: | Patient Identification #: |
|---|---|

### Shands HealthCare

‖‖‖‖‖‖‖‖‖‖‖ **AC0001**

*FACILITY* ___**Shands at UF**___
*please print facility name*

*This form provided by Shands at UF as a courtesy to patients and their physicians*
**Operative / Invasive Procedure Informed Consent** *(page 2 of 2)*
*If printed electronically, pages 1 & 2 must be stapled.*

Rev. 3/23/07                                        PS55435

**FIGURE 5-3b** Informed Consent (back side).

## Patient Reporting and Telemonitors

Many patients with chronic conditions are monitored at home using devices such as blood pressure monitors, glucose meters, and Holter monitors. Some of these devices store the readings and transfer the data to the doctor's system either by using a modem and phone line or by downloading from the device during a patient encounter. For blood pressure monitoring, if the device does not store the readings, the patient may keep a log, which is then entered into the patient's medical record at the doctor's office.

One example of a telemonitor is the Holter monitor, a device the patient wears for 24 to 72 hours to measure and record information about the patient's heart. The data is then transferred either remotely or in person to the doctor's computer where it is reviewed. Figure 5-11 shows a patient wearing a Holter monitor.

When a patient is seen in a doctor's office, measurements of vital signs, a glucose test, or even an ECG reflect only the patient's condition at that particular time. The advantage of telemonitoring is that it allows the provider to study these values measured many times over the course of the patient's normal daily activity.

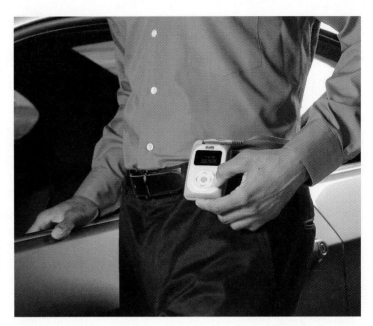

**FIGURE 5-11**

**An IQholter™ worn by the patient gathers cardio data.**

(Courtesy of Midmark Diagnostics Group.)

## E-Visits

One of the key technologies impacting our society is the Internet. It has changed the way people communicate, research, shop, and do business. It is also influencing changes in healthcare. While the banking, brokerage/investing, and travel industries have made Internet-based transactions readily available to consumers, healthcare as a whole has not. That seems to be changing.

One of the developments brought about by the Internet that offers interesting possibilities for enhancing the efficiency of providers and improving the quality of healthcare for the patients is the E-visit. An E-visit allows the patient to be treated by a clinician for nonurgent health problems without having to come into the office.

Although communication between provider and patient using e-mail is insecure or must be encrypted as required by HIPAA, an E-visit has advantages that e-mail lacks. Not only is the message secure, but the E-visit gathers symptom and HPI information, creating a documented medical record. When this information is integrated with the EHR, the E-visit becomes a part of the patient's chart, just like any other visit.

Also, e-mail is sent to a particular individual and therefore not likely to be accessible by another provider. In contrast, E-visits can be handled by the "doctor on-call," allowing practicing partners to share E-visit duty, just like they share other on-call services.

Equally as important to the clinician, the E-visits are reimbursed as a legitimate visit by Blue Cross/Blue Shield plans and other private insurance carriers in some states. A study by PricewaterhouseCoopers predicted that more than 20% of all office visits could be replaced by an online equivalent by 2010.[7]

**WORKFLOW OF AN E-VISIT** To use E-visits, the patient must be an established patient with the practice whose medical records are on file. E-visits would not be appropriate for a new patient who has never been seen at the practice. Here is an example of the basic workflow of an E-visit:

- A patient accesses the physician's website and signs on. The patient is already registered as an established patient of the practice.

- The patient answers a few simple questions and selects the reason for the visit from a list. From this information the software asks a set of questions appropriate to the complaint.

[7]*HealthCast 2010: Smaller World, Bigger Expectations* (PricewaterhouseCoopers, November 1999).

## A REAL-LIFE STORY

## Telemedicine at Mayo Clinics

### By Marvin P. Mitchell and Ron Rea

*Marvin P. Mitchell is the division chair of Media Support Services, Mayo Clinic, and Ron Rea is an analyst for Systems & Procedures, Mayo Clinic. Mayo Clinic is the largest and most prestigious not-for-profit group practice in the world. Its headquarters is in Rochester, Minnesota, with clinics in Jacksonville, Florida, and Scottsdale, Arizona.*

I think Mayo Clinic did its very first telemedicine consultation via satellite back in the 1960s as a demonstration project with Australia. When we opened our clinics in Jacksonville, Florida, in 1986 and Scottsdale, Arizona, in 1987 we got into it in a much bigger way.

Our goal was to be able to provide all the services that the Mayo Clinic in Rochester, Minnesota, offers to all of our patients, regardless of whether they came to Rochester, Jacksonville, or Scottsdale. We put into place the best technology available in the 1980s. That was a very high resolution satellite broadcasting system equivalent to what they now have at NBC or CBS, but with the transmission encrypted for privacy and security.

We had our first telemedicine consultation two days after Jacksonville opened their doors. We continued to do consultations by this method, but one area we struggled with was getting x-rays and larger diagnostic images to transmit with enough resolution for what we do.

Our practice at Mayo is largely tertiary and quaternary care; that is, very sick patients who have already been to family physicians and specialists; they are coming here for a subspecialist or sub-sub-specialist consultation. When you get to that level of care, the quality of imaging is absolutely critical.

We eventually found that face-to-face consultations via television didn't work very well. First, because there are a lot of things the consulting physician needs to go along with that: lab reports, diagnostic images, other examination records, and so forth. Second, it was disruptive to our physicians because they had to leave their practice and go to a special video studio. It was very difficult to get two or more physicians on the video link at the same time; if another opinion was needed, that specialist might not be available. So we began to phase the video out of telemedicine because it just wasn't working and we began looking for a different approach.

In 1996 we were approached by the UAE (United Arab Emirates) about doing telemedicine with their clinics. However, they were 10 time zones from Rochester, so doing real-time, face-to-face consultation would be almost impossible. Dr. George Gura (who is the medical director for the project) had the idea of creating a physician-to-physician, second-opinion service using what we call store-and-forward telemedicine.

To use store-and-forward telemedicine, they package up the case with all its inherent images, lab data, history, demographics, and transmit it to Mayo. This allows us to use a data network to send images in their original high-resolution form. It may take an hour for the image to get here, but it is an absolute perfect image, not like you would get shooting it with a video camera and sending them over video link.

The workflow is illustrated in Figure 5-12. The physician on the other end does the necessary examinations and tests they would normally do. If at some point they determine that they need a subspecialty consult, they get high-resolution images, scanned paper documents, motion image capture, angiography, and those types of things that they can generate on their end. That is packaged in an electronic format and transmitted with a consultation request to the Mayo telemedicine office.

We tried to design a system that works as if the patient were here. If, when Mayo's telemedicine office receives the electronic package, the patient has never been here before, we actually register this patient as though the person walked in the door. The patient is given a Mayo Clinic number and an electronic medical record is created.

When a patient comes to a Mayo clinic, we assign a personal physician to handle the patient's care; in most telemedicine cases that will be Dr. Gura. He will review the case and forward the information to the appropriate Mayo physician(s) following our processes here. For example, if they sent a CT scan, we actually create an order in the ordering system and the images are actually passed on to our PAC system for handling; a notification is sent to the techs to say there is a case waiting. They get the case up on the screen for the radiologist to view; the radiologist interprets it; dictates a report. Similarly with other specialties, neurology for example, they would look at the neurologist's reports, they would look at other information that was sent, and they dictate their second opinion into our clinical notes system. If a surgical consult is needed those are done as well.

When all the subspecialists' reports have been completed, a second-opinion document is compiled from them and sent back to the physician who requested the consult. That physician then has a second opinion that can be worked into the diagnostic and treatment planning for the patient. A real-time interaction between the physicians is not necessary.

One of the principal advantages of this workflow is that it is as transparent to the Mayo physicians as possible. They don't have to learn a new system; they don't have to change their practice model to accommodate telemedicine. They see the patient's records in the same system they use everyday.

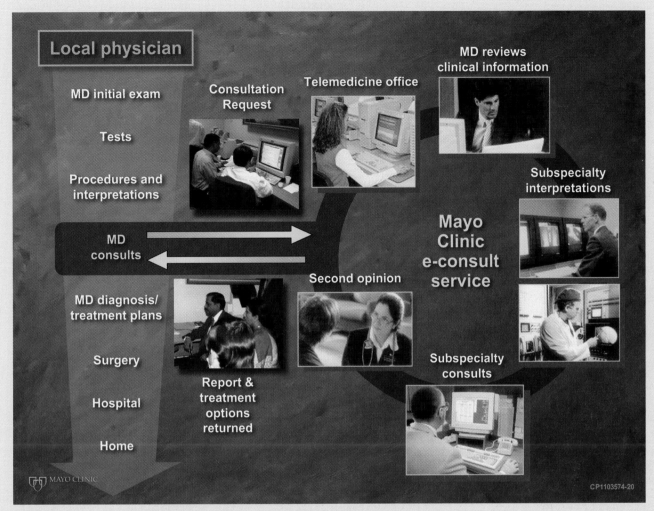

**FIGURE 5-12    Workflow of the Mayo Clinic telemedicine system**

(Courtesy of Mayo Clinic.)

One thing we require is that the physician on the other end ask a specific question, rather that ask for a general opinion. For example, "Is this Bell's palsy? Has the patient had a stroke?" That way we can make sure we are targeting exactly what the physician needs. Mayo provides value to the requesting physician, because we do have that subspecialty expertise that they don't.

This solution also solves the problem of licensure that has hindered telemedicine in the United States. Currently, most states require a physician to be licensed by that state to treat patients in that state. The regulations apply to telemedicine as well. Therefore, either out-of-state patients must travel to Mayo or our doctor must hold licenses in multiple states.

At Mayo, the telemedicine consultation is physician to physician; we are not giving advice to the patient, we are a resource for their doctor. Therefore, no laws are broken. This has the additional advantage of keeping the patient's home physician in control of the patient care at all times.

Telemedicine provides easy access to Mayo Clinic subspecialty care. It is like adding 1,600 subspecialists to the hospital with very little impact to them. It has a positive impact on the patients, improves the patient satisfaction with the hospitals, and avoids unnecessary travel and costs. I think similar savings could be realized using telemedicine more in the United States.

Mayo Clinic has a model of care that we try to adhere to at all times; it is just how we practice medicine. Over time we felt that the store-and-forward model of telemedicine worked best with our Mayo model of care and its multi-specialty integration, how we treat patients when they come through in that multi-specialty environment, and being able to ask other colleagues. That works best with store-and-forward. It didn't work well with video.

The patient answers the questions and can add free-text clarification at various points in the interview.

- E-visits are only used for nonurgent visits. If the condition seems urgent, the software advises the patient to seek immediate medical care and the provider is notified to determine the proper course of action.
- If the software determines that the condition is not urgent but the patient needs to be seen in the office, the patient is given a message to that effect and automatically offered a choice of available appointments.

- When the interview is complete, the clinician is notified that an E-visit is ready to review.

- The clinician reviews the patient-entered data and any relevant patient medical records and then replies to the patient. The system allows the provider and patient to continue to exchange messages, much like a question-and-answer session in the exam room, except for the factor of time, which is sometimes delayed by one or both parties' responses.

- The clinician can also prescribe electronically during the E-visit just as he or she would during an office visit. When patients receive the clinician's reply to the E-visit, they are prompted to select their preferred pharmacy from a list (if it is not already known to the EHR) and the prescription is electronically transmitted to the pharmacy by the doctor's system.

- The doctor's response can also include patient education material and comments or care instructions from the doctor, all of which are recorded in the care plan as well.

- Data from the E-visit can be merged into the doctor's EHR to become part of the patient's medical record. The doctor's practice management system can verify the patient eligibility for the E-visit and submit the claim electronically.

In an independent study sponsored by Blue Shield of California,[8] most patients and doctors in the study preferred a web visit to an office visit for nonurgent medical needs. Providers found that the E-visit gathered the important details and eliminated multiple messages back and forth that occur when trying to provide patient care via e-mail. The patients found that the time spent scheduling, driving, parking, and waiting was eliminated with an E-visit. The reality of online medical visits with your doctor is not a question of *if*, but *when*.

---

# Chapter 5 Summary

### Understanding Healthcare Records

Healthcare records have many purposes, the most important of which is the patient's care.

- The patient health record is the repository of data and information about a patient, the condition of the patient's health, the care and treatments the patient received, and the outcome of that care.
- The term *patient health record* has replaced the term *patient medical record* because it encompasses a holistic view of patient care. Though the terms are used almost interchangeably, an acute care patient record is usually concerned with one stay or episode, whereas an outpatient medical record is usually limited to one group or clinic.

- Data and information is not the same thing. Data are records of facts. Information is data in a useful form that conveys meaning.

### Functions of Healthcare Records

- A patient's health record serves as the principal communication document among various providers who might care for the patient at different times in different departments.
- The patient record provides the basis for all billing and reimbursement. Medical claims will not be paid by an insurance company if the patient record does not have enough detail about the encounter or treatment to support the claim.

---

[8]*The RelayHealth Web Visit Study: Final Report* (RelayHealth, January 2003), www.relayhealth.com. ©2002–2003 RelayHealth Corporation.

- The health record is a legal document; relevant portions of the patient's record may become evidence in a court of law.
- Healthcare records provide the basis for improvements in health.
  - Individually, a patient's record is evaluated and used to develop care plans for the patient.
  - Collectively, health records can be used by a healthcare facility to improve the quality and processes of healthcare delivery.
- Public health departments, Homeland Security, and law enforcement officials use information from health records.
- Researchers use patient records from *clinical trials* to monitor the effectiveness and safety of new drugs.
- De-identified health records are analyzed by researchers to find health trends in our society and measure which treatments seem to have the best outcomes.

## Primary and Secondary Records

Health information professionals classify health records as primary and secondary records:

- Primary records are those that are gathered directly from the patient and his or her providers and from devices and diagnostic tests. Primary records are used for patient care and as legal documents.
  - Examples of primary records include admission and discharge reports, nursing notes, physician examinations and notes, all orders, test results, operative reports, pathology and radiology reports, and administrative and demographic forms.
- Secondary records are those that are created later, by analyzing, summarizing, or abstracting from the primary records. Secondary records are used in billing, research, and quality improvement.
  - Examples of secondary records include insurance claims, master patient index, and ALOS reports.

## Contents of Health Records

Patient health record data consists of *administrative and demographic* data and *clinical* data. Administrative data includes a number of legal documents signed by the patient or their representative. These may include:

- HIPAA consent to use and disclose PHI
- Consent to treatment
- Medicare patient rights statement
- Assignment of benefits
- Informed consent
- Refusal of treatment
- Advance directives
- Organ donor
- Personal property list
- Disclosure records.

Demographic data is often gathered on paper forms, then transferred into the computer by the registration clerk. In a paper-based system, this principal document will be called a *face sheet*. In an electronic system, the forms may be scanned into a document image system.

Clinical data include documents created by the patient, nurses, clinicians, and other providers. Some standard types of clinical documents include:

- Medical history
- Physical exam
- Diagnostic and therapeutic orders
- Diagnostic and therapeutic reports
- Diagnostic images
- Operative records
- Nursing notes
- Referral consults
- Case management
- Discharge summary
- Obstetrical records
- Pediatric records
- Problem list
- Medication list
- Public health records.

## Documentation Standards

HIM professionals seek to ensure uniform quality patient records. Some of the ways to accomplish this are to use standardized data elements, data sets, and HIM policies and procedures.

- Data elements define specific units of information that may consist of several fields. For example, the patient name element would typically include first, middle, and last name and a suffix.
- Standard data sets are a collection of data elements determined to be the minimum necessary for a particular purpose.
- HIM policies and procedures establish documentation requirements for health records and are typically included in the rules medical staff must follow.

## Continuity of Care Records

Clinical data in the patient record helps provide a *continuity of care* as the patient is seen at different times by different healthcare workers.

- In an inpatient facility, the patient moves through different departments of a facility, for example, admitting, radiology, or surgery. Because providers record their findings, actions, and orders in the chart, subsequent caregivers can read what the previous nurses, doctors, or therapists have observed and what has been done.
- In an outpatient setting, a lapse of months or even a year between doctor visits is not uncommon. The exam notes from each visit, test results, and reports from consulting physicians and outside facilities are filed in

the patient's chart. This information about the patient's previous visits and treatments enables the clinician to provide continuity of care over a longer period of time.

However, because patients do not always go to the same doctors, the same medical practice, nor use just one pharmacy, a complete health record for the patient does not exist in any one place. A regional health information organization (RHIO) is one way for different providers to share patient records. One issue for a RHIO is who owns the data? Historically, the provider, group practice, or facility considered itself to be the owner of a patient's health record, but information sent via a RHIO is merged into the receiving facility's patient records, clouding the issue. Though the provider owns the patient record, HIPAA gives patients the right to review, copy, and amend their health record.

Patients are also creating personal health records through neutral online entities that allow them to make their records available to different providers they visit.

### Telemedicine

Telemedicine uses communication technology to deliver medical care to a patient in another location. Telemedicine can provide high-level medical expertise to remote and rural areas.

Telemedicine can be practiced in real time or in a store-and-forward manner.

- Real-time telemedicine requires the presence of all parties at the same time, for example, a conference call.
- Store-and-forward telemedicine allows one party to send information that is saved and then reviewed and responded to later.

Teleradiology is telemedicine specifically concerned with the transmission of diagnostic images from one location to another. Usually this is for the purpose of having the images "read" by a radiologist at the receiving end.

Telemonitoring allows doctors to study vital signs or tests measured many times in the course of the patient's normal daily activity using devices such as blood pressure monitors, glucose meters, and Holter monitors. The devices store the readings and transfer the data to the doctor's system either by using a modem and phone line or by downloading from the device during a patient encounter.

E-visits are being used in some states to allow the patient to be treated by a clinician for nonurgent health problems without having to come into the office. E-visits are conducted over the Internet.

## Critical Thinking Exercises

1. CMS takes the position that "if it isn't documented, it wasn't done." What does this mean and why would it matter to CMS?
2. Chapters 4 and 5 discussed data sets. Design a basic demographic data set. Make a list of just the fields you would need for the patient information. (You do not need to include insurance information.)

## Testing Your Knowledge of Chapter 5

1. Health records are classified as primary or secondary records. Give an example of each type.
2. List two ways in which healthcare records provide the basis for improvements in health.
3. Provide an example of patient health record data that is administrative or demographic data.
4. Provide two examples of types of clinical data in a patient's chart.
5. What is a RHIO?
6. What are some differences between the contents of patient records at an inpatient facility versus a doctor's office?
7. What does the acronym PHR stand for?
8. There are two methods of telemedicine. Which method is used by the Mayo Clinic?
9. Describe the difference between a data element and a data set.
10. How do HIM policies and procedures help ensure quality patient records?
11. Name three functions of patient health records.
12. The patient record provides the basis for all billing and reimbursement. What will happen if the patient record does not have enough detail?
13. What is the difference between data and information?
14. Provide an example of how the patient record helps provide continuity of care.
15. What is an E-visit?

# Organization, Storage, and Management of Health Records

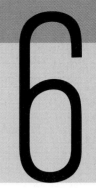

## LEARNING OUTCOMES

After completing this chapter, you should be able to:

- Explain the various ways in which paper records are organized and stored
- Differentiate source-oriented, problem-oriented, and integrated records
- Compare different methods of filing numeric charts
- Describe the workflow of charts in the HIM department
- Calculate the space requirements for filing paper charts
- Explain the processes involved in document imaging
- Discuss the HIM responsibilities of the legal health record
- Describe the AHIMA code of ethics

## ACRONYMS USED IN CHAPTER 6

Acronyms are used extensively in both medicine and computers. The following are those which are used in this chapter.

| | | | |
|---|---|---|---|
| **AHIMA** | American Health Information Management Association | **HIPAA** | Health Insurance Portability and Accountability Act |
| **ALOS** | Average Length of Stay | **OCR** | Optical Character Recognition |
| **CD** | Compact Disk | **OSHA** | Occupational Safety and Health Administration |
| **CMS** | Centers for Medicare and Medicaid Services | | |
| **COP** | Conditions of Participation | **PACS OR PAC SYSTEM** | Picture Archiving and Communication System |
| **DVD** | Digital Video Disk | **PDF** | Portable Document Format |
| **EHR** | Electronic Health Record | **PHI** | Protected Health Information |
| **EPHI** | Electronic Protected Health Information | **SOAP** | Subjective, Objective, Assessment, Plan |
| **ER** | Emergency Room | **VPN** | Virtual Private Network |
| **FTE** | Full-Time Equivalent Employee | | |

## Managing Health Records

By this point in the course, you have an idea of the types of information contained in a health record, who uses health records, and the importance of health records being complete and readily accessible. This chapter will discuss how the contents of those records may be organized, various ways they are stored, and the process and ethics of managing them.

While most healthcare facilities today use at least some computer technology to manage patient records, the reality is that healthcare is in transition and paper records are still prevalent at many locations. You could very well find employment at a facility that still uses paper medical records or is in the process of converting from paper to electronic records. Therefore, this chapter will introduce fundamental concepts for organizing and filing paper charts. These concepts will also be useful when working with electronic record systems because many EHR systems present information in a structure organized similar to that of traditional paper charts.

This chapter also covers the management of patient charts (whether electronic or paper) and the issues of record retention, long-term storage, records workflow, and HIM ethics.

### Understanding the Scope of the Problem

To understand why a system for the organization and storage of patient health records is necessary, it is helpful to understand the scope of the problem. Let's use a relatively small group medical practice, with three providers seeing a combined total of 80 patients per day, as an example:

- Each patient visit will have—at the least—an encounter form, a patient history form, and the doctor's SOAP note. That is three documents per patient, multiplied by 80 patients, equals 240 documents per day.

- Assume 25% of the patients require a registration form to change their demographic or insurance information or because they are new patients. That will add 20 additional pages, bringing the total to 260 per day.

- If half the patients are prescribed a medication, that will add 40 prescription records. The total is now 300 per day.

- If the office is open 5 days a week, that is $300 \times 5 = 1,500$ documents per week; in a year that is $52 \times 1,500 = 78,000$ documents to be organized, filed, stored, and retrieved.

These 78,000 records do not even include test orders and results, consults, referrals, problem lists, medication lists, and the myriad other documents in an ambulatory chart. The actual number of records would be much larger.

Now consider a large acute care hospital where charts typically have a 100 or more pages per patient. If the ALOS is 3.5 days and the hospital has 1,000 discharges per week, that results in more than 5 million documents per year the HIM department must manage ($100 \times 1,000 \times 52 = 5,200,000$).

These examples make it easy to see why the manner in which health records are handled, organized, and filed is of importance to healthcare organizations of all sizes.

## How Paper Charts Are Organized

Paper records usually consist of one or more file folders containing handwritten notes, transcribed reports, test results, demographic information sheets, patient history forms, and referral letters about the patient. Ambulatory practices may also store HIPAA authorizations, privacy notices, and other documents signed by the patient in the same folder. Acute care hospitals will store all of the documents described in Chapter 5 in the chart, but may have a separate chart for each visit.

Later we will explore how charts are identified, filed, and stored, but first let us look at how the documents are arranged within the chart itself. The organization of the documents within the paper chart should be standard across the practice, but may be different from one type of practice to another. There are several standard schemes for organizing a paper chart.

## Source-Oriented Record

A method called the *source-oriented record* method organizes the contents of the chart according to the source of the document. For example, physician notes are grouped in one section, radiology reports in another, lab results in another, nursing notes in another, and so on. Often the sections are separated by labeled dividers within the folder (as shown in Figure 6-1). This makes it easy to locate a particular group of documents, for example, to review all physician orders.

The source-oriented type of chart is frequently used at inpatient facilities because it works well when many different individuals are providing care to a patient for a particular problem. The drawback is that to review all records for a particular day or disease, the clinician must flip through each section looking for possible entries for that date.

## Problem-Oriented Record

A problem-oriented record organizes the patient's chart by diagnosis or medical problem. For example, a patient with several chronic diseases would have separate sections of the chart for each condition. A problem list at the front of the chart serves as an index to the record, listing each problem with a number. As problems are managed or resolved, the problem list is updated. If new problems occur, they are added to the list.

Though a problem list is used as an index to a problem-oriented record, the problem list is also a typical component in an ambulatory chart even where an outpatient facility organizes charts by a different method.

## Integrated Record

The integrated record intermingles documents from various sources arranged sequentially in order by date. This is called chronological order. Reverse chronological order is also date order, but with the newest documents at the front of folder and the oldest document at the back. Figure 6-2 illustrates pages arranged in reverse chronological order.

Integrated records, in reverse chronological order, is the type of record most frequently used in medical practices and ambulatory clinics. Because the newest documents are at the front of the chart, it is easy for the clinician to review the most recent patient visit or test result.

The advantage of an integrated chart (in reverse chronological order) is that the most recent progress notes and reports are on top. Because outpatient charts tend to include years of patient visits, it is likely that the more recent notes are the more relevant. It is also easier to add pages to the chart; the file clerk simply adds new documents to the front of the folder.

One disadvantage of the integrated chart is that to find a particular item you must know the date it was recorded or peruse the entire chart. It is also more difficult to compare reports or results from tests that were given weeks or month apart because other types of documents are interwoven between them.

Some inpatient facilities that use the source-oriented method for the overall chart may organize one or more sections within the chart using the integrated or problem-oriented method. For example, the sections for physician and ancillary therapy progress notes may be organized as an integrated record. Similarly, the nursing notes section may be organized using the problem-oriented method.

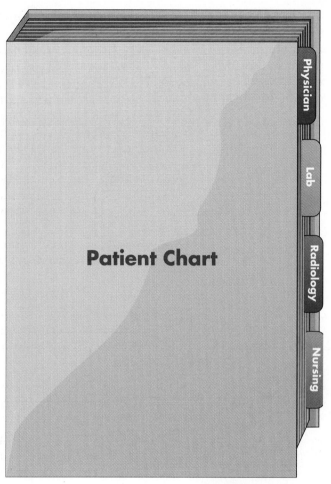

**FIGURE 6-1**

**Source-oriented record tabs separate documents by source.**

**FIGURE 6-2**

**Reverse chronological integrated record with newest documents on top**

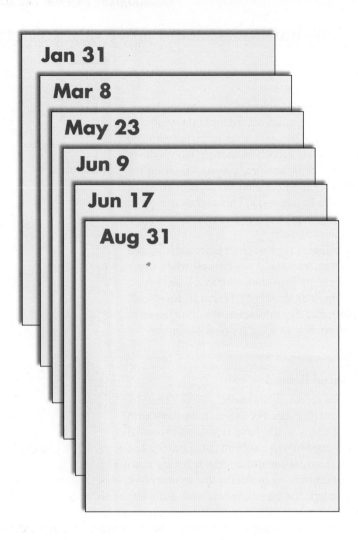

## Electronic Views

As just discussed, paper charts are organized using a source-oriented, problem-oriented, or integrated method. The data remains fixed in the order in which the chart was assembled. It would be very difficult to change methods later because all of the charts would have to be disassembled and reassembled.

EHR systems do not have that limitation. Computer databases store records in a method called random access. When the data is retrieved, it can be instantly organized to display in many different ways. These are sometimes referred to as *views* or reports. Using different views, EHR systems can reorganize the patient chart on demand for different providers or different purposes. Using the same data, an EHR can display a source-oriented chart, problem-oriented chart, or integrated chart.

The left panel of the computer screen in Figure 6-3 shows an EHR display of a problem-oriented view. The tabs above the list allow the user to switch to a source-oriented view, for example, surgical history or family history.

## Hybrid Health Records

As discussed earlier, healthcare is in the midst of transitioning to electronic systems. AHIMA has coined the term *hybrid health records* to describe systems that use both paper and electronic records. The ability of EHR systems to instantly switch views works best when the majority of data is in fielded records. However, for many facilities the transition to electronic records involves the continued use of paper forms, which are subsequently scanned into the chart. In these instances, the EHR can reorganize the document images by date, type, or other criteria, but

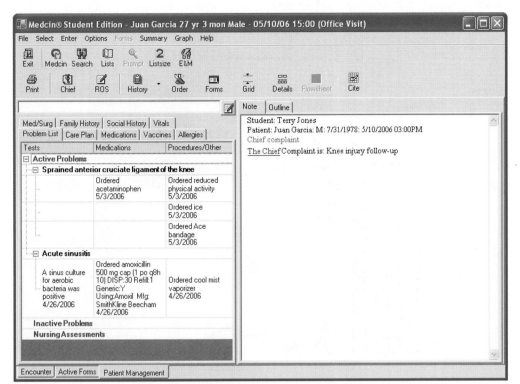

**FIGURE 6-3**

**Problem-oriented view in an electronic chart.**

not by the data written on the page. The term *hybrid health* record is also used where facilities keep a portion of the chart electronically and a portion of it in paper files.

Regardless of whether the patient chart remains on paper or consists of paper forms scanned into a document imaging system, paper records have some drawbacks: Handwritten records are often abbreviated, cryptic, or illegible. Paper records are not easily searchable. For example, if a practice is notified that all patients on a particular drug needed to be contacted, the only way of finding those patients is to literally open every chart and look at the medications lists.

## Loose Sheets

Whether the type of chart you use is a hybrid chart or a paper chart, a number of documents often need to be added to the chart at various times. Examples are lab reports delivered to a nursing unit after the patient has been discharged or transcription documents that arrive at doctor's offices days after the patient visit.

When loose sheets arrive after the inpatient chart has been assembled and processed, the chart must be located and the loose sheets added to the proper section of the chart. In some large hospitals, the handling and processing of loose sheets may require a full-time HIM position.

In an outpatient facility, documents such as transcription, lab, and consult reports will not arrive until days or weeks after the patient's visit, and so must be treated as loose sheets to be filed. This will consist of pulling the paper chart and integrating the pages in the proper sequence.

Even inpatient and outpatient facilities that scan all incoming paper documents into an EHR must establish a systematic procedure for handling loose sheets and ensuring the documents are properly scanned and cataloged into the computer.

# Filing Paper Records

As we discussed earlier, one of the primary purposes of the patient health record is to facilitate the continuity of care for the patient. This requires various providers to have access to the records of previous conditions, test results, current medications, problems, and treatments. To be useful, the chart must be accurate, complete, and up to date. It also must be available. To ensure availability,

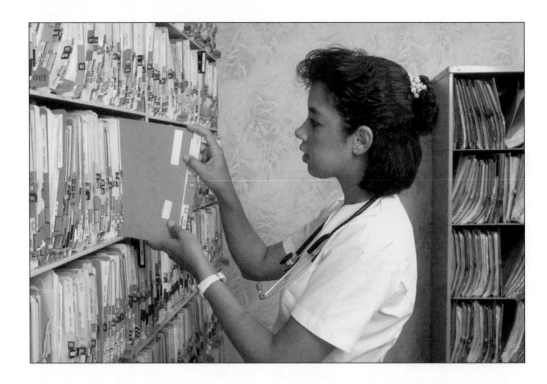

the HIM department must be able to quickly find a chart when it is needed and to track its location when it is not in the file room.

Just as there are various methods of organizing the documents within a paper chart, there are also different methods of organizing the folders in the file room. Filing systems are either alphabetic by the patient's last name or numeric, based on a unique number assigned to each patient chart. Figure 6-4 shows a medical assistant working with an alphabetical filing system.

Different filing systems are used because some work better in smaller than larger facilities and some work better for inpatient or outpatient facilities. Healthcare organizations select the filing method that best suits their needs. However, the various methods share the same goals:

- Ensure the files can be quickly located when needed.
- Easily detect where charts are misfiled or missing.
  - Expedite the daily retrieval and filling of charts.
  - Expansion of the system can occur with minimal reorganization of the files.

### Paper Chart Filing Systems

Paper charts consist of documents stored in a file folder. The folders are usually manufactured with a pronged metal clip that fastens the pages to the folder. One edge of the folder will have a large tab that protrudes. The HIM department will attach labels to the tab that identify the patient and are used to file the chart. Often the labels are different colors. Color coding the labels helps to minimize and detect filing errors. Figure 6-5 shows two folders designed to hold pages with a clip at the top. The chart label is attached to the large tab at the bottom of the folder.

In alphabetical systems, charts are filed by the patient's last name, first name, and middle initial or name. Some facilities using alphabetical systems add large block letters to the label representing the first three letters of the last name. These help the file clerk quickly find the right section of the charts when filing or retrieving patient records.

**FIGURE 6-5**

**Medical record folders**

(Courtesy of Ames Color-File.)

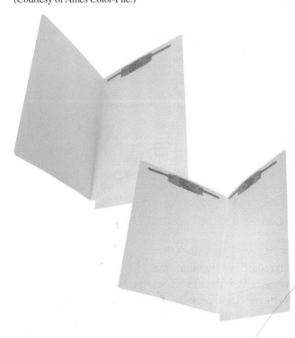

The advantages of an alphabetical filing system are that it is the easiest system to learn and charts can be located knowing only the patient's name. The disadvantage is that alphabetical charts are more prone to being misfiled than numbered charts. Also, because some letters of the alphabet have more surnames than others, alphabetical systems tend to grow unevenly and require frequent reorganization of the file room to make more space for certain parts of the alphabet.

Numeric systems assign each patient a medical record number and file charts by number. A master list of patients is used to find a patient's record number. However, as the length of the chart number grows, filing errors can occur, especially with longer chart numbers. Therefore, organizations with large chart numbers often use hyphens to divide the medical record number into several easy-to-read sequences. Facilities may also use a different color label for each digit 0 through 9 to prevent filing errors.

## Systems for Filing Numbered Charts

Patients are assigned sequential medical record numbers as new patients come to the facility or as new charts are required. Charts are labeled with the medical record number. All numeric methods of filing require the user to know the patient's chart number to find the chart. Typically a master patient index is used to look up the patient's chart number.

ALPHANUMERIC FILING    Alphanumeric systems attempt to combine both alphabetical and numeric filing methods by preceding the record number with one or two letters of the surname; for example, patient Garcia's chart might be labeled GA467801. This is called *alphanumeric* numbering because it contains both letters and numbers. This antiquated filing method has the disadvantage of alphabetical filing systems, as the file space grows unevenly, and also the disadvantage of numeric systems in that an index is still necessary to find a particular chart.

STRAIGHT NUMERIC FILING    Ambulatory facilities and smaller hospitals may file patient charts in a straight numeric sequence. The charts are filed in ascending numeric order; that is, the first chart in the file system will be the lowest number and the last chart will be the highest number.

One advantage of this file system is that it can grow without ever being reorganized because the most recently assigned number will always be added to the last shelf. The disadvantage, mentioned previously, is that as the numbers become longer filing errors increase.

To make it easier to correctly file numeric charts, hyphens can be used to separate long medical record numbers into three sets; for example, 467801 may be labeled as 46-78-01. This makes the number easier to read and easier to file. Six-digit numbers can be used for up to 1 million charts (00-00-00 to 99-99-99.) When a facility has more than a million charts, one of the sets is increased to three digits, for example, 123-00-00.

To further reduce errors, two variations of numeric filing may be used: *terminal digit filing* and *middle digit filing*. Both of these methods use chart numbers divided into three sets by hyphens. The file room shelves are divided into labeled sections reserved for each primary set of numbers. Within each section are subsections for each secondary set of numbers.

Terminal Digit Filing    Terminal digit filing uses the last set of the hyphenated record number (called the terminal digits) as the primary set of numbers for filing. For example, with chart number 46-78-01, the last set of digits (01) will be used as the primary set of numbers for filing purposes; the middle set of digits (78) will be the secondary set of numbers for filing order.

In Figure 6-6, the file clerk, reading the chart number sets from right to left, will go to the file area labeled section 01, locate subsection 78, and file the chart between charts 45 and 47. Charts are filed in ascending numerical order, but only within the proper section and subsection of the file shelf area.

While the rest of the hospital staff see the patient record number as 46-78-01, the HIM department sees it as the key to its filing location. All patient charts ending in 01 will be in the file room section labeled 01, all charts with the middle digits of 78 will be on the shelf for subsection 78. Charts ending in 01 but with the middle digits of 79 will be filed in subsection 79, as shown in Figure 6-7.

**FIGURE 6-6**

**Chart 46-78-01 being filed in Section 01, Subsection 78**

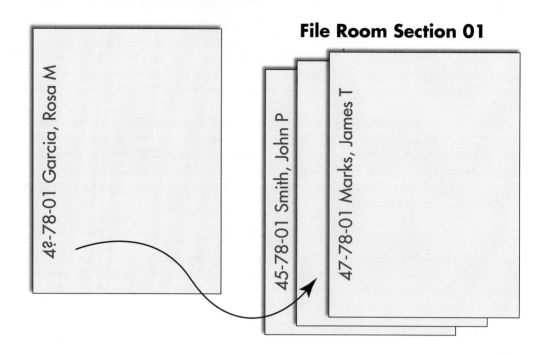

Figure 6-7 shows two subsections within section 01 of the file room. Notice the chart numbers on the folders, and notice how the charts are filed in two different subsections. Terminal digit filing reduces the chance of filing errors by limiting the number of charts in each subsection. Using this method, one million charts could be filed, yet there would never be more than 100 charts in any subsection.

**Middle Digit Filing** The middle digit filing method is similar to the terminal digit method except that the middle set of numbers is the primary set for filing purposes. In middle digit filing, the numbers of the middle set correspond to the numbered sections of the file room. Using the previous example, chart number 46-78-01 would be filed in section 78 of the file room. The middle digit system is only used where medical record numbers are six digits or less; facilities with record numbers greater than a million use terminal digit filing or straight numeric filing.

**FIGURE 6-7**

**Files in Section 01, Subsections 78 and 79**

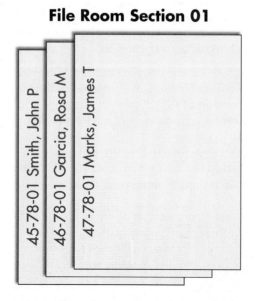 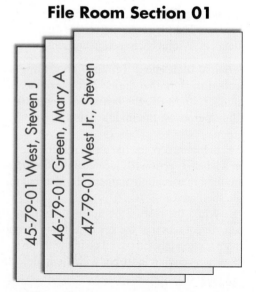

## Color Coding

To more easily detect misfiled paper charts, both alphabetical and numeric systems may use different colored labels for different letters or numbers. For example, on the label in Figure 6-8, the number 4 is purple, 6 is yellow, and 7 is brown. With a color-coded system, a folder filed in the wrong section or subsection will quickly stand out because its numbers will break the visual pattern created by the sequence of colored labels. For example, if the number 3 is orange, then subsection 33 should visually appear to have a consistent line of orange throughout the subsection. If a chart belonging in subsection 34 were accidentally misfiled there, a spot of purple in the midst of the row of orange labels would stand out.

## How Charts Are Numbered

Facilities that use numeric filing assign medical record numbers based on several different methods. In all cases, the patient's medical record number is unique. Ideally, there is only one number per patient.

**SERIAL NUMBERING** Some hospitals sequentially number their records, assigning a new number for each admission or ER visit. This allows the hospital to easily assemble and track every record and service related to that stay under one number. The disadvantage is that patients who have been in the hospital several times have several different medical record numbers.

**UNIT NUMBERING** Most ambulatory and inpatient facilities use unit numbering. A single medical record number is assigned the first time a patient is registered and the same number is used every time the patient returns. This results in a single chart for the patient. The Joint Commission recommends that unit numbering be used where feasible; when it is not feasible, the facility should have a system that makes available all of the patient's previous records when care is provided.

**SERIAL-UNIT NUMBERING** Serial-unit numbering is an alternative that allow facilities that use serial numbering to comply with the Joint Commission. As with straight serial numbering, a new number is assigned for each patient stay or visit; however, the records from the previous chart number are brought forward into the new one. The patient index is updated to reflect the new number. If this is practiced consistently, then records from all previous visits are always in the current folder.

**FAMILY NUMBERING** Some medical practices use numbers from their practice management systems as medical record numbers. Family numbering is useful for administrative tasks, because it makes it easy to bill parents for several children or to schedule spouses and children on the same days. However, it is not useful as a system of medical record numbers.

Family numbering ties the family records together by adding decimal numbers to the primary account number. Using account number 100, for example, the head of the household would be assigned number 100.0, the spouse 100.1, the first child 100.2, the second child 100.3, and so on.

The problem with using accounting numbers as medical record numbers occurs as families change. When the children grow up and leave home, when divorce occurs—any event that requires a new separate account to be set up is going to cause a change in the medical record number. Although family numbering is useful for accounting, an independent number should be assigned to each family member for their medical records.

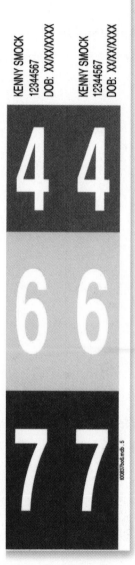

**FIGURE 6-8**
**Color-coded label**

(Courtesy of Ames Color-File.)

# Record Circulation and Storage

Paper charts are typically filed and retrieved by a clerk or other member of the HIM team. A list of charts that will be needed for the day is used to pull charts in advance. An *outguide* is put in the place where the chart was filed. An outguide is a paper or plastic placeholder that indicates a chart has been removed. Information on the outguide includes the chart number, when the chart was pulled, and the provider or department where it was sent. Figure 6-9 shows an outguide with a pocket to hold the requisition slip.

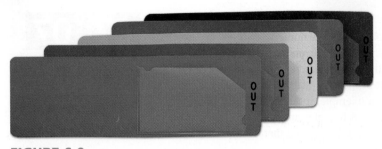

**FIGURE 6-9**

**An outguide**

(Courtesy of Ames Color-File.)

Charts that are needed for unscheduled patients, emergency admissions, or walk-in patients are requested either verbally or using a written form. Charts that are needed for administrative purposes, such as billing, chart review, or audits, are requested via a written form or computer-generated "pull list."

Charts are batched together by provider or department and delivered to a nurse or provider's staff.

If a patient is new and does not have a chart, a medical record number will be assigned and added to the patient index. A new folder will be created and labeled with the chart number. This process may occur in the registration department, but it is the responsibility of the HIM department to ensure that each patient is assigned a unique chart number.

When the patient has been checked out or discharged, the record is returned to the chart room for filing. Any additional documents belonging to the record are added in the appropriate places and the chart is refiled.

In acute settings, the medical record must be examined after the patient's discharge to ensure that all required documents are present, complete, and signed by a provider where required. As shown in Chapter 2, Figure 2-1, a hospital chart may pass through many stages and departments before it is filed.

In a doctor's office, the chart is sometimes filed after the patient encounter, then pulled and updated later as new documents, such as transcription and lab results, arrive.

Historically, both acute care and ambulatory care facilities stored x-ray films and other radiology records separate from the chart in large envelopes called *jackets* (shown in Figure 6-10). The jackets were filed in the radiology department or a filing location separate from the paper chart's location.

Many hospitals and radiology offices now store x-ray and other diagnostic images electronically in a PAC system. This eliminates the need to store x-ray films in jackets and provides improved accessibility.

## Problems with Paper Charts

Chart deficiencies and late arriving reports are an issue for both inpatient and outpatient facilities. When a change must be made or a report filed, the chart must be located and pulled to add the additional material, then filed again.

**FIGURE 6-10**

**X-Ray jacket**

(Courtesy of Ames Color-File.)

In addition, providers may hold onto charts, fail to return them in a timely fashion, or hand them off to another department without notifying HIM that they have been moved elsewhere. This results in the chart being unavailable to another user who may need it.

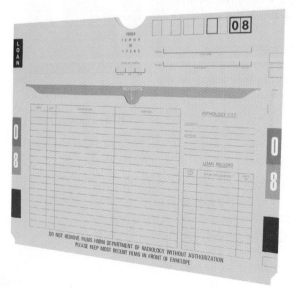

If an ambulatory practice has multiple locations, the chart must be transported from one office to another when a patient is seen at a different location than usual.

**DUPLICATE CHARTS** If a patient has more than one chart at a medical practice or inpatient facility, the charts must be identified and the information merged into one chart. Duplicate charts are undesirable because one or both charts will be incomplete, which can result in medical errors and endanger the patient.

A second chart for a patient might be started for any of several reasons:

- The registration clerk does not find the record of an existing patient in the master patient index and therefore creates a new patient record.
- The patient's name has changed through marriage or divorce and the demographic record has not been updated, so a new patient record is started.

- An inpatient facility uses serial numbering or serial-unit numbering, generating a new record number for each encounter, but the previous records were not located and brought forward.

- In an ambulatory practice, if a patient's chart cannot be located at the time of a visit or if the chart is at another location, a temporary folder may be created, which eventually must be merged with the original.

- Emergency department patients who arrive without ID, in a comatose condition, must have temporary charts created for them until the patient can be identified.

## Chart Tracking Systems

One of the principal HIM department responsibilities for paper charts is tracking and locating them. As mentioned earlier, the outguide will indicate the person or department to whom the chart was checked out. Unfortunately, charts for current patients are sometimes passed from department to department without informing HIM, so the whereabouts of the chart listed on the outguide may not be accurate.

Inpatient facilities and ambulatory facilities with a large number of providers use computer systems to track paper charts. One such system is shown in Figure 6-11. These systems let a provider or scheduling person request charts that will be needed. A list of charts to be pulled is printed in an order that optimizes pulling the charts.

Some computerized chart tracking systems use barcodes of the chart numbers (printed on the chart label) to automate identification of the chart. When the charts are returned to the file room, a barcode on the chart folder can be used to quickly check the chart back in. Where charts have barcodes, facilities may also be able track the movement of the chart between departments, allowing HIM to always know the chart's current location.

Where computerized chart tracking is not used, three-part paper requisition forms are used to request patient records and keep track of who has them. The first part of the form goes into a tracking system file, another part is placed in the outguide, and the other part is attached to the chart folder for delivery. In the case of unscheduled or emergency visits, chart requests are made by telephone and the requisition form is completed by the HIM personnel.

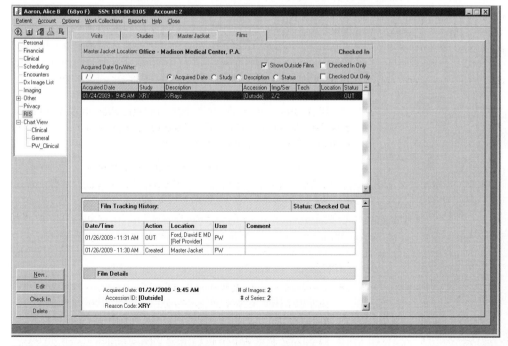

**FIGURE 6-11    Computerized chart tracking system**

**FIGURE 6-12**

**A large file room with mobile shelving units**

(Courtesy of Ames Color-File.)

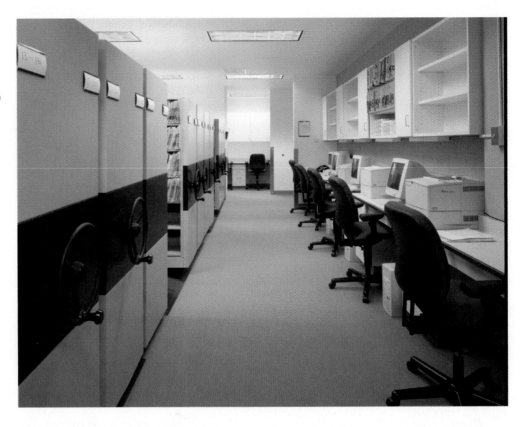

## Storage for Paper Records

In addition to the work involved in manually handling and filing paper charts, a vast amount of office space is consumed to accommodate their storage. Paper charts are stored in metal filing cabinets or shelving units. Figures 6-12 to 6-14 show several different types of storage units. Not only do shelves for filing paper charts occupy floor space, they also require aisle space for the file clerk to open the cabinet or walk between the units.

**FIGURE 6-13**

**Doors cover and lock file shelves.**

(Courtesy of Ames Color-File.)

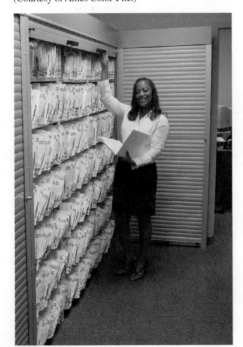

The amount of extra space required varies by the type of filing unit selected. The Occupational Safety and Health Administration (OSHA) has specified the amount of space required for filing areas. For example, the aisle between filing or shelving units must be at least 3 feet wide. Figure 6-12 shows a large file room where aisle space has been saved by using movable filing units.

Filing systems must comply with HIPAA and other regulations to ensure the records are secure. The filing cabinets and/or the file room must have locks to ensure privacy of the records. Access to the files must be controlled at all times. Pull-down doors cover and lock the file shelves shown in Figure 6-13.

The files must be secure from water and fire damage. Fire extinguishers in the file room should be chemical or halogen to minimize water damage to the files. The storage units must have a cover at the top to protect the records and the top of the unit must have at least 18 inches of clearance from the ceiling so that fire system sprinklers will not be blocked. In communities prone to flooding, file rooms should be located on the second floor or higher.

Facilities that have replaced paper charts with electronic systems have found that the valuable floor space once occupied by the file room and storage units can be repurposed for additional offices or treatment areas.

**CALCULATING STORAGE FOR PAPER RECORDS**   How much space do paper files take up? AHIMA estimates that the file for an average inpatient stay contains 100 pages. One hundred sheets of standard weight paper measures

1/2 inch thick. A manila folder (including the metal clip) and several dividers to separate sections adds 1/8 inch. Using this example, you would need 5/8 inch for each paper chart.

- A shelving unit for medical records that is 36 inches wide will have about 34 inches of filing space per shelf. Shelving is also available in widths of 42 or 48 inches.
- The standard depth of a shelf is 12 inches.
- Shelving units usually have six, seven, or eight shelves spaced about 10 inches apart. The number of shelves may be limited by the height of the ceiling (to allow clearance for the sprinkler system).

Using the example of 5/8-inch-thick charts, a 36-inch-wide unit with seven shelves can store approximately 378 patient charts. A facility will require 200 such units to store paper records for 75,000 patients.

Weight is also a factor to be considered. One inch of charts (folder, dividers, and papers) weighs approximately 2.5 pounds. Using the previous example, that is 590 pounds of paper. The shelving unit with lockable doors weighs 210 pounds; the total weight of each unit when filled with charts is 800 pounds. The combined weight for 200 units filled with files is 80 tons!

In an outpatient setting, patients visit the doctor's office multiple times over a number of years. Because the content of the chart varies by patient based on frequency of visits and the complication of their conditions, ambulatory patient charts can vary from 1/4 inch to more that 1 inch thick. In addition to medical records, doctor's offices also tend to store patient correspondence and insurance documents in the patient's chart; this also causes them to vary in size. Figure 6-14 shows another style of locking file cabinet. This style might be found in a small medical practice.

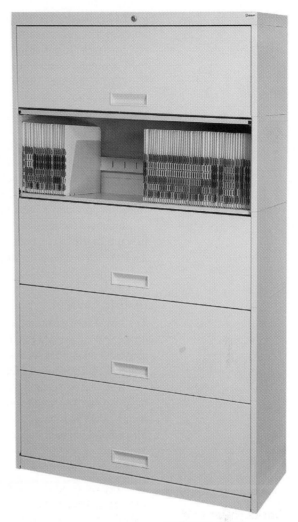

**FIGURE 6-14**

**File cabinet with locking doors**

(Courtesy of Ames Color-File)

## Critical Thinking Exercises

### Calculate the Size of an Outpatient Chart Filing System

A group medical practice has 40,000 patients. Charts vary in thickness from 1/4 to 1 inch thick. The average of all charts is 1/2 inch thick.

1. Using the average 1/2-inch thickness, how many inches of shelf space will be required for 40,000 charts?
2. The medical practice uses 48-inch-wide shelving units, which hold 46 inches of files per shelf. There are eight shelves. This means each unit can hold 8 × 46 inches = 368 inches. How many shelving units does the practice need to store its patient records?

## Document Imaging Systems

Though sometimes an EHR is referred to as a paperless chart, creating electronic health records does not necessarily eliminate paper copies of the records. However, the goal is to eliminate paper as the *only* copy of a patient's medical record.

Even with the implementation of a codified EHR, there will always be some paper. Obviously there are all the old paper charts of established patients, but there is also a continuing influx of referral letters and other medical documents from outside sources.

Many healthcare organizations choose to bring paper documents into the EHR as scanned images. Though document images do not offer the benefits of fielded, codified medical records, they do provide widespread accessibility and a means to include source documents for a complete electronic chart.

Most document imaging systems have a computer program to associate various ID fields and keywords with scanned images. This is called *cataloging the image*. Cataloged data adds the capability to search for the electronic document images in multiple ways.

Scanning old charts into the EHR can be daunting for established group practices and hospitals where hundreds of thousands of old charts may exist. The easiest strategy is to only scan the charts of patients who are scheduled to be seen. Thus, if the practice sees 100 patients a day, only 100 charts are scanned, not the thousands that are looming in the file room. This method also increases the likelihood that any chart the provider wants is already scanned in the system, since the provider is most likely interested in upcoming and recently seen patients.

Inpatient facilities may use a similar strategy, scanning charts of previous patients only when they return. However, once the document image system becomes part of the normal workflow for the HIM department, the hospital may decide to scan older charts to recoup the floor space that storing them requires.

## Quality Control

The process of scanning documents into an imaging system includes not only capturing the image, but cataloging the image, tying it to the correct patient, and entering data in the computer about the document such as the date, provider, type of image, and so on. Figure 6-15 shows an example of a document imaging management component of an EHR system.

It is during scanning and cataloging that quality control is most important. Once a document has been scanned and cataloged, the original may be shipped to a remote storage facility or shredded. In either case, the original document may no longer be available for comparison. Though the scanned document image is stored safely on the computer, if it has been incorrectly

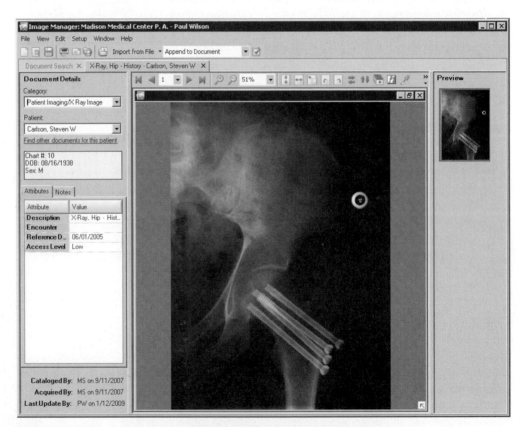

**FIGURE 6-15**   **Intergy document image management screen**

cataloged, it may not be easy to locate. The problem is equivalent to that of a paper system where, for instance, a file clerk misfiled a document in the wrong patient's folder, then refiled the folder.

Similar problems that must be avoided include cataloging documents as the wrong type, or *improper batching*. For example, a lab result grouped with the billing forms could cause it to be missed by a provider reviewing the chart. Also, some systems keep documents of the same type in the order in which they are scanned. If pages of a particular section are scanned out of order, it could make it difficult for the clinician to later review the chart chronologically.

For the most part, the cataloged data is entered by hand, but in some instances the image cataloging can be automated. Here are some examples of automated image cataloging:

- Paper forms can include a barcode on the form containing cataloged data; the scanning software interprets the barcode and creates the cataloged record. For example, a HIPAA authorization form that was printed for obtaining a patient's signature might also include a barcode identifying the patient, date, and document type, allowing automatic cataloging of the signed copy. In Chapter 3, Figure 3-4 shows an example of a form that has a barcode used for document scanning.

- Optical character recognition (OCR) software can recognize text characters in images. Some document imaging systems can be programmed to find and use the text contained in the scanned document to populate the fields in the cataloged records. Typically, only a few types of documents are processed this way because each document type requires custom programming. However, when an organization images thousands of the same type of document, it can be worth it. For example, your bank keeps an image of the front and back of each check it processes. Because the account number and check number are in a consistent place at the bottom of the check, the bank computers can automatically catalog each image to the correct account as they are scanned.

Even when cataloging is automated, manually preparing the chart for scanning is a necessary HIM function. This is called "prepping" the chart. Prepping steps include the following:

- Staples and paper clips must be removed.

- The health information technician then verifies that all the documents in the chart belong to the patient.

- At some facilities with EHR systems, portions of the paper chart may be printouts of information already imported or scanned. Those pages are omitted from the batch to prevent duplicates.

- Pages are examined and batched in the correct order, usually by document type and date.

- Wrinkled or damaged documents are either scanned individually on a flatbed scanner, or copied, and the copy is used in the batch.

- Where documents are scanned in large batches, barcoded divider sheets are printed and inserted between groups of pages. The scanning software recognizes the divider pages and uses the information on them to change the catalog information as the batch is processed.

The batch is then scanned. A high-volume scanner is shown in Figure 6-16. Once the scanning is completed, HIM personnel examine the scanned images to ensure they are legible, and then enter or verify the catalog information. When everything has been checked, the pages are returned to the chart, archived, or shredded (depending on the policy of the HIM department.)

## Microfilm

An older method of archiving paper records is to store them on microfilm. Each page of the chart is photographed on film. The images are then stored on rolls of film called microfilm or on small sheets of film called microfiche. The photographic images are very small but can be viewed at

**FIGURE 6-16**

**A high-volume scanner for scanning batches of documents.**

(Courtesy of IBML.)

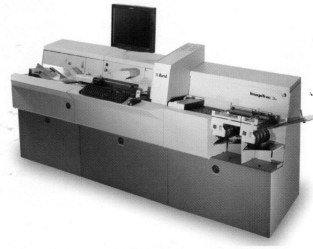

## Automating HIM Workflow

### By Shannon Welchi and Shelly Wymer

*Shannon Welchi, RHIA, is HIM department manager, and Shelly Wymer, RHIT, CCS, is electronic records coordinator at Allegiance Health Hospital in Jackson, Michigan.*

Our Health Information Management department is pretty well computerized, though a portion of our records are still in paper; these are scanned into a document imaging system. About 70% of our inpatient record is now imported data; therefore, it does not have to be scanned.

We usually receive the patient's chart the same day the patient is discharged or the day after. We want to get the material scanned in as quickly as we can, because once the documents are in our system they are secure and accessible to those who need them.

When we receive paper records in our department, our first step is to prep the record. We pull out any paper copies of documents that have already been imported; those we won't need to scan. For example, nursing notes originate in our CIS system; any paper copies are just printouts of what is already in the system. The same thing is true of lab results and many other reports.

Records are cataloged by patient and then by account number. (In our hospital every visit is a new account number. Though patients have one medical record number their whole life, every time they come in, a new account number is assigned. Some would call this a visit number.)

Next the documents are categorized with a document type for retrieval purposes. Each document type has a designated code. There are barcodes on some forms that automatically identify them. When we scan it, the scanner software automatically catalogs as much about the document as it can and then we key the rest. The barcodes are specific to the document type, but not the patient or account.

We also have documents that we don't want barcodes on, because the barcode causes the software to automatically split the batches. It has to do with how we want to organize the records; for example, we don't barcode our physician orders. If we had 10 pages of orders with barcodes on them, the system would create 10 sections labeled physician orders with one order in each. Since our users want to click one thing and view all the orders, we group orders ourselves during the document prep.

We handle 1,500 discharges per month. We have 3½ FTEs (full-time equivalent employees) to index and 1 person in prep. We scan documents in batches of about 1,000 to 2,000 pages. Prepping allows us to do that. When we put those 1,200 pages in the scanner, they are organized the way we want them.

The indexing scheme is minimal on our end, but gives users enough detail to locate what they want. We help our users get to the documents they want more quickly by giving them subsets [similar to *electronic views* discussed earlier in this chapter]. Subsets limit a particular user's view to the type of documents that are pertinent to them. However, if something they want isn't in their subset, it is easy for them to switch to a view of the entire chart.

For example, when a physician signs in to complete his discharge summary, he receives a subset that will give him a list of documents pertinent to dictating his discharge summary. Generally these subsets are task or role based. For example, a billing coder would see what billing would typically need, but our system allows subsets to be customized by user, so a particular user can set up subsets specific to them.

Though nearly everybody has a customized subset that fits their needs, we don't have a lot of maintenance of the subsets once they are set up. For example, when new physicians come on board, we will start them with the physician subset, and then if they want any customization we will do that for them. Sometimes this is based on specialty, because a certain specialty might need documents that another physician wouldn't require.

One thing our system does for us is to automate much of the workflow. We can define and automate workflow by document type. Certain documents need to go to coding, but not until the chart is ready for coding. For example, a one-day surgery patient's chart that needs to go to coding won't be released until the operative notes are done. So our system waits until that operative note is there before it sends the chart to coding. It also sends it to analysis. They can see the surgeon hasn't dictated his note yet and remind him to do that. All these things happen concurrently. Now that the record is online, it can be in 50 different places. Instead of having somebody constantly watching and determining "Do we have an operative note?" the system does that for us.

Physicians now complete records online. We also have a physician portal so physicians can complete records from off-site, from their home or offices. They can log on through a VPN to sign their records. The effect that this had on our delinquency rate was outstanding. We had a low delinquency rate before, but once we created the portal, we cut it by two-thirds.

We used to look at stacks of records to know what had to be done. We don't do that anymore. We have workbaskets online; you can see how many records are in there to be coded and how many are in there to be analyzed. We also handle our release of information forms online. We get about 60 requests a day for patient records, whether that is from the patient or other healthcare organizations. We make sure it's a valid request; we do all our HIPAA verification. Then we can fulfill requests by just highlighting what they need and it's done. It is a rare thing that we would need to print paper.

We can fax directly from our system; so if a physician office calls for records, we can fax those right to them. Of course now that we have the physician portal, they don't call us as much as they used to. They now can log on, look at the record, and they're done. It's more efficient for them and it has drastically changed what we do and how the department operates.

full size using a projector called a microfilm reader. An index is used to locate the microfiche or microfilm roll containing the patient records.

At one time, microfilm was a popular alternative, but it has waned with the advent of computer document imaging.

# Legal and Ethical Management of Health Records

Having explored what a *health record* is, we now turn our attention to what a *legal* health record is. The patient record serves not only as a record of patient care, but as the business and legal record of the services provided. For example, the patient health record is abstracted by the HIM department, and then coded and released to the business office/billing department for charge posting and submission of insurance claims. Furthermore, the patient's record itself is subject to audit by CMS and third-party payers to substantiate insurance claims.

The patient record may also be required in legal proceedings, for example, for cases involving automobile collisions, worker injuries, and liability. The records may also be required to prove regulatory compliance or used in medical malpractice cases by a provider or facility.

AHIMA defines the legal health record as the record that is "generated at or for a healthcare organization as its business record and is the record that would be released upon request."[1]

Ensuring that complete and accurate legal health records are maintained is the responsibility of the HIM professional. The first step in this process is to ensure that all of the information required by the facility's HIM policies are present and all items requiring signatures have been signed or authorized (electronically signed). For example, the HIM department for an inpatient facility processes a patient's chart at discharge. If the facility uses any paper records, the first step is collection of the information from the floor/ unit and assembly of the records into a specified order. Whether the records are paper or electronic, they are analyzed for deficiencies, such as missing items that should be present or any missing signatures or electronic authorizations.

A deficiency report listing the missing items is prepared and providers are notified. Once all the missing documents or signatures have been obtained, the records can be abstracted and coded for billing. Finally, the record is reviewed for completeness, and if the chart is paper it is filed.

The order in which the steps in the above process are performed may vary by facility. For example, some facilities may scan documents as soon as they are received, making them immediately available online. Other organizations may begin abstracting and coding records before the patient is even discharged. Some EHR systems automatically detect records that require electronic signatures and alert the responsible clinician without requiring a deficiency report to be generated.

## Record Retention

Patient health records must be kept by the provider not only for patient care, but to meet regulatory and accreditation requirements. To facilitate secondary use of the records, such as research, education, and quality improvement, organizations may choose to keep them even longer than legally required.

The length of time that health records must be retained can vary by state law, contractual obligations, and even the age of the patient. Record retention is usually a matter of policy. Taking into consideration the legal requirements and desired uses for the information, the healthcare organization establishes a record retention schedule, which then simplifies decision making for the workforce.

The CMS conditions of participation (COP) stipulate minimum time periods that health records must be maintained. State laws can vary widely and sometimes require longer retention periods. The table in Figure 6-17 shows AHIMA's recommended minimum retention periods for various types of health records.[2]

---

[1]"Update: Guidelines for Defining the Legal Health Record for Disclosure Purposes," *Journal of AHIMA,* 76, no. 8 (September 2005): 64A–G.
[2]Adapted from Donna M. Fletcher and Harry B. Rhodes, *Retention of Health Information (Updated),* AHIMA Practice Brief (Chicago: AHIMA, 2002), www.ahima.org.

**FIGURE 6-17**
**AHIMA'S minimum retention periods for various types of health records**

| Sample Health Record Retention Schedule | |
|---|---|
| **Hospital Health Information** | **Recommended Retention Period** |
| Adult Patients' health records | 10 years after the most recent encounter |
| Children's health records | 10 years after child reaches the age of majority (or longer if required by state law) |
| Fetal heart monitor records | 10 years after child reaches the age of majority (or longer if required by state law) |
| Registers of births and deaths | Permanently |
| Register of surgical procedures | Permanently |
| Master patient/person index | Permanently |
| Disease index | 10 years |
| Comprehensive outpatient rehabilitation facilities (CORF) | 5 years after patient discharge |
| Laboratory Pathology tests | 10 years after date of results report |
| Diagnostic images (such as x-ray film) | 5 years |
| Mammography | 5 years if subsequent mammograms are performed on the patient at the facility 10 years if no additional mammograms are performed |

The retention of records of inactive cases and former patients brings us to the discussion of archiving. Paper records, in particular, consume vast amounts of storage space. Most facilities eventually have to move some of their paper files elsewhere. Archiving consists of selecting the patient files that are least likely to be needed again and storing them in another place or in another form that requires less floor space.

- *Microfilm* is sometimes used for archiving medical records. The records are photographed and stored on microfilm. Microfilm, described earlier in this chapter, was used extensively during the last century.

- *Document imaging* consists of scanning each page of the chart with a device that resembles an office copier called a scanner. The scanner sends digital information to a computer to store as a digital image.

- *Off-site storage,* as the name implies, means that paper records are boxed up and shipped elsewhere to be kept in a controlled environment. These are typically records that must be kept for legal reasons, but which the facility is relatively sure will not be needed again or at least not in the near future. Some large healthcare organizations own warehouses to store older medical records, while others use the service of a commercial record storage company.

As health records become computerized, the issue of storage space no longer becomes a question of floor space but of disk space. By simply adding more disk drives to a computer network or by moving older records to CD, DVD, or Blu-ray disks, a vast amount of healthcare data can be kept indefinitely.

## Destruction of Health Records

When health records have passed the scheduled retention period or when paper records have been converted to digital images or microfilm, it may be the policy of the healthcare organization to destroy them. In some facilities that use only electronic health records, paper documents that are received from outside the facility are immediately scanned, verified by HIM, and then destroyed.

Paper records are usually destroyed by shredding the documents and/or incinerating them. The destruction of health records is the responsibility of the HIM department and should be done under the supervision of an HIM employee. If the task is contracted to an outside entity, there must be a signed HIPAA business associate agreement to protect the patient privacy and organization's legal liability.

It is not usually necessary to destroy electronic health records at the end of the retention period, because disk storage space is relatively cheap. Also, electronic health records are usually backed up onto optical disks or magnetic tape to ensure their preservation. However, computers or disks that once held EPHI must be purged of health information before they are disposed of (as described in the HIPAA regulations in Chapter 3).

## Release of Information

As custodian of the health record, HIM professionals are not only responsible for the health record but also for managing the release of the information contained in it. As we discussed in Chapter 3, HIPAA regulations require the patient's authorization to release health information, except to authorized government agencies. Prior to release, the HIM professional must ensure that the proper release documents have been signed, decide what portions of the record should be disclosed, and keep track of those disclosures.

HIPAA consent permits the sharing of PHI for treatment, payment, or operation of the healthcare facility, so if a consulting physician needs a portion of the chart, the HIM department will locate and copy, print, or fax the requested pages. Similarly, HIPAA grants patients access to their chart, but the HIM professional will often help the patient determine which portions they need. For example, consider a patient who lives elsewhere who was treated for a broken bone. The patient requests a copy of the x-ray of the bone to take to his or her doctor back home; the HIM professional might also suggest the patient take a copy of the radiologist's report as well.

Anytime a copy of the chart is made, the HIM department keeps track of it. Disclosure records are kept for at least six years. Patient's have a right to request a list of disclosures each year. Though these requests will usually come through the privacy officer, the HIM department will prepare the report.

## Producing Legal Health Records

When copies of a patient's chart are requested for use in a legal matter, HIM department guidelines should be followed exactly. HIM departments should have a written policy listing the types of documents that constitute the legal record and how the copies are to be prepared.

Though EHR systems have the benefit of being able to present the same data in various formats, it is important that attorneys for both sides receive identical copies. For example, lab software prints lab reports in a different format than the EHR software, even though the data is the same. One attorney cannot be sent the lab software report and the other attorney the EHR software report; they must both receive the exact same report. Also, upgrades or enhancements to the EHR software can cause records printed on one date to look different from the same records printed at a later date.

For these reasons, some facilities produce a PDF document in response to legal requests. The PDF file, if retained, can be reprinted at anytime to consistently produce the same exact copies for all the parties involved.

# HIM Ethics

The professional standards by which health information professionals conduct themselves are called *ethics*. Healthcare facilities create policies and procedures to provide guidance in the care and handling of confidential records. The policies and procedures tell employees when and how to do something for which they are responsible. A code of ethics provides guidance in how to act in a professional capacity and helps to guide those who create policies and procedures for their facilities.

Many of the professional organizations discussed in Chapter 2 have adopted a code of ethics for their members. A good example for HIM professionals to follow is the AHIMA Code of Ethics, a portion of which is reprinted here.

## Preamble

The ethical obligations of the health information management (HIM) professional include the protection of patient privacy and confidential information; disclosure of information; development, use, and maintenance of health information systems and health records; and the quality of information. Both handwritten and computerized medical records contain many sacred stories—stories that must be protected on behalf of the individual and the aggregate community of persons served in the healthcare system. Healthcare consumers are increasingly concerned about the loss of privacy and the inability to control the dissemination of their protected information. Core health information issues include what information should be collected; how the information should be handled, who should have access to the information, and under what conditions the information should be disclosed.

Ethical obligations are central to the professional's responsibility, regardless of the employment site or the method of collection, storage, and security of health information. Sensitive information (genetic, adoption, drug, alcohol, sexual, and behavioral information) requires special attention to prevent misuse. Entrepreneurial roles require expertise in the protection of the information in the world of business and interactions with consumers.

## Professional Values

The mission of the HIM profession is based on core professional values developed since the inception of the Association in 1928. These values and the inherent ethical responsibilities for AHIMA members and credentialed HIM professionals include providing service, protecting medical, social, and financial information, promoting confidentiality; and preserving and securing health information. Values to the healthcare team include promoting the quality and advancement of healthcare, demonstrating HIM expertise and skills, and promoting interdisciplinary cooperation and collaboration. Professional values in relationship to the employer include protecting committee deliberations and complying with laws, regulations, and policies. Professional values related to the public include advocating change, refusing to participate or conceal unethical practices, and reporting violations of practice standards to the proper authorities. Professional values to individual and professional associations include obligations to be honest, bringing honor to self, peers and profession, committing to continuing education and lifelong learning, performing Association duties honorably, strengthening professional membership, representing the profession to the public, and promoting and participating in research.

These professional values will require a complex process of balancing the many conflicts that can result from competing interests and obligations of those who seek access to health information and require an understanding of ethical decision-making.

## Purpose of the American Health Information Management Association Code of Ethics

The HIM professional has an obligation to demonstrate actions that reflect values, ethical principles, and ethical guidelines. The American Health Information Management Association (AHIMA) Code of Ethics sets forth these values and principles to guide conduct. The code is relevant to all AHIMA members and credentialed HIM professionals and students, regardless of their professional functions, the settings in which they work, or the populations they serve.

The AHIMA Code of Ethics serves six purposes:

- Identifies core values on which the HIM mission is based.
- Summarizes broad ethical principles that reflect the profession's core values and establishes a set of ethical principles to be used to guide decision-making and actions.
- Helps HIM professionals identify relevant considerations when professional obligations conflict or ethical uncertainties arise.
- Provides ethical principles by which the general public can hold the HIM professional accountable.
- Socializes practitioners new to the field to HIM's mission, values, and ethical principles.
- Articulates a set of guidelines that the HIM professional can use to assess whether they have engaged in unethical conduct.

The code includes principles and guidelines that are both enforceable and aspirational. The extent to which each principle is enforceable is a matter of professional judgment to be exercised by those responsible for reviewing alleged violations of ethical principles.

## The Use of the Code

Violation of principles in this code does not automatically imply legal liability or violation of the law. Such determination can only be made in the context of legal and judicial proceedings. Alleged violations of the code would be subject to a peer review process. Such processes are generally separate from legal or administrative procedures and insulated from legal review or proceedings to allow the profession to counsel and discipline its own members although in some situations, violations of the code would constitute unlawful conduct subject to legal process.

Guidelines for ethical and unethical behavior are provided in this code. The terms "shall and shall not" are used as a basis for setting high standards for behavior. This does not imply that everyone "shall or shall not" do everything that is listed. For example, not everyone participates in the recruitment or mentoring of students. A HIM professional is not being unethical if this is not part of his or her professional activities; however, if students are part of one's professional responsibilities, there is an ethical obligation to follow the guidelines stated in the code. This concept is true for the entire code. If someone does the stated activities, ethical behavior is the standard. The guidelines are not a comprehensive list. For example, the statement "protect all confidential information to include personal, health, financial, genetic and outcome information" can also be interpreted as "shall not fail to protect all confidential information to include personal, health, financial, genetic, and outcome information."

A code of ethics cannot guarantee ethical behavior. Moreover, a code of ethics cannot resolve all ethical issues or disputes or capture the richness and complexity involved in striving to make responsible choices within a moral community. Rather, a code of ethics sets forth values and ethical principles, and offers ethical guidelines to which professionals aspire and by which their actions can be judged. Ethical behaviors result from a personal commitment to engage in ethical practice.

Professional responsibilities often require an individual to move beyond personal values. For example, an individual might demonstrate behaviors that are based on the values of honesty, providing service to others, or demonstrating loyalty. In addition to these, professional values might require promoting confidentiality, facilitating interdisciplinary collaboration, and refusing to participate or conceal unethical practices. Professional values could require a more comprehensive set of values than what an individual needs to be an ethical agent in their personal lives.

The AHIMA Code of Ethics is to be used by AHIMA and individuals, agencies, organizations, and bodies (such as licensing and regulatory boards, insurance providers, courts of law, agency boards of directors, government agencies, and other professional groups) that choose to adopt it or use it as a frame of reference. The AHIMA Code of Ethics reflects the commitment of all to uphold the profession's values and to act ethically. Individuals of good character who discern moral questions and, in good faith, seek to make reliable ethical judgments, must apply ethical principles.

The code does not provide a set of rules that prescribe how to act in all situations. Specific applications of the code must take into account the context in which it is being considered and the possibility of conflicts among the code's values, principles, and guidelines. Ethical responsibilities flow from all human relationships, from the personal and familial to the social and professional. Further, the AHIMA Code of Ethics does not specify which values, principles, and guidelines are the most important and ought to outweigh others in instances when they conflict.

## Code of Ethics 2004

**Ethical Principles:** The following ethical principles are based on the core values of the American Health Information Management Association and apply to all health information management professionals.

Health information management professionals:

I. Advocate, uphold and defend the individual's right to privacy and the doctrine of confidentiality in the use and disclosure of information.

II. Put service and the health and welfare of persons before self-interest and conduct themselves in the practice of the profession so as to bring honor to themselves, their peers, and to the health information management profession.

III. Preserve, protect, and secure personal health information in any form or medium and hold in the highest regard the contents of the records and other information of a confidential nature, taking into account the applicable statutes and regulations.

IV. Refuse to participate in or conceal unethical practices or procedures.

V. Advance health information management knowledge and practice through continuing education, research, publications, and presentations.

VI. Recruit and mentor students, peers and colleagues to develop and strengthen professional workforce.

VII. Represent the profession accurately to the public.

VIII. Perform honorably health information management association responsibilities, either appointed or elected, and preserve the confidentiality of any privileged information made known in any official capacity.

IX. State truthfully and accurately their credentials, professional education, and experiences.

X. Facilitate interdisciplinary collaboration in situations supporting health information practice.

XI. Respect the inherent dignity and worth of every person.

### Acknowledgement

Adapted with permission from the Code of Ethics of the National Association of Social Workers.

### Resources

National Association of Social Workers. "Code of Ethics." 1999. Available at http://www.naswdc.org.

Harman, L. B. (Ed.). Ethical challenges in the management of health information. Gaithersburg, MD: Aspen, 2001.

AHIMA Code of Ethics, 1957, 1977, 1988, and 1998.

Revised & adopted by AHIMA House of Delegates July 1, 2004.

# Chapter 6 Summary

In this chapter we discussed how the contents of health records can be organized, various ways they are stored, and the process and ethics of managing them. The large quantities of records that must be dealt with make the issues of how health records are handled, organized, and filed important to healthcare organizations of all sizes.

## How Paper Charts Are Organized

Although many healthcare organizations are transitioning to electronic records, paper records are still prevalent at many locations. In this chapter we discussed several standard schemes for organizing a paper chart:

- *Source-oriented charts* organize the contents according to the source of the document. Sections are separated by labeled dividers within the folder. For example, physician notes are grouped in one section, radiology reports in another, lab results in another, nursing notes in another, and so on. The source-oriented type of chart is found more frequently in inpatient than ambulatory settings.

- *Problem-oriented records* organize the patient's chart by diagnosis or medical problem. For example, a patient with several chronic diseases will have separate sections of the chart for each condition. A problem list at the front of the chart serves as an index to the record, listing each problem with a number.

- *Integrated records* intermingle documents from various sources sequentially in order by date. Usually the order is from the oldest dated document at the back to the newest documents at the front. This scheme is often used in physician practices. Inpatient facilities may use it within the subdivided physician and ancillary therapy sections of a source-oriented chart.

Electronic health records are not restricted to any one of these methods of chart organization. Because the electronic chart is composed of data records, they may be displayed in many different *views*, according to the need of the provider at the time.

When a portion of a chart is stored electronically and a portion of it is on paper, the type of record is a *hybrid health record*. Most often the paper records are subsequently scanned into the electronic record after the patient is discharged.

The term *loose sheets* refers to documents that need to be added to a chart at various times after the patient encounter. With paper charts, these may be documents that arrive after the chart has been assembled. With electronic health records, these may be patient records received from other facilities that are waiting to be scanned into the EHR.

## Filing Paper Records

This chapter also discussed several methods by which paper charts are filed.

*Alphabetical filing* systems using the patient's name are the easiest to learn, but they are more prone to misfiling. Also, because some letters of the alphabet have more surnames than others, alphabetical systems tend to grow unevenly and require frequent reorganization of the file room.

*Numeric filing* systems assign sequential medical record numbers to the chart. This eliminates the need to frequently reorganize the file room but does require a master patient index to find the patient's chart. However, filing errors can occur, especially with numbers longer than six digits.

To reduce recognition errors, some numeric systems use hyphens to divide long record numbers into three sets of numbers, for example, 12-34-56. To reduce numeric filing errors, two variations of numeric filing may be used. These are *terminal digit filing* and *middle digit filing*. Both of these methods use chart numbers divided into three sets by hyphens. The file room shelving units are divided into labeled sections reserved for each primary set of numbers. Within each section are subsections for each secondary set of numbers.

- *Terminal digit filing* uses the last set of the hyphenated record numbers (called the terminal digits) as the primary set of numbers for filing purposes. For example, with chart number 12-34-56, the last set of digits (56) will be used as the primary set of numbers for filing; the middle set of digits (34) will be the secondary set of numbers for filing. In this example, the chart would be filed in section 56, subsection 34.

- The *middle digit filing* method is similar to the terminal digit method except that the middle set is the primary set of numbers for filing purposes. In middle digit filing, the numbers of the middle set correspond to the numbered sections in the file room. Using the previous example, chart number 12-34-56 would be filed in section 34 of the file room. The middle digit system is only used where medical record numbers are six digits or less; facilities with record numbers greater than a million use terminal digit filing or straight numeric filing.

*Color coding* of chart labels can be used for both alphabetical and numeric systems. Different colored labels are used for different letters or numbers. With a color system, a folder filed in the wrong section or subsection will quickly stand out because its numbers will break the color sequence of the labels.

Medical record numbers are assigned by several different methods:

- *Serial numbering* sequentially assigns a new number for each admission or ER visit. This allows the hospital to easily assemble and track every record and service related to that stay under one number. The disadvantage is that patients who have been in the hospital several times have several different charts.

- *Unit numbering* assigns a single medical record number the first time a patient is registered and the same number is used every time the patient returns. This results in a single chart for the patient. Most ambulatory and inpatient facilities use unit numbering because it is recommended by the Joint Commission.
- *Serial-unit numbering* is an alternative that allow facilities that use serial numbering to comply with the Joint Commission. As with serial numbering, a new number is assigned for each patient stay or visit; however, the records from the previous chart number are brought forward into the new one. The patient index is updated to reflect the new number. If this is practiced consistently, then records from all previous visits are always in the current folder.
- *Family numbering* is used in some pediatric and family medical practices. A primary account number is assigned to the family, then a decimal number extension is assigned for each family member. For example, using account number 100, the head of the household would be assigned record number 100.0, the spouse 100.1, the first child 100.2, the second child 100.3, and so on. Family numbering is useful for administrative tasks because it makes it easy to bill parents for several children or to schedule spouses and children on the same days. However, it is not useful as a system for medical record numbers because as family members change (children grow up, parents divorce, etc.), the chart numbering becomes disrupted.

## Record Circulation and Storage

Medical record circulation and storage is the responsibility of the HIM department. Paper charts are filed and retrieved by a member of the HIM team.

- A list of charts that will be needed for the day is used to pull charts in advance.
- Charts that are needed for unscheduled patients, emergency admissions, or walk-in patients are requested either verbally or using a written form.
- A paper or plastic placeholder called an *outguide* is put in place of the chart when it is pulled.
- Charts are batched together by provider or department and delivered to a nurse or provider's staff.
- When the patient has been checked out or discharged, the chart is returned to the chart room for filing.
  - In acute settings, the chart must be examined after the patient's discharge to ensure that all required documents are present, complete, and signed where required before it is filed.
  - In a doctor's office, the chart is usually filed immediately, then pulled and updated later as transcription and other documents arrive.

Inpatient facilities and ambulatory facilities with a large number of providers may use computer systems to track paper charts. These systems let a provider or scheduling person request charts that will be needed. A list of charts to be pulled is printed in an order that optimizes pulling the charts. Some computerized chart tracking systems use barcodes of the chart numbers to automate identification of the chart.

Where computerized chart tracking is not used, three-part paper requisition forms are used to request patient records and keep track of who has them.

In both acute care and ambulatory care facilities, x-ray films and other radiology records are typically stored separate from the chart in large envelopes called *jackets*. The jackets are filed in a separate department or filing location than the paper chart.

Paper charts and x-ray jackets are stored in metal filing cabinets or shelving units. Securely storing paper records takes up a significant amount of space. Standard size medical records storage units are typically 36-, 42-, or 48-inch-wide shelves. The shelves are 12 inches deep. Units usually have six, seven, or eight shelves spaced about 10 inches apart.

AHIMA estimates that inpatient charts have 100 pages. This would make the average chart about 5/8 inch thick. Outpatient charts vary in thickness, depending on how many years the patient has been coming to the practice and how frequently the patient visits the doctors. Outpatient charts can vary in thickness from 1/4 to 1 inch or more.

It is estimated that a paper medical record 1 inch thick weighs approximately 2.5 pounds. Therefore, a shelf with 34 inches of filing space must be able to support 85 pounds of weight.

Not only do the file units occupy floor space, but additional floor space must be reserved for aisles so the files can be accessed. File rooms and file storage units must provide security and fire protection.

### Document Imaging Systems

Document imaging management systems are computer systems that scan and store images of paper documents. Facilities use document imaging systems to complement EHR systems and to replace or eliminate paper charts.

When documents are scanned into an imaging system, they must be cataloged. This involves entering data in the computer about the document, such as the patient ID, date, provider, type of image, and so on. For the most part, the cataloged data is entered by hand, but in some instances the image cataloging can be automated. During scanning and cataloging, quality control is important.

Some scanners have the capability to scan documents in batches rather than individually. To prepare a chart for scanning, HIM personnel examine the pages; remove staples, paper clips, and duplicate pages; replace or manually scan torn or damaged pages; and, if necessary, ensure that documents are assembled in the correct order.

When scanning is completed, the images are checked for quality and cataloged information is verified or entered manually. Once the process is completed, the pages are returned to the chart, archived, or shredded (depending on the policy of the HIM department).

## Legal and Ethical Management of Health Records

Legal and ethical management of health records is an important function of the HIM department. Patient records serve not only the care of the patient, but as the business and legal record of the services provided. The legal health record may be required for audit by government or accrediting agencies or in legal proceedings.

Ensuring the existence of complete and accurate legal health records is the responsibility of the HIM professional. The first step is to ensure that all of the information required is present and that all items requiring signatures have been signed or authorized (electronically signed). If any item is missing or incomplete, the second step is to prepare a deficiency report and notify the affected provider. Once the record is complete, the final step is to review the file for completeness and if it is a paper chart, to file it.

Patient health records must be retained by the provider not only for patient care, but to meet regulatory and accreditation requirements. The length of time that health records must be retained can vary by state law, contractual obligations, and even the age of the patient. Record retention is usually guided by each facility's HIM policy, which takes these and other factors into account. Review Figure 6-17, which lists AHIMA's recommended minimum retention periods for various types of health records.

When health records have passed the scheduled retention period or when paper records have been converted to digital images or microfilm, it may be the policy of the healthcare organization to destroy the paper records. Paper records are usually destroyed by shredding the documents and/or incinerating them.

The destruction of health records is the responsibility of the HIM department and should be done under the supervision of an HIM employee. If the task is contracted to an outside entity, there must be a signed HIPAA business associate agreement to protect the patient's privacy and the organization's legal liability.

It is not usually necessary to destroy electronic health records at the end of the retention period because disk storage space is relatively cheap. However, computers or disks that once held EPHI must be purged of health information before they are disposed of, as required by HIPAA regulations.

HIM professionals are not only responsible for the health record but also for managing the release of the information contained in it. HIPAA regulations require the patient's authorization to release health information, except to authorized government agencies. Prior to release, the HIM professional must ensure that the proper authorization documents have been signed, decide what portions of the record should be disclosed, and keeps track of these disclosures. The disclosure records will be kept for at least six years.

When copies of a patient's chart are requested for use in a legal matter, HIM departments should have a written policy listing the types of documents that constitute the legal record and how the copies are to be prepared.

## HIM Ethics

The professional standards by which health information professionals conduct themselves are called *ethics*. Healthcare facilities create policies and procedures to provide guidance in the care and handling of confidential records. The policies and procedures tell employees when and how to do something for which they are responsible. A code of ethics provides guidance in how to act in a professional capacity and helps to guide those who create policies and procedures for their facilities. Review the AHIMA code of ethics provided earlier in this chapter.

# Testing Your Knowledge of Chapter 6

1. List the three ways in which documents can be organized in paper charts.

2. What is reverse chronological order?

3. What is a hybrid health record?

4. According to AHIMA, how many pages are in the average inpatient file?

5. When charts are filed alphabetically, the file system must be reorganized periodically. Why is this necessary?

6. What are loose sheets?

7. List the three types of numeric filing systems.

8. What is an outguide?

9. A group medical practice adds 100 patients per month. The average thickness of a new patient's chart is 1/4 inch. If each file room shelving unit can hold 368 inches of files, how many new shelving units must be added per year just to accommodate new patient charts?

10. A facility has numbered each section of its file room to use terminal digit filing. In which section of the room would you locate patient chart 46-78-03?

11. When pages are scanned into a document imaging system, what is the purpose of cataloging the image?

12. What is a deficiency report?

13. What is the minimum record retention period for adult health records?

14. Name at least four of the ethical obligations of HIM professionals listed in the AHIMA Code of Ethics preamble.

15. The AHIMA Code of Ethics serves six purposes. Name at least three of them.

# 7

# Electronic Health Records

After completing this chapter, you should be able to:

- Define electronic health records
- Explain why electronic health records are important
- Discuss what forces are driving the adoption of electronic health records
- Describe the functional benefits derived from using an EHR
- Compare different forms of EHR data
- Describe different methods of capturing and recording data
- Explain why patient visits should be documented at the point of care
- Explain how electronic signatures work
- Describe the workflow of an office fully using EHRs

## ACRONYMS USED IN CHAPTER 7

Acronyms are used extensively in both medicine and computers. The following acronyms are used in this chapter.

| | | | |
|---|---|---|---|
| **ABN** | Advance Beneficiary Notice | **HIPAA** | Health Insurance Portability and Accountability Act |
| **AHRQ** | Agency for Healthcare Research and Quality | **Hx** | History |
| **CDC** | Centers for Disease Control and Prevention | **ICU** | Intensive Care Unit |
| **CDR** | Clinical Data Repository | **IOM** | Institute of Medicine of the National Academies |
| **CMS** | Centers for Medicare and Medicaid Services | **LOINC®** | Logical Observation Identifiers Names and Codes |
| **CPOE** | Computerized Physician Order Entry; Computerized Provider Order Entry | **OB** | Obstetrics |
| | | **PACS OR PAC SYSTEM** | Picture Archiving and Communication System |
| **CPRI** | Computer-Based Patient Record Institute | **PIN** | Personal Identification Number |
| **CT SCAN** | Computerized Tomography Scan | **Px** | Physical Examination |
| | | **RHIO** | Regional Health Information Organization |
| **DUR** | Drug Utilization Review | **Rx** | Therapy (Including Prescriptions) |
| **Dx** | Diagnosis | | |
| **ECG OR EKG** | Electrocardiogram | **SNOMED-CT®** | SNOMED Stands for Systematized Nomenclature of Medicine; CT stands for Clinical Terms |
| **EHR** | Electronic Health Record | | |
| **HHS** | Department of Health and Human Services | | |

| **SOAP** | Subjective, Objective, Assessment, Plan | **Tx** | Tests (Performed) |
| | | **URI** | Upper Respiratory Infection |
| **Sx** | Symptoms | | |

# Evolution of Electronic Health Records

The idea of computerizing patients' medical records has been around for more than 30 years, but only in the past decade has it become widely adopted. Prior to the EHR, a patient's medical records consisted of handwritten notes, typed reports, and test results stored in a paper file system. Though paper medical records are still used in many healthcare facilities, the transition to electronic health records is under way.

Beginning in 1991, the IOM (which stands for the Institute of Medicine of the National Academies) sponsored studies and created reports that led the way toward the concepts we have in place today for electronic health records. Originally, the IOM called them *computer-based patient records*.[1] During their evolution, EHRs had many other names including electronic medical records, computerized medical records, longitudinal patient records, and electronic charts. All of these names referred to essentially the same thing, which in 2003, the IOM renamed as the electronic health record or EHR.

## Institute of Medicine

The IOM report[2] put forth a set of eight core functions that an EHR should be capable of performing:

### Health Information and Data:

- Providing a defined data set that includes such items as medical and nursing diagnoses, a medication list, allergies, demographics, clinical narratives, and laboratory test results; providing improved access to information needed by care providers when they need it.

### Result Management:

- Computerized results can be accessed more easily (than paper reports) by the provider at the time and place they are needed.
  Reduced lag time allows for quicker recognition and treatment of medical problems.
  The automated display of previous test results makes it possible to reduce redundant and additional testing.
  Having electronic results can allow for better interpretation and for easier detection of abnormalities, thereby ensuring appropriate follow-up.
  Access to electronic consults and patient consents can establish critical links and improve care coordination among multiple providers, as well as between provider and patient.

### Order Management:

- Computerized provider order entry (CPOE) systems can improve workflow processes by eliminating lost orders and ambiguities caused by illegible handwriting, generating related orders automatically, monitoring for duplicate orders, and reducing the time required to fill orders.
  CPOE systems for medications reduce the number of errors in medication dose and frequency, drug allergies, and drug–drug interactions.
  The use of CPOE, in conjunction with an EHR, also improves clinician productivity.

---

[1] R. S. Dick and E. B. Steen, *The Computer-Based Patient Record: An Essential Technology for Health Care* (Washington, DC: Institute of Medicine, National Academy Press, 1991, revised 1997, 2000).
[2] Ibid.

### Decision Support:

- Computerized decision support systems include prevention, prescribing of drugs, diagnosis and management, and detection of adverse events and disease outbreaks.

    Computer reminders and prompts improve preventive practices in such areas as vaccinations, breast cancer screening, colorectal screening, and cardiovascular risk reduction.

### Electronic Communication and Connectivity:

- Electronic communication among care partners can enhance patient safety and quality of care, especially for patients who have multiple providers in multiple settings that must coordinate care plans.

    Electronic connectivity is essential in creating and populating EHR systems with data from laboratory, pharmacy, radiology, and other providers.

    Secure e-mail and web messaging have been shown to be effective in facilitating communication both among providers and with patients, thus allowing for greater continuity of care and more timely interventions.

    Automatic alerts to providers regarding abnormal laboratory results reduce the time until an appropriate treatment is ordered.

    Electronic communication is fundamental to the creation of an integrated health record, both within a setting and across settings and institutions.

### Patient Support:

- Computer-based patient education has been found to be successful in improving control of chronic illnesses, such as diabetes, in primary care.

    Home monitoring by patients is accomplished by means of electronic devices; examples include self-testing by patients with asthma (spirometry), glucose monitors for patients with diabetes, and Holter monitors for patients with heart conditions. Data from monitoring devices can be merged into the EHR, as shown in Figure 7-1.

**FIGURE 7-1**

**Data from digital spirometer transfers to EHR.**

(Courtesy of Midmark Diagnostics Group.)

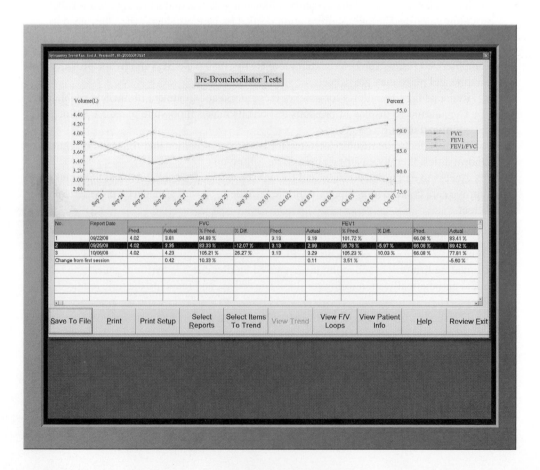

**Administrative Processes and Reporting:**

- Electronic scheduling systems increase the efficiency of healthcare organizations and provide better, timelier service to patients.

    Communication and content standards are important in the billing and claims management area.

    Electronic authorization and prior approvals can eliminate delays and confusion; immediate validation of insurance eligibility results in more timely payments and less paperwork.

    EHR data can be analyzed to identify patients who are potentially eligible for clinical trials, as well as candidates for chronic disease management programs.

    Reporting tools support drug recalls.

**Reporting and Population Health:**

- Public and private sector reporting requirements at the federal, state, and local levels for patient safety and quality, as well as for public health, are more easily met with computerized data.

    Eliminates the labor-intensive and time-consuming abstraction of data from paper records and the errors that often occur in a manual process.

    Facilitates the reporting of key quality indicators used for the internal quality improvement efforts of many healthcare organizations.

    Improves public health surveillance and timely reporting of adverse reactions and disease outbreaks.

In addition to the IOM, ideas from CPRI and HIPAA help us define the EHR.

## Computer-based Patient Record Institute

Another early contributor to the thinking on EHR systems was the Computer-based Patient Record Institute (CPRI), which identified three key criteria for an EHR:

- Capture data at the point of care.
- Integrate data from multiple sources.
- Provide decision support.

## HIPAA Security Rule

The HIPAA Security Rule did not define an EHR, but perhaps it broadened the definition. The Security Rule established protection for *all* personally identifiable health information stored in electronic format. Thus, everything about a patient stored in a healthcare provider's system is protected and treated as part of the patient's EHR.

## EHR Defined

In *Electronic Health Records: Changing the Vision,* authors Murphy, Waters, Hanken, and Pfeiffer define the EHR to include "any information relating to the past, present or future physical/mental health, or condition of an individual which resides in electronic system(s) used to capture, transmit, receive, store, retrieve, link and manipulate multimedia data for the primary purpose of providing health care and health-related services."[3] EHRs can include dental health records as well.

The core functions defined by the IOM and CPRI suggest that the EHR is not just what data is stored, but what can be done with it. In the broadest sense, *EHRs are the portions of a patient's medical records that are stored in a computer system as well as the functional benefits derived from having an electronic health record.*

## Social Forces Driving EHR Adoption

Visionary leaders in medical informatics have been making the case for EHRs for a long time. However, the combination of several important reports caught the public's attention and set in motion economic and political forces that are driving the transformation of our medical records systems.

---

[3]Gretchen Murphy, Kathleen Waters, Mary A. Hanken, and Maureen Pfeiffer, eds., *Electronic Health Records: Changing the Vision* (Philadelphia: W. B. Saunders Company, 1999), 5.

**HEALTH SAFETY**   The IOM published a report stating:

> "Health care in the United States is not as safe as it should be—and can be. At least 44,000 people, and perhaps as many as 98,000 people, die in hospitals each year as a result of medical errors that could have been prevented, according to estimates from two major studies.
>
> Beyond their cost in human lives, preventable medical errors exact other significant tolls. They have been estimated to result in total costs (including the expense of additional care necessitated by the errors, lost income and household productivity, and disability) of between $17 billion and $29 billion per year in hospitals nationwide. Errors also are costly in terms of loss of trust in the health care system by patients and diminished satisfaction by both patients and health professionals.
>
> A variety of factors have contributed to the nation's epidemic of medical errors. One oft-cited problem arises from the decentralized and fragmented nature of the health care delivery system—or 'non-system,' to some observers. When patients see multiple providers in different settings, none of whom has access to complete information, it becomes easier for things to go wrong."[4]

These statements got the attention of the press and public. They also got the attention of 150 of the nation's largest employers.

**HEALTH COSTS**   Employers who sponsored employee health insurance programs had become frustrated by the increasing costs of health insurance benefits for which they had little or no say about the quality of care. Following the release of the IOM report, these employers formed the Leapfrog group.

A study by the Center for Information Technology Leadership found more than 130,000 life-threatening situations caused by adverse drug reactions alone. The study suggested that $44 billion could be saved annually by installing computerized physician order entry systems in ambulatory settings.

Leapfrog created a strategy that tied purchase of group health insurance benefits to quality care standards. It also promoted CPOE as a means of reducing errors.

**GOVERNMENT RESPONSE**   The response to the IOM report was swift and positive, within both the government and private sectors. Almost immediately, President Bill Clinton's administration issued an executive order instructing government agencies that conduct or oversee healthcare programs to implement proven techniques for reducing medical errors, and creating a task force to find new strategies for reducing errors. Congress appropriated $50 million to the Agency for Healthcare Research and Quality (AHRQ) to support a variety of efforts targeted at reducing medical errors.

President George W. Bush followed through by establishing the position of the National Coordinator for Health Information Technology, under the U.S. Department of Health and Human Services (HHS) to "develop, maintain, and direct the implementation of a strategic plan to guide the nationwide implementation of interoperable health information technology in both the public and private health care sectors that will reduce medical errors, improve quality, and produce greater value for health care expenditures."[5]

President Barack Obama identified the EHR as a priority for his administration and signed into law the Health Information Technology for Economic and Clinical Health (HITECH) Act. The act promotes the widespread adoption of EHRs and authorizes Medicare incentive payments to doctors and hospitals using a certified EHR and eventually financial penalties for physicians and hospitals that don't.[6]

---

[4]Linda T. Kohn, Janet M. Corrigan, and Molla S. Donaldson, eds., *To Err Is Human: Building a Safer Health System* (Washington, DC: Committee on Quality of Health Care in America, Institute of Medicine, 1999).

[5]President George W. Bush, Executive Order #13335, April 27, 2004.

[6]H. R. 1 American Recovery and Reinvestment Act of 2009, Title XIII Health Information Technology for Economic and Clinical Health, February 17, 2009.

**CHANGING SOCIETY**   Changes in the way we live have also made paper medical records outdated. In an increasingly mobile society, patients relocate and change doctors more frequently and thus need to transfer their medical records from previous doctors to new ones. Additionally, many patients no longer have a single general practitioner who provides their total care. Increased specialization and the development of new methods of diagnostic and preventive medicine require the ability to share exam records among different specialists and testing facilities.

The Internet, one of the strongest forces for social change in the past decade, also affects healthcare. Consumers are becoming accustomed to being able to access very sensitive information securely over the web. They are beginning to ask "Why can't I access my health records online?" Additionally, there are literally millions of health-related pieces of information on the web. Patients are arriving at their doctor's office armed with questions and sometimes answers. Medical information previously unavailable to the average consumer is now as easy to access as searching Google™ or WebMD®.

# Functional Benefits of an EHR

The ability to easily find, share, and search patient records makes an EHR superior to a paper record system. However, remember the definition of EHR as not just stored data but the *functional benefits* that can be derived from having that data accessible. Four benefits derived from EHR data that cannot easily be achieved with paper records are health maintenance, trend analysis, alerts, and decision support. These will be described in a moment. First it is necessary to review the various forms in which EHR data is stored before exploring how these and other functional benefits are derived from it.

## Form Affects Functionality

An EHR with any form of data offers improved accessibility over a paper chart, but to achieve its full functional benefits, the computer must be able to quickly and accurately identify the information in the record. The form in which the data is stored determines to what extent the computer can use the content of the EHR to provide additional functions that improve the quality of care.

Chapter 4 discussed various forms in which medical records are stored in the database. These may be broadly categorized into three forms:

- *Digital images:* This category includes scanned documents, diagnostic images, digital x-rays, and even annotated drawings or sound recordings.

   Images can be retrieved and displayed by the computer, but a human is required to interpret the meaning of the content.

- *Text:* The second type of data includes word processing files of transcribed exam notes and also text reports. It is principally obtained in the EHR by importing text files from outside sources.

   The text files are useful for doctors and nurses to read and can be searched by the computer for research purposes. However, text data is seldom used for generating alerts, trend analysis, decision support, or other real-time EHR functions, because the search capability is slow and the results often ambiguous.

- *Discrete data:* This third form of stored information in an EHR is the easiest for the computer to use. It can be instantly searched, retrieved, and combined or reported in different ways. Discrete data in an EHR may be subcategorized into *fielded data* and *coded data.*

**CODED DATA**   Coded data is fielded EHR data that goes a step further. By associating a code with each medical term and storing the appropriate code in the medical record, ambiguities about the clinician's meaning are eliminated.

Within medicine, many different terms are used to describe the same symptom, condition, or observation. Additionally, clinicians often use short abbreviations to document their observations in a patient chart. This makes it difficult for a computer to compare notes from one physician to another. For example, exam notes by two different providers might phrase a knee injury problem differently:

> Dr. 1: "knee injury"
>
> Dr. 2: "knee trauma"

A search of medical records for "knee injury" might not find the second record. To realize the full benefits of an EHR, it is necessary to record a code identifying the clinical information in addition to the text description.

When a code is stored in the medical record, the record is considered codified. A codified EHR is more useful than a text-based record because it precisely identifies the clinician's finding or treatment. The more parts of a medical record that can be codified, the more useful the data becomes to support additional functional benefits.

**STANDARD EHR CODING SYSTEMS**   EHR data stored in a fielded, codified form adds significant value, but using a national standard code set instead of proprietary codes to codify the data will better enable the exchange of medical records among systems, improve the accuracy of the content, and open the door to the functional benefits derived from having an electronic health record.

EHR coding systems are called *nomenclatures*. EHR nomenclatures differ from other code sets and classification systems in that they are designed to codify the details and nuance of the patient–clinician encounter. EHR nomenclatures are different from billing code sets in this aspect. For example, a procedure code used for billing an office visit does not describe what the clinician observed during the visit, just the type of visit and complexity of the exam. EHR nomenclatures need to have a lot more codes to describe the details of the exam; for this reason, they are said to be more granular.

Two prominent nomenclatures for EHR records are SNOMED-CT and Medcin®. Another prominent coding system, LOINC, is used for lab results. Unfortunately, many hospital systems use none of these standard systems, having instead developed internal coding schemes applicable only to their facilities. These work within the organization but create problems when trying to integrate other software or work with a RHIO.

**SNOMED-CT** SNOMED stands for Systematized Nomenclature of Medicine; CT stands for Clinical Terms. SNOMED-CT is a medical nomenclature developed by the College of American Pathologists and United Kingdom's National Health Service. It is a merger of two previous coding systems, SNOMED and the Read codes.

**Medcin** Medcin is a medical nomenclature and knowledge base developed by Medicomp Systems, Inc., in collaboration with physicians on staff at the Cornell, Harvard, Johns Hopkins, and other major medical centers. The purpose of the Medcin nomenclature and the intent of the design differentiate it from other coding standards. SNOMED-CT and other coding systems were designed to classify or index medical information for research or other purposes. Medcin was designed for point-of-care usage by the clinician. Medcin is not just a list of medical terms, but rather a list of *findings* (clinical observations) that are medically meaningful to the clinician.

An EHR system based on Medcin enables the clinician to select fewer individual codes and to quickly locate other clinical findings that are likely to be needed. This difference reduces the time it takes to create exam notes and allows a physician to complete the patient exam note at the time of the encounter.

**LOINC** LOINC stands for Logical Observation Identifiers Names and Codes. LOINC was created and is maintained by the Regenstrief Institute, which is closely affiliated with the Indiana University School of Medicine. LOINC standardizes codes for laboratory test orders and results, such as blood hemoglobin and serum potassium, and also clinical observations, such as vital signs or EKG.

LOINC is important because currently most laboratories and other diagnostic services report test results using their own internal, proprietary codes. When an EHR receives results from multiple lab facilities, comparing the results electronically is like comparing apples and oranges. LOINC provides a universal coding system for mapping laboratory tests and results to a common terminology in the EHR. This then makes it possible for a computer program to find and report comparable test values regardless of where the test was processed.

## Functional Benefits from Codified Records

Because coded data is nonambiguous, the computer can use it for health maintenance, trend analysis, alerts, decision support, orders and results, administrative processes, and population health reporting. We will now explore four of the functional benefits that can be derived from using a codified EHR.

**HEALTH MAINTENANCE**   One of the best ways to maintain good health is to prevent disease, or if it occurs, to detect it early enough to be easily treated. Two important components of health maintenance are preventive care screening and immunizations.

**Preventive Care**  The simplest example of health maintenance is a card or letter reminding the patient that it is time for a checkup. In a paper-based office, creating this reminder is a manual process. However, when a medical practice has electronic records, preventive screening can become more dynamic and sophisticated.

Health maintenance systems, also known as preventive care systems, can go beyond simple reminders for an annual checkup. When an EHR has codified data, it can be electronically compared to the recommendations of the U.S. Preventive Services Task Force.

---

### U.S. PREVENTIVE SERVICES TASK FORCE

The U.S. Preventive Services Task Force is an independent panel of experts in primary care and prevention that systematically reviews the evidence of effectiveness and develops recommendations for clinical preventive services.

The task force makes recommendations about preventive services based on age, sex, and risk factors for disease. Research has shown that the best way to ensure that preventive services are delivered appropriately is to make evidence-based information readily available at the point of care. The task force recommendations have been incorporated in EHR systems from several vendors.

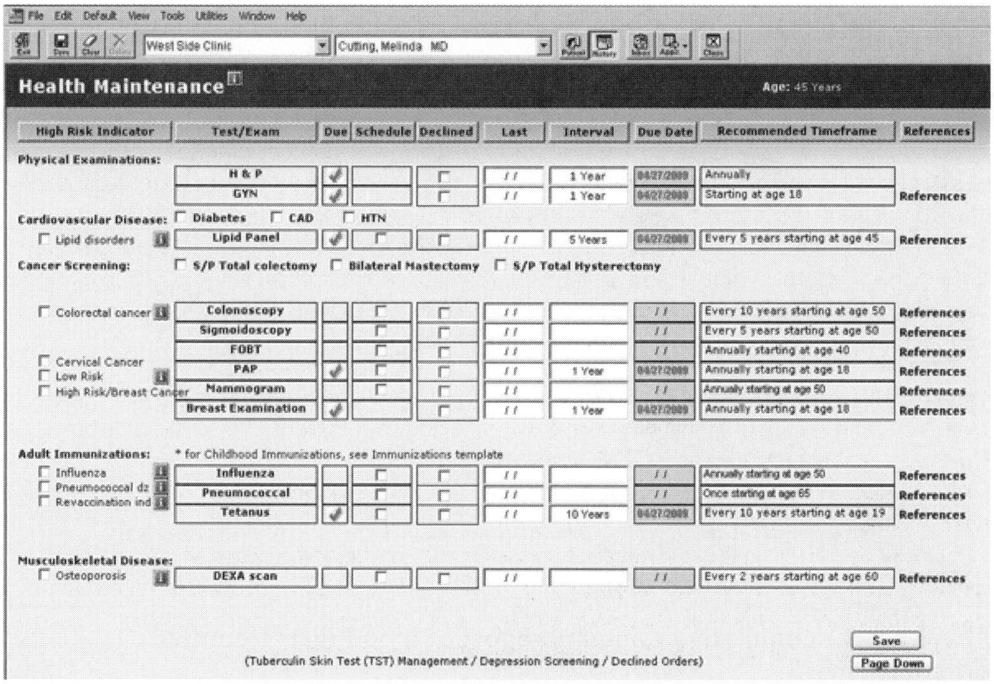

---

**FIGURE 7-2**

**Health Maintenance screen.**

(Courtesy of NextGen.)

Using a sophisticated set of rules, the EHR software compares the list of tests recommended for patients of a certain age and sex to previous test results stored in the EHR. It also calculates the time since the test was last performed and compares that to the recommended interval for repeat testing. A guideline unique to the patient is generated and displayed on the clinician's computer. Using this information, the clinician can order tests, discuss important healthcare options, and recommend lifestyle changes to the patient at the point of care. Figure 7-2 shows the Health Maintenance screen from EHR vendor NextGen.

It would be difficult to create standardized rules for the preventive care system if the tests were not coded using a standardized coding system. Preventive care screening guidelines are not

```
********************************************* Blood Gases ********************************************

DATE:             [-----------------------12/18/07---------------------]  12/17/07
TIME:             2132        1920        1720        1506        1615        NORMAL       UNITS

pH-Arterial       7.30 L      7.36        7.38        7.47 H      7.48 H      7.35-7.45
PCO2-Arterial     47.4 H      41.1        38.3        34.8 L      33.0 L      35-45        mm Hg
PO2-Arterial      90.2        189.0 H     187.0 H     188.0 H     227.0 H     90-105       mm Hg
HCO3-Arterial     22.8        22.8        22.0        24.9        24.4        21-27        mEq/L
Base Excess-A                                         1.7         1.6         0-3          mEq/L
Base Deficit-A    3.2 H       1.9         2.3                                 0-3          mEq/L
O2 Sat Dir-A      96.0        99.3 H      99.5 H      99.6 H      99.9 H      95-99        % Saturation
O2 Content-A      15.9        15.3        14.6 L      10.3 L      14.4 L      15-17        vol %
Hemoglobin-BG     12.0        10.8        10.3        7.2         10.1                     g/dL
CarboxyHb-A       1.1 H       1.0 H       1.2 H       0.9         1.6 H       0.0-0.9      % Saturation
MetHb-A           0.9         0.4         0.7         0.4         0.8         0.0-0.9      % Saturation
FIO2                          .55         .56         0.54        .65                      %


****************************************** Whole Blood Chemistries ******************************************

DATE:             [-----------------------12/18/07---------------------]  12/17/07
TIME:             2209        2132        1920        1720        1506        1615        NORMAL       UNITS

Sodium-WB                                 142         142         142         139         135-145      mEq/L
Potassium-WB      3.5                     3.3         3.0 L       2.9 L       2.7 L       3.3-4.6      mEq/L
Calcium Ionized               1.21        1.05        0.99 L      1.07        1.08        1.05-1.30    mmol/L
Lactic Acid-WB                1.3         0.8         1.1         0.8         0.5         0.3-1.5      mmol/L
Glucose-WB                    197 H       156 H       165 H       118 H       90          65-99        mg/dL
Hematocrit-WB                 37          34 L        32 L        22 L        31 L        36-46        %


****************************************** General Chemistry ******************************************

DATE:             12/23/07 [-----12/22/07-----] [----------12/21/07----------] 12/20/07
TIME:             *0620    0653    0327    1835    0915    0532    2048        NORMAL       UNITS

Sodium            140                                     143                 136-145      mmol/L
Potassium         2.7 L   3.0 L          2.9 L   3.0 L   2.7 L               3.3-5.1      mmol/L
Chloride          101                                     100                 98-107       mmol/L
Carbon Dioxide    32 H                                    36 H                22-30        mmol/L
Urea Nitrogen     10                                      7                   6-20         mg/dL
Creatinine        0.54                                    0.60                0.40-0.90    mg/dL
Glucose           115 H                                   96                  65-99        mg/dL
Calcium           8.4                                     8.0                 8.0-10.6     mg/dL
Magnesium         1.9                                     2.3         1.8     1.5-2.8      mg/dL
Phosphorus Inorg  2.3 L                                   2.8         1.8 L   2.7-4.5      mg/dL
CK Total                          165                                 273 H   30-170       U/L


--------------------------------------------------------------------------------------------------
     H=Abnormal High          L=Abnormal Low          H*=Critical High            L*=Critical Low
   Date Printed: 12/28/2007            Admit Date: 12/16/2007         Discharge Date: 12/23/2007
                           INPATIENT MEDICAL RECORDS COPY                    Page: 1
```

**FIGURE 7-3** Cumulative summary report of blood tests from five different times.

limited to lab tests; other examples include mammograms, hearing and vision screening, and certain elements of the physical examination.

**Immunizations** The other important component of preventive care is immunizations. Immunization slows down or stops disease outbreaks. Vaccines prevent disease in the people who receive them and protect those who come into contact with unvaccinated individuals.

Immunizations must be acquired over time. Vaccines cannot be given all at once. Several require repeated applications over a period of time, and some such as the measles vaccine cannot be given to children under the age of 1 year. Therefore, the CDC and state health departments have designed a schedule to immunize children and adolescents from birth through 18 years. The CDC also publishes a recommended immunization schedule for adults. Adult immunizations are different from those given to a child.

Using the codified data in an EHR, computers can compare a patient's immunization history with the CDC-recommended vaccines and intervals and identify which immunizations the patient needs. EHR systems can also scan the data and generate letters to patient who haven't been in recently but may need to renew their immunizations.

**TREND ANALYSIS** In healthcare, laboratory tests are used to measure the level of certain components present in specimens taken from the patient. When the same test is performed over a period of time, changes in the results can indicate a *trend* in the patient's health.

With a paper chart, the clinician must page through the reports and mentally remember the values to compare them. With an electronic health record, the computer can find matching results in the data and generate a cumulative summary report or a graph, making it easier to compare test results from different times and dates.

The cumulative summary report shown in Figure 7-3 has three sections of results: blood gases, whole blood chemistries, and general chemistry. Within each section are the results from tests performed five different times; the date and time is printed above each column of data.

The report is read from left to right; each row contains the name of the test component followed by result values for each of the five times. The right two columns are informational; they contain the range of values considered normal for each particular test and the unit of measure.

A simple graphing tool can turn numeric data in the EHR into a powerful visual aid that would be impractical to create from a paper chart. Figure 7-4 provides an example of how data

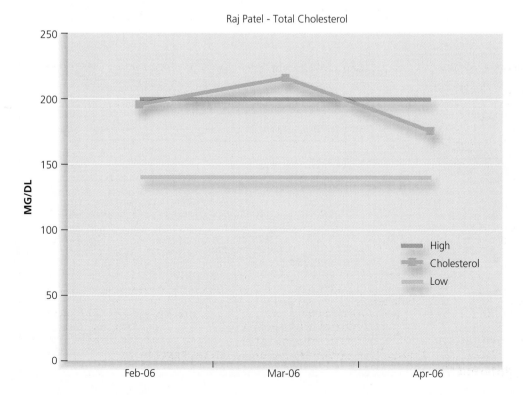

**FIGURE 7-4**

**Graph of total cholesterol from codified lab results.**

from multiple lab tests can be quickly extracted and graphed for the clinician. The value of the total cholesterol results over a three-month period of time is trended with the green line. The reference ranges of normal high (200) and low (140) values are shown in the graph as red and blue lines, respectively.

The computer is able to generate this graph because the data is fielded and the different tests and components have unique codes. From all the possible tests a patient might have had, the computer can quickly find those coded as "total cholesterol." Using a graph, the clinician can easily see the trend of this patient's total cholesterol.

Trend analysis is not limited to lab test results. Graphs of patient weight loss or gain are used as patient education tools. Effects of medication can be measured by comparing changes in dosage to changes in blood pressure measurements. Flow sheets (shown later in Figure 7-15) are another type of trend analysis tool.

**ALERTS**   One of the important reasons for the widespread adoption of EHRs is the potential to reduce medical errors. Paper charts and even electronic charts that are principally scanned images depend on the clinician noticing a risk factor about the patient. However, when an EHR consists primarily of fielded and codified data using standard nomenclature, rules can be set up that allow the computer to do the monitoring.

*Alert* is the term used in an EHR for a message or reminder that is automatically generated by the system. Alerts are based on programmed rules that cause the EHR to alert the provider when two or more conditions are met. For example, an electronic prescription system generates an alert when two drugs known to have adverse interactions are prescribed for the same patient.

Alerts can be programmed for just about anything in the EHR. However, the most prevalent alert systems are those implemented with electronic prescription systems. Interactions between multiple prescription drugs, allergic reactions to certain classes of drugs, and patient health conditions that contraindicate certain drugs can all contribute to suffering, additional illness, and in extreme cases even death.

To prevent this, most physicians consult the patient medication list, allergy list, and the *Physicians' Desk Reference* (for interactions) before writing a prescription. As a further precaution, the pharmacy checks for drug conflicts and provides the patient with warning materials about the drug. When prescriptions are written electronically, however, the computer can quickly and efficiently check for drug safety and present the clinician with warnings, alerts, and explanatory information about the risks of particular drugs. Figure 7-5 shows a clinical warning alert generated by the Allscripts EHR system.

**FIGURE 7-5**

**Electronic prescription DUR alert.**

(Courtesy of Allscripts, LLC.)

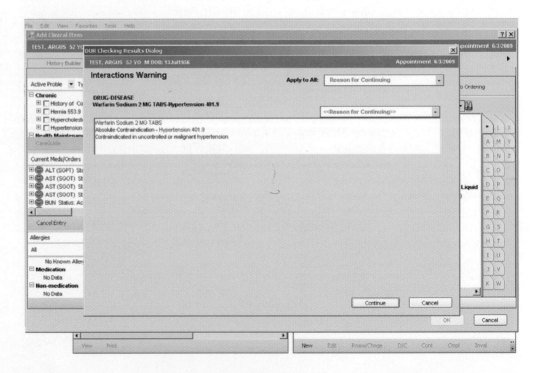

**Drug Utilization Review**  When the clinician writing an electronic prescription selects a drug and enters the Sig[7] information, the EHR system scans the patient chart for allergy information, past and current diagnoses, and a list of current medications. This information is then passed to a drug utilization review (DUR) program that compares the prescription to a database of most known drugs. The database includes prescription drugs as well as over-the-counter drugs, and even nutritional herb and vitamin supplements. The DUR program performs the following functions:

- The drug about to be prescribed is checked against the patient medication list to determine if there is a conflict with any drug the patient is already taking. Certain drugs remain in the body for a period of time after the patient has stopped taking it. This latency period is factored in as well.

- Ingredients that make up the drug are checked against the ingredients of current medications to see if they conflict or would hinder the effectiveness of the drug.

- Drugs are checked for duplicate therapy, which occurs when a patient is taking a different drug of the same class that would have the effect of an overdose.

- Allergy records are checked for food and drug allergies that would be aggravated by the new drug.

- Some drugs cannot be given to patients with certain medical conditions; the patient's diagnosis history is checked to see if such a situation would occur.

- A patient education alert is created when the drug might be affected by certain foods or alcohol interactions.

- If the Sig has been entered at the time of the DUR, then it is also checked to see if it matches recommended guidelines for the drug. Too much, too little, too many days, or too many refills could cause overdosing, underdosing (causing it to be ineffective), or abuse.

If the DUR software finds any of these conditions, the clinician is given an alert message explaining the conflict. The clinician can then alter the prescription or select a new drug, having never issued the incorrect one.

**Formulary Alerts**  Another type of alert found in many EHR prescription systems warns the clinician if the drug about to be prescribed is not covered by a patient's pharmacy benefit insurance. This is important because if a patient's insurance won't pay for it, the patient may choose not to fill the prescription or to take less than the amount prescribed.

Insurance plans provide formularies indicating preferred, nonpreferred, and noncovered drugs. If the clinician prescribes a drug that is not on the list, then when the patient tries to have the prescription filled, the pharmacy will call and ask the physician to change it. This causes an inconvenience to the patient and wastes the doctor's time. Instead a clinician using an EHR can select from a list of therapeutically equivalent drugs that are on the formulary of the patient's insurance plan and avoid writing an incorrect prescription. Figure 7-6 shows an Allscripts Therapeutic Alternatives alert.

**Other Types of Alerts**  Electronic lab order systems can provide alerts as well. For example, certain tests are not covered by Medicare. CMS requires that patients sign a waiver indicating that they were notified that a test would not be covered. The waiver is called an Advance Beneficiary Notice (ABN). When certain tests are ordered, the clinician is alerted if an ABN is required. Another example is an alert that monitors changes in values of certain blood tests and pages a doctor whenever the value is outside of a certain range.

Alerts can be generated by nonactions as well. Task list systems can notify an administrator when medical items are not handled in a timely fashion. CPOE systems can generate alerts when results for a pending test order have not been received within the time that it would normally require for that type of test.

Once an EHR system contains codified data, an alert system is just a matter of programming a rule to watch for a certain event or detect a finding with a value above or below the desired limit.

---

[7]Sig, from the Latin *signa,* are the instructions for labeling a prescription.

**FIGURE 7-6**

**Electronic prescription formulary alert.**

(Courtesy of Allscripts, LLC.)

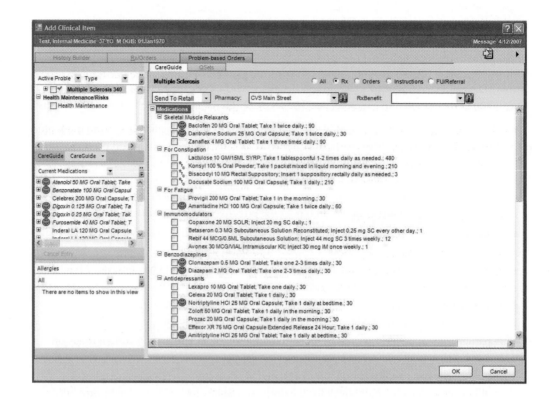

**DECISION SUPPORT**   Physicians are trained to analyze information from a patient's history, physical exams, and test results for a medical decision. They are also accustomed to researching the medical literature when faced with an unusual case. However, the quantity of information available to clinicians regarding conditions, disease management, protocols, case studies, and treatments far exceeds their available time to read it.

*Decision support* refers to the ability of EHR systems to store or quickly locate materials relevant to the findings of the current case. These might include defined protocols, results of case studies, or standard care guidelines prepared by specialists, medical societies, or government organizations.

Decision support is not about "artificial intelligence" replacing a physician with a computer; it is instead about providing help just when the clinician needs it. There are many examples of decision support systems, but let us look at four:

**Prescriptions:**

- Decision support can include the drug formularies mentioned earlier. Formularies can be used to look up drugs by name or therapeutic class. Electronic prescription systems provide decision support to the clinician by comparing alternative brands that are therapeutically equivalent. They can also provide information on costs, indications for use, treatment recommendations, dosage, guidelines, and prescribing information.

**Medical References:**

- Decision support systems can provide quick access to medical references directly from the EHR. This can make access to evidence-based guidelines or medical literature as easy as clicking on a link in the chart.

**Protocols:**

- Protocols are one form of decision support that can ultimately speed up documentation of the patient exam and improve patient care. Protocols are standard plans of therapy established for different conditions. With a decision support system, when a doctor has diagnosed a patient with a particular condition, the appropriate protocol appears on the EHR screen and all therapies are ordered with a click of the mouse.

**Medication Dosing:**

■ Many medications have serious side effects, some of which must be monitored by regular blood tests. When both the medications and lab results are stored in the EHR as codified data, it is possible for decision support software to compare changes in medication dosing with changes in the patient's test results. This assists the clinician in adjusting the patient's medication levels to obtain the maximum benefit to the patient.

Each of the functional benefits we have discussed—health maintenance, trend analysis, alerts, and decision support—are products of EHR systems that store medical records as codified, fielded data. It is only when these functional benefits are added to the clinical practice that the EHR approaches the vision of the IOM discussed at the beginning of this chapter.

## Capturing and Recording EHR Data

The value of having an EHR is evident, but how does the data get into the EHR? In addition to scanning paper documents (discussed in Chapter 6) and the direct data entry of the exam note (discussed later in this chapter), there are additional sources of EHR data that can be imported directly into the system:

■ Lab test orders and results represent a significant portion of the pages in a paper chart. Most reference labs have computerized both the orders and results and have interfaces to their systems available. Electronic lab order and results systems can be interfaced to merge the test results directly into the patient's chart.

   One benefit of electronic lab results described earlier is that the numerical data that makes up many lab results lends itself to trend analysis, graphs, and comparison with other tests. The ability to review and present results in this manner allows providers to see the immediate, tangible benefits of using an EHR. Not only is the practice eliminating paper, but providers also should begin to realize the potential of conducting trend analyses with an EHR.

■ If some providers continue to use dictation/transcription of exam notes, the word processing files in which that transcription is saved can be imported directly as EHR text records. Also if a practice formerly used dictation/transcription and has retained those files, importing them as EHR text records may be more efficient than scanning the printed versions of those documents. Although these text records are not codified like those created when clinicians enter actual data, they are at the very least more accessible and searchable than scanned materials.

■ Radiology studies are often dictated and transcribed. If the word processing files are available, they can be imported into the EHR as text records. In some systems, digital images such as x-rays can be directly incorporated into the EHR and associated with the radiology report; or in facilities where a PAC system is used, diagnostic images can be made to appear as part of the record, even though they are on a separate system.

■ Vital signs are numerical in nature and therefore eminently applicable to trend analysis and graphing. These are especially useful for creating growth charts in pediatric practices and assisting adolescent and adult patients with weight loss goals. Some of the modern devices used to take blood pressure readings, temperature, pulse, and respiration can automatically transfer the readings to an EHR. Unfortunately, this level of automation is more prevalent in hospitals and ICU systems than in medical offices. The average medical office uses common instruments such as a scale, thermometer, and blood pressure cuff. The measurements are manually taken and recorded by a medical assistant. However, even without automated equipment, the medical assistant could enter the data in the computer instead of writing it on a sheet of paper.

■ The patient's problem list (acute conditions for which the patient was recently seen as well as chronic conditions such as high blood pressure or diabetes) may be able to be generated automatically from patient history and past visits, then simply updated by a nurse or doctor each time the patient is seen.

**FIGURE 7-7**

**Nurse enters data at patient's bedside.**

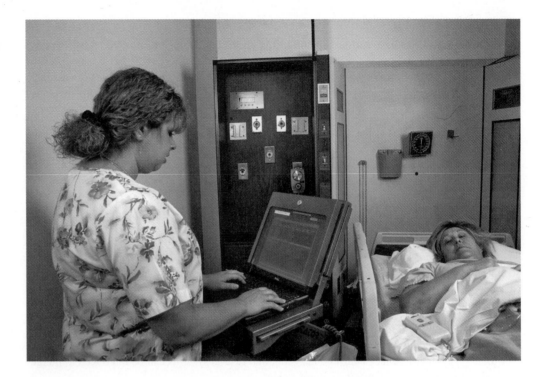

- History and symptom information can be entered directly by the patient on a computer in the waiting room instead of on a paper form on a clipboard. The patient-entered data is reviewed by the doctor during the exam and then merged into the EHR. This will be discussed in more detail later in the chapter.

- When clinicians use the EHR to write prescriptions, the orders are also automatically recorded in the EHR as part of the workflow. Another benefit of having the patient's past prescriptions in the computer is that it makes renewing prescriptions much faster for the provider.

## Documenting at the Point of Care

A goal of most EHR systems is to improve the accuracy and completeness of the patient record. One way to achieve this is to record the information in the EHR at the time it is happening. This is called *point-of-care documentation*. In a physician's office, this means completing the SOAP note before the patient ever leaves the office. In an inpatient setting, this means that nurses enter vital signs and nursing notes at bedside, not at the end of their shift. Figure 7-7 shows a nurse entering notes while seeing the patient.

**BENEFITS OF REAL-TIME DOCUMENTATION**   Leading physician experts on the EHR, Allen R. Wenner, an M.D. in Columbia, South Carolina, and John W. Bachman, an M.D. at the Mayo Clinic, wrote:

> Documenting an encounter at the point of care is the most efficient method of practicing medicine because the physician completes the medical record at the time of a patient's visit. Dictation time is saved and the need for personal dictation aides is eliminated. Thus, point-of-care documentation is less expensive than traditional dictation with its associated high cost of transcription. In addition, the physician can sign the note immediately.
>
> Patient care is improved because the patient can leave with a complete copy of the medical record, a step that stimulates compliance. The delivery process is improved with point-of-care documentation because referrals can be accomplished with full information available at the time that the referral is needed. For these benefits to occur,

the clinical workflow changes to improve efficiency, increase data accuracy, and lower the overall cost of healthcare delivery.[8]

The EHR system strives to improve patient healthcare by giving the provider and patient access to complete, up-to-date records of past and present conditions; it also enables the records to be used in ways that paper medical records could not. The sooner the data is entered, the sooner it is available for other providers and the patient.

## Nurse and Medical Assistant-Entered Data

In hospitals of all sizes, nurses enter nursing notes, nursing assessments, and vital signs into the medical record. In ambulatory settings, the nurse or medical assistant takes the vital signs and discusses with the patient the reason for the visit, and possibly reviews allergy or medication information. Using an EHR, the nurse or medical assistant can initiate an exam record for the visit, enter the chief complaint, update any allergy records, make note of any medications the patient may have had prescribed elsewhere as well as any over-the-counter medications being taken. In this way, a nurse or medical assistant helps to build the EHR note without impacting the clinician's time with the patient.

## Patient-Entered Data

There are several things about documenting an encounter that become evident when the workflow is studied.

- Only the patient has the information about what symptoms were present at the outset of the illness and what the outcome of medical treatment of those symptoms was.

- The patient is also typically the source of past medical, family, and social history, which is also recorded in the medical record.

- Up to 67% of the nurse or clinician's time with the patient is spent entering the patient's symptoms and history into the visit documentation.

In the late 1980s, Dr. Allen Wenner wondered if a medical history couldn't be taken by a computer. The medical literature was replete with academic efforts at patient computer dialogue beginning with Warner Slack at Harvard[9] and John Mayne at Mayo Clinic.[10] If the patients entered their own data, it would free up clinical staff and allow more of the physician's time to be focused directly on the important issues identified by the patient. Dr. Wenner confirmed the theories of the academics—if given the opportunity, adding information to their medical chart while waiting was readily accepted by most patients. Working with his colleagues at Primetime Medical Software, he developed Instant Medical History™, an automated patient data-entry component for the EHR. It is available in many commercial EHR systems today.

**WORKFLOW USING PATIENT-ENTERED DATA**    Several workflows are compatible with Instant Medical History. Instant Medical History can be administered on a kiosk or pen-tablet device in the waiting room, in a subwaiting area, in the exam room, or at home via the web.

Figure 7-8 shows a sample interview screen for Instant Medical History. To the patients, it represents a replacement of the clipboard with questions that the receptionist used to hand patients on arrival at medical offices. The difference is that the questions are asked one at a time and can dynamically branch to other question sets based on the answers provided by the patient.

Patients complete the computer program at their own pace. The computer calculates well and can use the answers to several questions to branch to standardized screening instruments published in the medical literature. Patients have an opportunity to change their answers.

---

[8]Allen R. Wenner and John W. Bachman, "Transforming the Physician Practice: Interviewing Patients with a Computer," Chap. 26 in *Healthcare Information Management Systems: Cases, Strategies, and Solutions,* 3rd ed., ed. Marion J. Ball, Charlotte A. Weaver, and Joan M. Kiel (New York: Springer Science+Business Media, Inc., 2004), 297–319. Copyright © 2004 Springer Science+Business Media, Inc. New York.

[9]W. V. Slack, G. P. Hicks, C. E. Reed, et al., "A Computer-Based Medical-History System," *New England Journal of Medicine* 274 (1966): 194–98.

[10]J. G. Mayne, W. Weksel, and P. N. Sholtz, "Toward Automating the Medical History," *Mayo Clinic Proceedings* 43 (1968): 1–25.

**FIGURE 7-8**

**Instant medical history on a kiosk in the waiting room.**

(Courtesy of Primetime Medical Software & Instant Medical History.)

**FIGURE 7-8**

**Instant medical history on a kiosk in the waiting room.**

(Courtesy of Primetime Medical Software & Instant Medical History.)

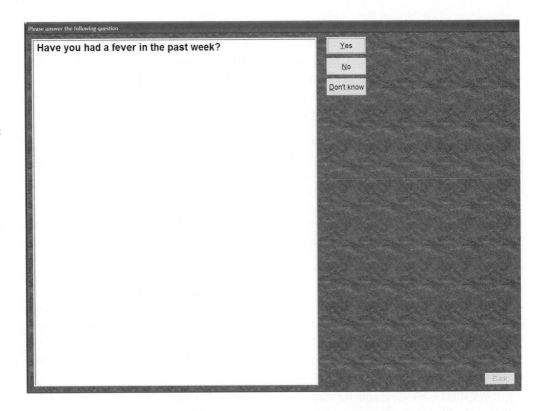

Patients can review their histories (as shown in Figure 7-9) and are better prepared to interact with the physician.

Because interview software records subjective information from the patient, the data represents a more complete and accurate reflection of a patient's complaints than a physician's dictation after the visit. Another important element of history taking is the depth to which a patient is asked questions. Dr. Wenner found that the use of computer interviews improves the quality of the information presented by the patient. Because the process gives the patient time to remember and record details, it is more complete.

**FIGURE 7-9**

**Summary screen allows patient to review answers.**

(Courtesy of Primetime Medical Software & Instant Medical History.)

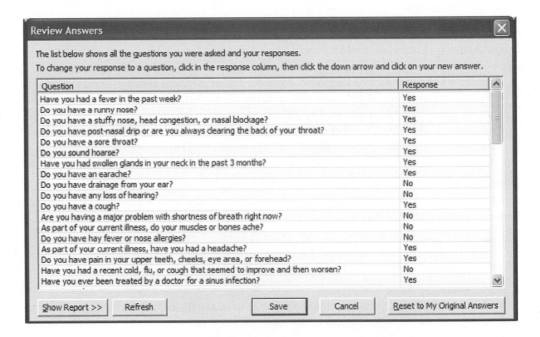

Once the patient has answered the questions, the information is organized for the provider in a succinct and easy-to-read format that becomes the starting point for the patient encounter. The clinician can review this output either on a computer screen or as a printout. After asking a few confirmatory questions, physicians can complete the medical history in the examination room while the patient is still present. The physician can add additional information as necessary and the exam note can be completed by the physician at the point of care.

Because patients want their physicians to arrive at the best diagnosis, Dr. Wenner found that patients are willing to answer questions. Also, because the clinician reviews the information entered by the patient instead of having to enter it, more time is available for explaining the diagnosis and educating the patient. Thus, the patient's time and effort to enter the data are rewarded. Allowing patients to enter their own history frees up the clinician's time while improving the depth and quality of the information gathered.

It is important to note that, although patients are entering their symptom and history information in the computer, they are not accessing the EHR so there are no HIPAA security concerns. The patient-entered data is separate from the EHR system until it is reviewed and made part of the exam note by the clinician or nurse.

**ALTERNATIVE WORKFLOW**    Some medical offices imbed Instant Medical History in their website so that patients can complete the symptom and history interview prior to their appointment using the Internet. In that case, the data will already be available to the clinician when the patient arrives at the office. In some instances, the clinician can make medical treatment decisions without a face-to-face visit; these are called E-visits (discussed in Chapter 5).

---

### PREVENTIVE HEALTH SELF-SCREENING

Patient interview software can also perform the health maintenance preventive screening discussed earlier in this chapter. Because most patients wait 15 minutes to see a physician, it is medically appropriate to screen patients for compliance with health maintenance guidelines while they wait.

In the course of a yearlong study, patients were invited to answer a few questions on the computer when they spoke to the triage nurse, but screening was completely voluntary. Over time, the software revealed the need for hundreds of tetanus shots, varicella vaccinations, Papanicolaou smears, and other preventive measures by asking patients simple questions about the duration since their last assessment. Preventive health screening is one of the identified benefits of an EHR.

---

## Clinician-Entered Data

The core of the true codified EHR comes when the provider begins to record the actual exam findings in a medical record program instead of dictating and having it transcribed later. Though it takes more of the provider's time to enter the information in the computer, some physicians see the time spent entering the EHR as a reasonable trade-off for the time spent dictating and reviewing transcribed documents.

Entering observations and findings as medical data into an EHR has many additional advantages for the provider than just the elimination of transcription. One of these is the correct calculation of billing and diagnosis codes. Government and private insurance claims have strict rules about what (evaluation and management) billing codes are allowed based on the documented level of an exam. Most EHR systems have built-in functions that help the provider select the correct billing code based on the data entered in the exam note. Many of these systems can automatically transfer the codes to the billing system when the exam is completed. This subject will be covered further in Chapter 9.

**SAVING CLINICIANS' TIME**    Because the physician's time with the patient is very valuable, the method used to document the exam must be optimized to be as efficient as possible. Usually this is achieved by a combination of features in the application software and the medical nomenclature.

**FIGURE 7-10**

**EHR systems use tabs to logically group findings.**

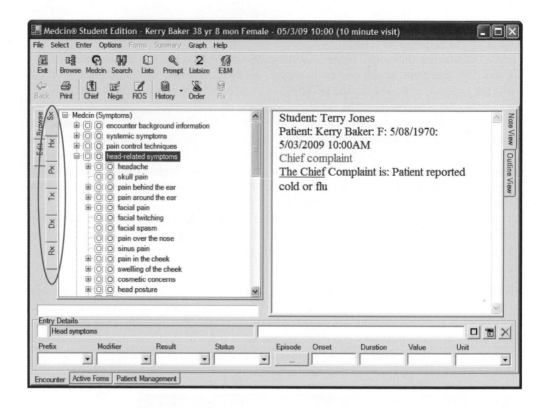

Most EHR systems designed for real-time data entry have the user select a *finding* (a medical term or phrase the clinician wants to record). However, to be successfully used in real time, an EHR must make it easy for the clinician to locate the correct finding.

EHR vendors work constantly with EHR users to devise means to locate and present findings when they are most likely needed. Most EHR systems designed for point-of-care data entry use some or all of the features discussed next to help speed up data entry.

**NOMENCLATURE**   Use of a standardized nomenclature allows the clinician to select the desired terminology, minimizes the need to type, and creates a codified medical record behind the scene. When the clinician selects a finding, the EHR may display several sentences describing the patient's condition in precise medical language.

EHR nomenclatures designed for point-of-care data entry, such as Medcin, also contain links between related findings, making possible the search-and-prompt features described below.

The EHR shown in Figure 7-10 is based on the Medcin nomenclature. The screen layout and functional behavior are similar to many EHR systems. The screen is divided into four functional sections. Two rows of icons across the top of the screen (called a toolbar) are used to quickly access special features. The center portion of the screen consists of two (white) panels. The left panel displays the Medcin nomenclature. The clinician records findings by clicking the red or blue button next to a finding. The text of that finding then appears in the right panel, which displays the actual patient exam note as it is being created (see Figure 7-11). The bottom portion of the screen contains two rows of fields for adding details about a finding.

EHR nomenclatures contain hundreds of thousands of findings. It would be extremely inefficient to have to scroll or search through the entire nomenclature each time the clinician wanted to record a finding. Therefore, it is more useful to present only a portion of the nomenclature at a time. Tabs in the left panel of Figure 7-10 (circled in red) are used to logically group the nomenclature into six broad categories. The tabs are organized to accommodate the SOAP format and labeled with abbreviations familiar to medical personnel:

- Sx which stands for symptoms
- Hx which stands for history

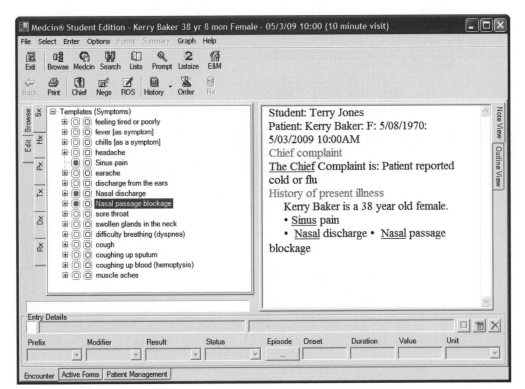

**FIGURE 7-11**

**List (in left panel) of symptoms typical for upper respiratory infections.**

- Px which stands for physical examination
- Tx which stands for tests performed
- Dx which stands for diagnosis and includes syndromes and conditions
- Rx which stands for therapy (including prescriptions).

Separating the nomenclature in this way limits the list to findings relevant to the task. For example, in Figure 7-10 the Sx tab is selected, limiting the list to symptoms. If the Dx tab were selected, only findings that would be used for diagnosis would be displayed.

**LISTS** Because many medical offices see a lot of patients with the same condition, physicians tend to perform the same type of exam, look for the same findings, order the same tests, and prescribe from a short list of treatments recommended for that condition. Therefore, it is logical for the practice to create shorter, quicker methods of locating the necessary findings, by the type of exam or condition.

This is not "canned medicine." These are templates to display findings that the doctor uses most frequently for different types of conditions or diseases, so that the exam can be documented with minimal navigation or searching. For example, a pulmonary specialist sees primarily respiratory cases, nephrologists see patients with kidney problems, and during the cold and flu season family physicians see many patients with upper respiratory infections (URIs).

Lists are just subsets of the full nomenclature. The full nomenclature remains available if the physician needs to record a finding not showing on the list. Figure 7-11 shows a list used for patients with URIs. Separate lists can be created for each type of exam and for each medical condition that the practice commonly sees.

Lists are dynamic and can contain an unlimited number of findings. Lists can include findings for every section of the SOAP note, so as to quickly document the complete visit.

**FORMS** The concept of forms is to display a desired group of findings in a presentation that allows for quick entry of not only positive and negative findings, but of any additional detail, such as the date of onset or a value such as the patient's weight.

**FIGURE 7-12**

**Short intake form speeds entry of past medical, family, and social history.**

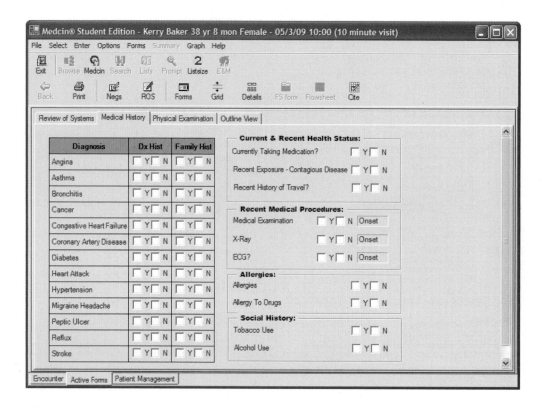

Forms are made up of the same nomenclature findings as are lists. In contrast to lists, which scroll dynamically, forms are static; that is, findings have a fixed position on the screen, and will remain in that location every time the form is used.

Another difference is that, whereas lists always arrange findings in the appropriate tab (Sx, Hx, Px, Tx, Dx, and Rx), this is not a requirement of forms. The form designer is free to put any finding anywhere on the form. This allows each form to be designed to for the quickest entry of data for a particular type of exam.

For example, Figure 7-12 shows a form that allows the nurse to quickly record the patient's medical history and the patient's family and social history on one page of the form, even though the findings will appear in three different sections of the note.

Because the findings are prearranged on forms, it is easier for the user to see that all the necessary findings have been checked. The form designer can even require the entry of certain fields before the user can close the page, thus ensuring important information has been recorded. Forms also offer many additional features to make recording the information even faster. These include check boxes, drop-down lists, pop-up calendars, and even free-text boxes to further comment on a finding.

The form method of data entry is found in systems from nearly every EHR vendor. Its similarity to paper forms makes it familiar to users. Compare Figure 7-12 with the patient history form shown in Chapter 5, Figure 5-4.

**FIGURE 7-13**

**Search for angina pectoris.**

**SEARCH** The search function provides a quick way for the clinician to locate a desired finding in the nomenclature. Search produces a list of the findings almost instantly. Search is a necessary feature because even when using a form or list for a routine exam it is not uncommon for the patient to ask about a second condition not related to the reason for the visit. In Figure 7-13, the search is for angina pectoris, a finding that would not be in the typical URI list.

Search functions are standard in most EHR systems. One advantage of a standardized nomenclature is that it includes synonyms that allow users to locate the correct finding even when searching by an alternative term for that finding.

Within medicine many different words are used to describe the same symptom, condition, or observation; standardized nomenclatures help in several ways. Here are search features available in many popular EHR systems:

1. The search function performs automatic word completion, so if you search for *knee* but the finding is for *knees,* it will still find it.

2. The nomenclature includes an extensive list of synonyms, which are used in an alternate word search. For example, if you search for *knee injury,* the search results will also include findings for *knee burns, knee trauma,* and *fractured patella,* among others.

3. The search function identifies related findings in the other (SOAP) sections of the nomenclature, so that when you search for a word or phrase in a particular tab, related findings are automatically available in the other tabs. This means that as the clinician proceeds through the exam, the other tabs may already have findings related to the searched term available for selection.

**PROMPT**    EHR systems that use the Medcin nomenclature have an additional feature called "Prompt with current finding." The prompt function allows the user to dynamically generate a list of clinical findings.

Figure 7-14 shows the result of using the prompt feature. In the previous example, the clinician searched for *angina pectoris.* Once the finding was displayed, the clinician highlighted the finding and then clicked the Prompt button (circled in red). A full list of all symptoms, history, physical exam, tests, medications, treatments, and diagnosis findings related to angina was then instantly available for the doctor to select from.

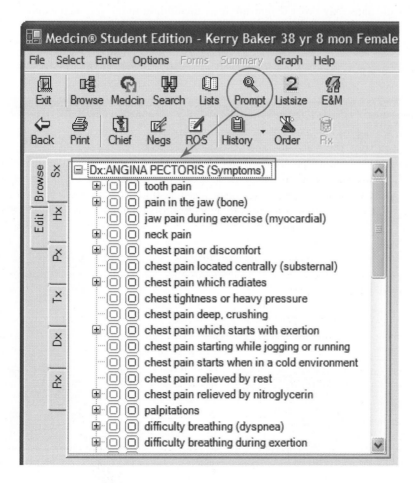

**FIGURE 7-14**

**Prompt changes list to findings related to angina pectoris.**

### Flow Sheets

Another important EHR feature is the ability for the provider to view and incorporate information from a previous visit to update it in the current exam. Flow sheets present data from multiple encounters in column form. The flow sheet format allows for a side-by-side comparison of findings over a period of time. A paper version of a nursing flow sheet was shown in Chapter 5, Figure 5-6.

Some clinicians prefer to view a patient chart this way. When outpatients are seen for follow-up visits to previous exams, this can be a real time saver for the provider. It is also ideal for chronic disease management, such as diabetes, or long-term conditions such as pregnancy. OB offices use flow sheets to monitor pregnancy, because it affords them a view of the previous visits while documenting the current one.

Many EHR systems generate flow sheets dynamically; however, not all EHR systems implement flow sheets in the same manner. EHR systems that do not have codified exam notes limit flow sheets to lab results or vital signs. When an EHR uses a codified nomenclature, it is possible to create clinical flow sheets that present findings from entire encounters in columns by encounter date. An example of a computerized flow sheet is shown in Figure 7-15.

The flow sheet in Figure 7-15 is made up of rows and columns of *cells*. The first column displays descriptions of findings for the current patient. The date of the current encounter is at the top of the column. The remaining columns to the right display encounter data from previous visits.

The cells within the column display the words POS (in red) or NEG (in blue), or a numerical value for the finding. A blank cell indicates no finding was recorded on that encounter date.

By comparing the values recorded for a finding over several dates, it is easier to spot trends in the patient's health conditions. It is also easier to remember to recheck the same items during the patient's current visit. Findings can be recorded for the current encounter in the first column of the flow sheet as the examination proceeds.

**ORDERS** Clinicians may order diagnostic tests in addition to the physical exam. In the plan section of the note, the clinician may order medications or therapy. When clinicians order lab tests and write prescriptions within the EHR system, those orders are automatically documented.

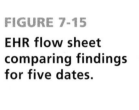

**FIGURE 7-15**

**EHR flow sheet comparing findings for five dates.**

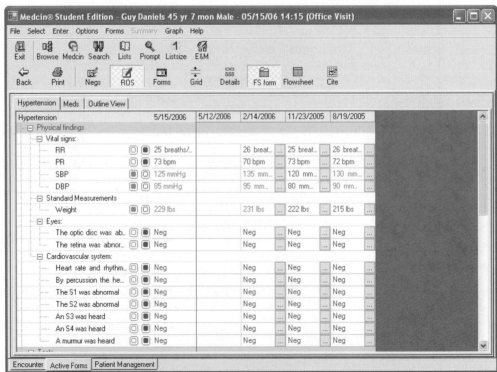

New orders can also be compared to previous tests and medications given to the patient to alert the physician if there is a conflict.

One time-saving feature that is typical in all commercial EHR systems is the concept of keeping a list of a clinician's frequently used orders. This allows the clinician to write the entire prescription or lab order with a single click of the mouse.

With thousands of tests that could be ordered and thousands of drugs to choose from, a clinician doesn't have the time to go through a search of medications or tests to write an Rx or order a lab. Many clinicians find that they order a fairly narrow range of tests (appropriate to their specialty and patient population) and write prescriptions for only a small group of medications. It makes sense for clinicians to keep a list of the items they most frequently use from which they can select when writing the order.

**PROTOCOLS**    Protocols, also sometimes called order sets, are lists of tests, treatments, therapy, or plans of care recommended for certain conditions. Once the clinician has diagnosed the patient in the assessment section, the EHR can present a list of orders from which to select. Unlike the list of frequently used orders discussed above, a protocol lists orders most appropriate to the patient's condition, even if they are not frequently ordered by the clinician. The use of protocols or order sets helps the clinician quickly order and document the plan of care for the patient. Chapter 5, Figure 5-5, showed a paper form of a postop neurosurgery order set.

# Electronic Signatures

Once the electronic medical record has been completed, it must be signed. All types of records in the patient's chart must be signed by an authorized individual. In EHR systems those signatures are electronic. An electronic signature is not a facsimile of the signature you create with a pen on paper, but rather a computer process that meets three criteria:

**Message Integrity:**
- Message integrity means the recipient must be able to confirm that the document has not been altered since it was signed.

**Nonrepudiation:**
- The signer must not be able to deny signing the document.

**User Authentication:**
- The recipient must be able to confirm that the signature was in fact "signed" by the real person.

The electronic signature process involves the successful identification and authentication of the signer at the time of the signature, binding of the signature to the document, and nonalterability of the document after the signature has been affixed. Only *digital signatures* meet all three of these criteria.

However, many of the records in an EHR system are not stored documents. As we discussed in Chapter 4, they are rows of fielded data. What is displayed on the screen as a physical exam note may be in fact hundreds of computer records. Therefore, most EHR systems do not produce a true digital signature for each note, but rather use a security mechanism within the software to authenticate the signer, and then lock that group of records as "signed," thereafter preventing further changes.

Beyond the pure mechanics of the EHR signature system are the responsibilities of the healthcare organization and providers to make electronic signatures work. The organization must have clear policies regarding who can sign what types of orders and documents. Further, there must be processes for authenticating that the users are who they say they are, and finally, there must be clear policies regarding who can set up, credential, and grant signing permission to the users.

Whether electronic signatures in a system are true digital signatures or a software mechanism for locking and protecting EHR system records, it is important for providers to follow the policies and procedures of their facility. Most EHR systems have an internal audit trail of who creates each document and medical record.

- Always log on to the EHR as yourself.
- Always log off when you are through.
- Keep your passwords or PIN numbers private.

This will prevent someone else from signing medical records under your ID.

## Flow of an Office Fully Using EHRs

Earlier in this chapter Dr. Wenner and Dr. Bachman stated that an EHR changes the workflow of a medical office. Figure 7-16 illustrates the workflow of a visit to an office that fully uses the electronic capabilities that are available in EHR systems today, including patient participation in the process and the capabilities of the Internet. Follow the arrows in the figure as you read the descriptions of the steps listed here:

1. An established patient phones the doctor's office and schedules an appointment.
   *Internet alternative:* Patients are increasingly able to request an appointment and receive a confirmation via the Internet.
2. The night before the appointment, the medical office computer electronically verifies insurance eligibility for patients scheduled the next day.
3. On the day of the appointment, the patient arrives at the office and is asked to confirm that the demographic information on file is still correct.

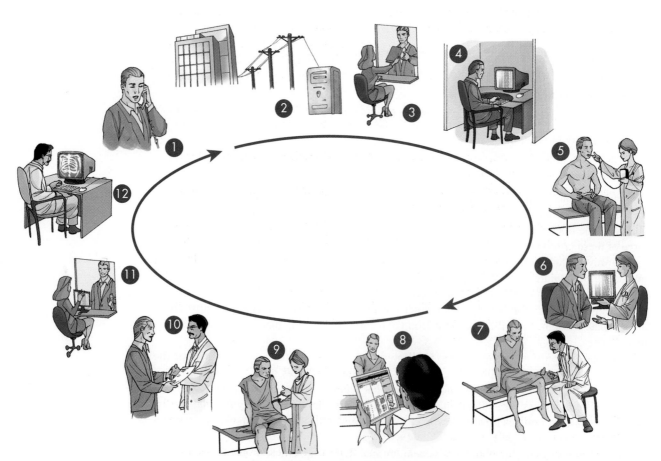

**FIGURE 7-16** **Workflow in a medical office fully using EHRs.**

4. A receptionist, nurse, or medical assistant asks the patient to complete a medical history and reason for today's visit using a computer in a private area of the waiting room. The patient completes a computer-guided questionnaire concerning his symptoms and medical history.

   *Internet alternative:* Some medical practices allow patients to use the Internet to complete the history and symptom questionnaire before coming to the office.

5. When the patient has completed the questionnaire, the system alerts the nurse that the patient is ready to move to an exam room.

   The nurse measures the patient's height and weight and records it in the EHR. Using a modern device, vital signs for blood pressure, temperature, and pulse are recorded and wirelessly transferred into the EHR.

6. *Subjective:* The nurse and patient review the patient-entered symptoms and history. Where necessary the nurse edits the record to add clarification or refinement.

   The physician enters the exam room and discusses the reason for the visit and reviews with the patient the information already in the chart.

7. *Objective:* The physician performs the physical exam. The clinician typically makes a mental provisional diagnosis. This is used to select a list or template of findings to quickly record the physical exam in the EHR.

   The EHR presents a list of problems the patient reported in past visits that have not been resolved. The physician reviews each, examining additional body systems as necessary, and marks the improvement, worsening, or resolution of each problem.

   *Assessment:* Applying his or her training to the subjective and objective findings, the clinician arrives at a decision of one or more diagnoses, and decides if further tests might be warranted.

8. *Plan of treatment:* The clinician prescribes a treatment, medication, and/or orders further tests using the EHR.

   If medication is to be ordered, the physician writes the prescription electronically. The prescription is compared to the patient's allergy records and current drugs. The physician is advised if there are any contraindications or potential problems. The prescription is compared to the formulary of drugs covered by the patient's insurance plan and the physician is advised if an alternate drug is recommended (thereby avoiding a subsequent phone call from the pharmacist to revise the prescription). The prescription is then transmitted directly to the patient's pharmacy.

   A built-in function of the EHR accurately calculates the correct evaluation and management code used for billing. The billing code is confirmed by the physician and automatically transferred to the billing system.

   When the visit is complete, so is the exam note. The physician signs the note electronically at the conclusion of the visit.

9. If lab work has been ordered, a medical assistant will obtain the necessary specimen and the order is sent electronically to the lab.

10. *Patient education:* Because of the efficiency of the EHR system, the physician has more personal time with the patient for counseling or patient education. In many systems the provider can display and annotate pictures of body areas for patient education, and print them so that the patient can take them home.

    When the patient is dressed, he or she is given patient education material, medication instructions, and a copy of the exam notes from the current visit. Allowing the patient to take away a written record of the visit enables better compliance with the doctor's plan of care and recommended treatments.

11. The patient is escorted to the checkout area.

    If x-rays or other diagnostic tests have been ordered at another facility, the office staff may call on behalf of the patient and schedule the tests.

    If a follow-up visit has been indicated, the patient will be scheduled for the next appointment.

12. If lab tests were ordered, the results are sent to the doctor electronically, are reviewed on screen, and automatically merged into the EHR.

    If radiology or other diagnostic reports are sent to the practice electronically as text reports, they are imported into the EHR and can be reviewed by the physician.

## A REAL-LIFE STORY

## Experiencing the Functional Benefits of an EHR
### By Henry Palmer, M.D.

*Henry Palmer, M.D., specializes in internal medicine and is affiliated with Rush University Medical Center.*

I am a physician practicing at two locations, neither of which is where my computers are. I have computers in the exam rooms and I am documenting with the patients, but the data is going over the Internet into the servers in real time.

Rush University Medical Center, like other large institutions, had many different computer systems in their departments. Trying to unite all these legacy systems was very difficult, but they wanted to be able to access all the information relatively easily from one system. Rush has a CDR or clinical data repository, which stores the data from various legacy systems. For example, the clinical notes section includes all of the radiology, ultrasound, stress testing, cardiology, and operative reports; these are transcribed reports, all text based.

Lab results, however, come in as data. The results are imported automatically. You can set how far back in time you want to default your view of them. This is very handy because you are able to see the trends. You can also graph it. You can rearrange the view to see your results horizontally or vertically.

It has demographic information for the patient, of course, and helpful information about admission and discharge. Let's say I want to look at the admission from two months ago. I can highlight it and find out who the providers were for that admission, the insurance information for that admission as well as the diagnosis.

Rush also has an order entry system. When you sign in, it automatically shows if you have a patient who is in the hospital. This is handy, particularly in the case of primary care physicians, because sometimes your patients get admitted without your knowledge. A patient may get admitted into the surgical service and you might never be called.

The order entry screen first shows if there are any orders approaching expiration. It also asks me to authenticate any verbal orders I had given over the phone, but had not yet countersigned.

I can pull up a patient and view results through the order system. I can look at results in different ways—results for the last five days, all the results since admission, or just the ones that were critical. I can see details about particular results, the normal ranges, and some additional information about how to interpret those results.

When I write a medication order, it goes electronically to the pharmacy. The order system will also provide alerts to drug interactions or areas of concern the hospital has identified with the drug. When ordering potassium, for example, the system would advise you that it should only be given in a certain quantity if the patient is on certain medications that tend to increase potassium levels anyway.

It is easy to order labs by just clicking one box. You can also order a consult. CPOE works. It's not perfect, but in a large institution like this it has to work or it wouldn't be used.

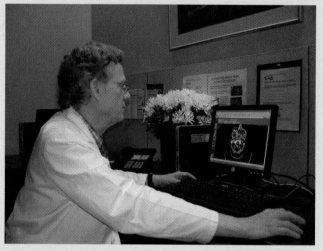

**FIGURE 7-17    Dr. Palmer reviews a CAT scan.**

Our PAC system eliminates the need to have to go down to radiology to see x-rays. On the average workstation you can view the images of the patients' x-rays with reasonable definition. If you want really fine detail, you can go to any of the high-definition monitors that are scattered around the hospital. You can also display the radiologist's report. Reading the report will guide you toward the areas of concern.

We also use an electronic signature program for signing off on charts. Basically this brings up the document, allows me to edit it, and I can finalize my signature. I can also indicate which doctors I want to receive copies of my document. The system will then automatically fax them to the doctors involved with the patient care.

Decision support includes access to the Rush medical library from inside our system. You enter your search term and it will retrieve an index of the article. You can go directly to what you wanted to read, for example, the treatment or the diagnostic approach to the disease.

One of the challenges as a primary care physician is that my patients are searching the Internet. They will often come in with research in hand and ask some very cogent questions. I think the downside can be that people assume that because they have read it on the Internet that it applies to them or that they know what to do with the information—and that is not always the case.

The biggest problem I see in health information technology today is the segregation of records, particularly between inpatient and outpatient systems. When patients are admitted, their outpatient records are not there. Synchronizing those, I think, would be a big step forward and also eliminate redundancy in testing.

Accessibility is not a problem in the EHR system because there is no chart to "refile." Multiple providers can access the patient's chart, even simultaneously; for example, a physician could review the previous lab results before entering the exam room, even if the nurse was currently entering vital signs in the chart.

---

# Chapter 7 Summary

## Evolution of Electronic Health Records

Though electronic health records have been called by various names for the past 30 years, the acronym EHR is currently used as shorthand for the electronic health record.

By EHR we mean the portion of a patient's medical records that is stored in a computer system *as well as the functional benefits* derived from having an electronic health record.

The IOM put forth a set of eight core functions that an EHR should be capable of performing:

- Health information and data
- Result management
- Order management
- Decision support
- Electronic communication and connectivity
- Patient support
- Administrative processes and reporting
- Reporting and population health

The CPRI has identified three key criteria for an EHR:

- Capture data at the point of care.
- Integrate data from multiple sources.
- Provide decision support.

Social changes driving the need for EHR include an increasingly mobile society, where patients move and change doctors more frequently. Additionally, patients today see multiple specialists for their care. This means their medical record no longer resides with a single general practitioner who provides their total care. Thus, the ability to share exam records and test results is important to the patient's continuity of care.

Healthcare organizations, medical schools, employers, and even the government have recognized the importance of computerizing the various components of the medical record. Studies from the IOM and others have shown that a large number of deaths occur from preventable medical errors; many are caused by not having access to the patient's medical information.

The EHR can help to improve patient health, the quality of care, and patient safety by providing access to complete, up-to-date records of past and present conditions. This enables EHR records to be used in ways that paper medical records cannot.

## Functional Benefits of an EHR

The form in which patient records are stored will affect the ability to achieve the functional benefits of EHRs identified by the IOM. The format of the data determines to what extent the data can be used dynamically by the computer to extend the EHR. The forms of data are broadly categorized into three types:

1. Digital image data (provides increased accessibility).
2. Text-based data (provides accessibility and text search capability and can be reformatted for display on different devices).
3. Discrete data, fielded and ideally codified (provides all of the above plus the capability to be used for alerts, health maintenance, and data exchange).

The term *codified* refers to the system of assigning standard codes to medical terms that underlie the description which is visible to the user. Codified records also make it easy to find, share, and search patient records.

EHR coding systems are called nomenclatures. EHR nomenclatures differ from billing codes in that EHR nomenclatures have many more codes used to describe the detail of the exam such as the symptoms, history, observations, and plan. SNOMED-CT and Medcin are EHR nomenclatures. LOINC is a nomenclature primarily used for lab tests.

EHR software allows clinicians to document the patient exam by selecting findings for symptoms, history, physical examination, tests, diagnoses, and therapy.

The functional benefits of an EHR include health maintenance, trend analysis, alerts and decision support:

- *Health maintenance* improves patient health through prevention and disease management. Immunizations, patient education, counseling on preventive measures, and early detection through appropriate screening help patients live healthier lives.

  Immunizations must be acquired over time. Using the data in the chart, the EHR compares the patient's immunization history to the schedule recommended by the CDC (or state health department) to determine what vaccine is due and when.

  Disease prevention through periodic screening and early detection can also save lives. Health maintenance programs generate patient-specific guidelines by comparing the electronic patient records to the recommendations of the U.S. Preventive Services Task Force. Using this information the clinician can order tests, discuss important healthcare options, and recommend lifestyle changes to the patient at the point of care.

- *Trend analysis* presents test results, vital signs, or other EHR data from several dates in a side-by-side comparison or graph that allows the clinician to spot trends in the patient's health records. Examples of data presentations that are useful for trend analysis include cumulative summary reports, graphs, growth charts, and flow sheets.

- *Alerts* are messages or reminders that are automatically generated by the EHR to make the provider aware of a special situation. For example an electronic prescription system generates a DUR alert when two drugs known to have adverse interactions are prescribed for the same patient. Other examples of alerts include drug formulary checking, alerts generated when lab results are outside the normal range, and alerts when an ordered test will require the patient to sign an ABN form.

- *Decision support* refers to the ability of EHR systems to quickly access evidence-based information relevant to the findings of the current case. These might include defined protocols, results of case studies, or standard care guidelines prepared by specialists, medical societies, or government organizations. Drug formularies and dosing guidelines are also forms of decision support.

These functional benefits are made possible by EHR data primarily consisting of codified records. When an EHR uses a national standard nomenclature for its codes, many other functional benefits can be realized, including reducing the time it takes for the clinician to document the exam and the ability to exchange data electronically in a RHIO.

## Capturing and Recording EHR Data

Completely documenting a visit before the patient ever leaves the office is the easiest way to use an EHR and provides the most rewarding benefits from the system.

A significant contribution of data into an EHR can come from sources other than direct entry by the clinic staff. Examples include word processed files from dictated exam notes that have been transcribed and electronic lab orders and results.

Many healthcare organizations scan paper documents into the EHR. Though document images do not offer the benefits of a codified medical record, they do provide widespread accessibility and a means to include source documents for a complete electronic chart.

Numerous studies have shown that patient-entered data can also become a significant contributor to the EHR for some of the following reasons:

- Only the patient has the information about what symptoms were present at the outset of the illness and what the outcome of medical treatment of those symptoms was.
- The patient is also the source of past medical, family, and social history.
- Patient-entered data is a more accurate reflection of a patient's complaints.

- Patients who can review their histories are better prepared for the visit.
- Patient-entered data is organized by the computer for the provider in a succinct and easy-to-read format that becomes the starting point for the patient encounter.
- Up to 67% of the nurse or clinician's time with the patient is spent entering the patient's symptoms into the visit documentation.
- It allows the clinician more time to discuss the treatment plan with the patient.

EHR systems use features such as lists, forms, search, and prompt to preload the findings that are likely to be needed for each type of patient.

- *Lists:* Lists allow the clinician or medical practice to view a subset of the nomenclature typically used for a particular condition or type of exam.

  Because shorter lists mean less scrolling, lists speed up data entry of routine exams. Lists are flexible and can contain as many findings as necessary to document a typical visit.

- *Forms:* Forms display a desired group of findings in a presentation that allows for quick entry of not only positive and negative findings but of entry details, such as a value or result. Forms also provide other features that lists cannot:

  1. Forms are static; findings have a fixed position on forms and will consistently remain in that position, every time the form is used.
  2. Findings from multiple sections of the nomenclature can be mixed on the same page of the form in any way to enable the quickest data entry.
  3. Forms may include check boxes, drop-down lists, pop-up calendars, and even free-text boxes for recording comments.
  4. Forms can control which findings are required and which are optional; every question on a form does not have to be answered for every visit.

- *Search:* The search function provides a quick way to locate a desired finding in the nomenclature. Search addresses semantic differences in medical terms in three ways:

  1. The search function performs automatic word completion, so if you search for *knee* but the finding is for *knees*, it will still find it.
  2. The nomenclatures includes an extensive list of synonyms, which are used in an alternate word search.
  3. The search function identifies related findings in other tabs, so that when you search for a word or phrase in a particular tab, related findings are automatically available in the other tabs.

- *Prompt:* This is short for "prompt with current finding." The prompt feature generates a list of findings that are clinically related to a finding that was highlighted when Prompt was clicked.

- *Flow sheets:* When clinicians treat patients with long-term conditions, they sometimes prefer to use flow sheets to view data from multiple encounters in columnar form. This format allows for a side-by-side comparison of findings over a period of time.
- *Orders:* Electronic ordering systems allow a provider to write an order and document it in the exam note in one step.
- *Protocols:* Sometimes called order sets, protocols are lists of tests, treatments, therapy, or plans of care recommended for certain diagnoses. The use of protocols or order sets helps the clinician quickly order and document the plan of care for the patient.

### Electronic Signatures

When the clinician has completed an exam note or signs an order in an EHR, it is signed electronically. A valid electronic signature must meet three criteria:

1. **Message Integrity:** Message integrity means the recipient must be able to confirm that the document has not been altered since it was signed.

2. **Nonrepudiation:** The signer must not be able to deny signing the document.
3. **User Authentication:** The recipient must be able to confirm that the signature was in fact "signed" by the real person.

### Flow of an Office Fully Using EHRs

Review Figure 7-16 and the associated description of the workflow of an office fully using an EHR. Notice how efficient it is when the patient, nurse, and doctor document the encounter at the point of care. Patient care is improved because orders and results transmitted electronically save time and can help prevent medication errors and duplicate tests. Patient compliance is improved when the patient can leave with a complete record of the visit and relevant patient education materials.

## Critical Thinking Exercises

1. The topic of electronic health records is frequently in the news. Describe something you have read or seen on TV about EHRs.
2. How would you react if your doctor asked you to fill out your medical history on a computer instead of a paper form? Do you think there are some people who would have difficulty with this? If so, give examples.

## Testing Your Knowledge of Chapter 7

1. What is the definition of an EHR?
2. What is advantage of codified data over document imaged data?
3. Name at least three forces driving the change to the EHR.
4. List the three criteria of an electronic signature.
5. List at least two ways codified data in the EHR can be used to manage and prevent disease.
6. What is a flow sheet?
7. What is a nomenclature?

*The tabs on the left of the EHR screen are used to logically group findings. The tabs have medical abbreviations. Write the meaning of each of the following:*

8. Sx _____

9. Hx _____

10. Px _____
11. Tx _____
12. Dx _____
13. Rx _____
14. Name at least two benefits of having patients entering their own symptoms and history into the computer.
15. Describe at least two differences between lists and forms.

# 8 Additional Health Information Systems

After completing this chapter, you should be able to:

- Describe departmental health record systems
- Explain how departmental health record systems contribute to the EHR
- Discuss the factors that cause facilities to use multiple information systems
- Describe patient registration and master patient indexes
- Describe the workflow of electronic lab orders and results
- Describe radiology information systems
- Describe workflow dictation and transcription
- Explain how speech recognition works
- Describe pharmacy, emergency department, and surgical information systems
- Compare implant and transplant registries
- Explain the concept of clinical trials

## ACRONYMS USED IN CHAPTER 8

Acronyms are used extensively in both medicine and computers. The following acronyms are used in this chapter.

| | | | |
|---|---|---|---|
| **ADT** | Admission, Discharge, Transfer System | **EHR** | Electronic Health Record |
| **CAP** | College of American Pathologists | **EMT** | Emergency Medical Technician |
| **CAT** | Computerized Axial Tomography | **ER** | Emergency Room or Department |
| **CD** | Compact Disk | **FDA** | Food and Drug Administration |
| **CDR** | Clinical Data Repository | **HIS** | Health Information System |
| **CIO** | Chief Information Officer | **HL7** | Health Level 7 |
| **CPOE** | Computerized Physician Order Entry; Computerized Provider Order Entry | **ICU** | Intensive Care Unit |
| | | **IOM** | Institute of Medicine of the National Academies |
| **CR** | Computed Radiography | **IV** | Intravenous |
| **CT SCAN** | Computed Tomography Scan | **LIS** | Laboratory Information System |
| **DICOM** | Digital Imaging and Communications in Medicine | **LOS** | Length of Stay |
| | | **MPI** | Master Patient Index |
| **DNR** | Do Not Resuscitate | **MRI** | Magnetic Resonance Imaging |
| **DR** | Digital Radiography | **NMDP** | National Marrow Donor Program |
| **DUR** | Drug Utilization Review | | |
| **ECG** | Electrocardiogram | **OR** | Operating Room |

| **PACS OR PAC SYSTEM**  Picture Archiving and Communication System | **RIS** | Radiology Information System |
| | **UNOS** | United Network for Organ Sharing |
| **PET**  Positron Emission Tomography | | |
| **RFID**  Radio-Frequency Identification | **VBC** | Visible Black Character |

# Departmental Information Systems

After reading the previous chapters, you might imagine that a hospital or doctor's office has one large health record computer system. The reality, however, is that health records originate from many separate systems. Some of these records are imported into the EHR or into a central clinical data repository (CDR). Others are retrieved and displayed from the EHR but actually remain stored on their respective systems.

The overall health information system (HIS) includes both clinical and administrative systems. This chapter will focus primarily on systems that are used by the various specialized departments as they perform their daily tasks and that act as the source of data for certain aspects of the EHR. Administrative, billing, and management systems will be discussed in Chapters 9 through 12.

The HIS and even the EHR system are typically not a single software package, but rather a complex arrangement of multiple individual systems contributing data to the whole patient record. It is not uncommon for an inpatient facility HIS to be comprised of 60 to 400 different software applications. Ambulatory facilities with an EHR may have 2 to 6 different systems. Hospitals have these disparate systems in place for many reasons. First, what is the overall philosophy of the IT selection committee?

*Integrated Systems Approach:*   An integrated systems approach biases decisions toward software compatibility. Insofar as possible, the approach calls for using one vendor's systems and where that isn't possible selecting systems that have been interfaced with the vendor's systems at other hospitals.

An integrated systems approach has the advantage that everything works together and there are fewer vendors to deal with. The disadvantage is that the preferred vendor's solution for certain departments may lack functionality offered by the competition, or the vendor may not offer software for those departments, forcing the hospital to select nonintegrated software anyway.

*Best-of-Breed Approach:*   The best-of-breed approach is to select systems that best meet a department's needs, regardless of the vendor. This ensures maximum software functionality for the individual departments. The disadvantage of this approach is that department software products may not work with the EHR or may require custom interfaces. This approach also requires IT to deal with more vendors and makes it more difficult to resolve software and interface issues.

Another reason hospitals sometimes have different software systems is because certain departments wield more influence with the hospital management and have the power to select their own software, even if it is incompatible with other systems. Another reason is that CAT scan, MRI, and PET equipment and even ICU monitors or other biomedical devices may come with their own software, which is required to operate the device. These systems must then be interfaced with the hospital registration, CPOE, and EHR systems.

Outpatient facilities that are not affiliated with hospitals, such as a doctor's office, tend to have fewer systems. Usually the doctors are the decision makers and typically a practice management system is already well established. If the practice management vendor offers an acceptable EHR system, that will be the system of choice. However, if the office has its own laboratory, a separate laboratory information system (LIS) will be used. Similarly, if the office has ECG or other diagnostic equipment, software supplied with the device may need to be interfaced. Specialists may have additional software important to their specialty. Radiologists may have a radiology information system (RIS) and a small PAC system. Cardiologists have many different diagnostic devices and, therefore, may have different software for each of them.

In summary, inpatient facilities generally consider the HIS to be the principal system and the various department systems to be ancillary systems that are integrated or interfaced with the HIS. Ambulatory facilities generally consider the practice management system to be the principal system and the EHR is often a component of it, from the same vendor. Other software in the doctor's office usually consists of programs for specific equipment that may or may not be interfaced to the EHR.

## Patient Registration

Though most of this chapter will discuss clinical departmental systems that contribute to the patient health record, one administrative system is key to both paper and electronic charts: the patient registration system and master patient index (MPI). In some facilities this is called the admission, discharge, transfer (ADT) system.

The patient registration system contains demographic information about the patient such as name, address, sex, date of birth, and next of kin. It also contains guarantor and insurance information used for billing. Figure 8-1 shows a patient registration screen from the Paragon Community Hospital information system.

ADT systems may also store some clinical data, such as the admitting and discharge diagnosis, LOS, and organ donor, DNR, consent, and other forms that have been signed by the patient. These will be discussed in Chapter 9.

Most important to the HIM department, the patient registration record contains the patient's medical record number. In an HIM department that files paper charts numerically, the patient registration or MPI system is necessary to find the chart. In a computerized facility, the patient registration record is used by the EHR and every departmental system to connect the electronic health records to the correct patient.

At one time the master patient index was manually kept on file cards. Today however, even paper-based facilities have computerized their patient registration and MPI processes.

The master patient index (MPI) may be a separate system or merely an index of the patient database, depending on the facility. Large healthcare organizations comprised of multiple

**FIGURE 8-1**

**Patient registration screen.**

(Courtesy of McKesson Corporation.)

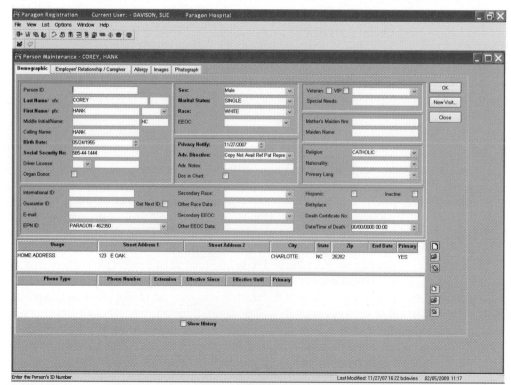

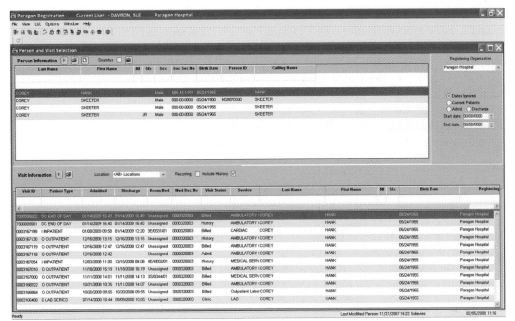

**FIGURE 8-2**

**Master patient index.**

(Courtesy of McKesson Corporation.)

facilities maintain the MPI as a separate database, combining the patient information from multiple registration systems. Facilities that are not affiliated with other entities may use the patient registration database as the MPI; this is especially true of group medical practices. If the MPI is a separate database, it will contain fewer fields than the registration system, typically first name, middle name, surname, suffix, date of birth, sex, and a unique ID field.

The main purposes of the MPI are to provide patient lookup and prevent duplicate registrations of the same patient. Figure 8-2 shows the master patient index for the Paragon Community Hospital information system.

The MPI or registration system may also include a *Soundex* field. Soundex[1] is used to codify the phonetic sounds of surnames. The Soundex code consists of the first letter of the surname followed by a three-digit numeric code, for example, P630. The code is determined according to the table shown in Figure 8-3. Soundex is used for driver's licenses, college student registration, genealogy searches, the U.S. Census Bureau, and healthcare organizations. The purpose of the Soundex

| Soundex | |
|---|---|
| Letters | Code |
| B, F, P, V | 1 |
| C, G, J, K, Q, S, X, Z | 2 |
| D, T | 3 |
| L | 4 |
| M, N | 5 |
| R | 6 |
| A, E, H, I, O, U, W, Y | Skipped |
| Zeroes are added if the code is less than 3 digits long | 0 |
| If code is longer than 3 digits extra digits are dropped | |

**FIGURE 8-3**
**Table for determining Soundex codes**

[1]Soundex was created and patented by Robert C. Russell in 1918.

lookup is to find surnames that sound phonetically alike when the user is unsure of the spelling. For example, the Soundex for Pardee is P630; Partie, Prat, and Parad are also P630. Soundex lookup provides the user with a list of similar sounding names from which they might locate the correct patient.

# Laboratory Services

A laboratory information system (LIS) receives orders and sends results of medical tests performed by the lab. Laboratory services consist of many sciences:

- Hematology
- Chemistry
- Immunology
- Blood bank (donor and transfusion)
- Pathology
- Surgical pathology
- Cytology
- Microbiology
- Flow cytometry

Automated laboratory instruments, which are used to analyze blood and other samples, typically have an electronic interface connected to the LIS. This enables the test equipment to transfer test results directly to the LIS database. The LIS can also send information about the equipment. For example, some instruments are capable of running several different types of tests. The LIS system can translate ordered test codes into instructions that it then sends to the test equipment.

The HL7 interface standard (discussed in Chapter 4) is used to connect the LIS with HIS, CPOE, EHR, and other healthcare systems.

Figure 8-4 shows a laboratory information system screen displaying a batch of instrument results for patients and quality control material. Color-coded alerts are used to draw the

**FIGURE 8-4**

**LIS display of results received from an automated instrument.**

(Courtesy of Sunquest Information Systems.)

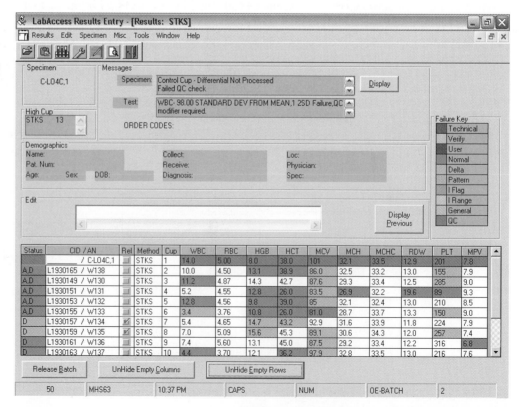

technologist's attention to those results that might need extra review or need to be repeated to verify high or low results or a significant change from the last time the patient had the same test run.

Not all lab work is performed by automated equipment. For example, some tests are performed by growing *cultures* and examining them, or by examining tissue or other samples through a microscope. The doctor who performs this work is a specialist called a pathologist. There are several areas of pathology:

- Clinical pathology uses chemistry, microbiology, hematology, and molecular pathology to analyze blood, urine, and other body fluids.
- Anatomic pathology performs gross, microscopic, and molecular examination of organs and tissues and autopsies of whole bodies. Surgical pathology performs gross and microscopic examination of tissue removed from a patient by surgery or biopsy.

Test results are first stored in the LIS and then transferred to the EHR. Test results that are not electronically transferred into the LIS are manually entered. The pathology report is usually a text report, but it is also stored in the LIS.

Figure 8-5 shows the workflow of a laboratory test. Review the figure as you read the following steps:

1. The clinician orders one or more tests for the patient. The order is recorded in the patient records and sent to the LIS system. The order is assigned a unique ID called a requisition or accession number.

2. A nurse, phlebotomist, or medical technician receives the order and obtains the required specimen from the patient. The specimen containers are labeled with the patient ID and requisition number. In many facilities the labels have barcodes. When several tests are

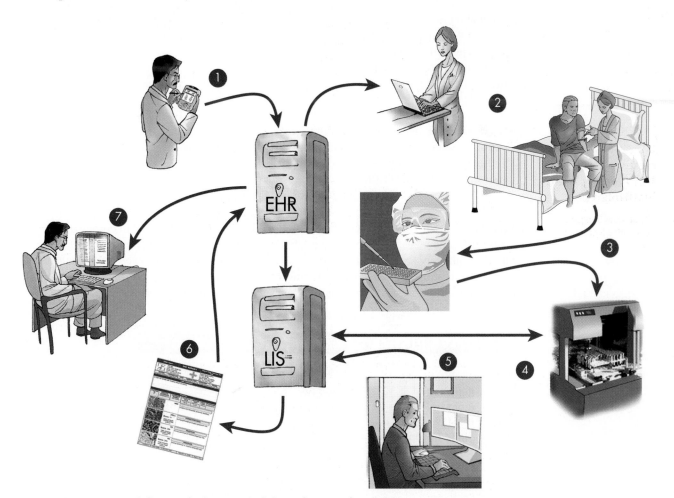

**FIGURE 8-5** **Workflow of electronic lab orders and results.**

ordered, multiple tubes of blood may be drawn, one for each type of test. In other instances the blood may be divided into separate samples at the lab.

3. The collected specimen is sent to the lab where its receipt is recorded in the LIS. Manual or automated testing begins with preparation of the specimen sample. The specimen labels and test orders are verified to ensure the right test is performed on the right patient.

4. If the testing will be performed by an automated analyzer, the order is downloaded to the instrument and the sample is placed in the analyzer. The equipment reads the barcode on the label, locates the downloaded information, and performs the ordered test(s).

5. When an automated test is complete, the analyzer sends the results to the LIS. Results are autoverified, verified by repeat analysis, and/or checked by the lab technician and pathologist. When a manual test is complete, the lab technician or pathologist enters the result manually in the LIS. Pathology reports may also be dictated; the transcribed report is then stored in the LIS and also sent to the EHR.

6. The lab report is generated by the LIS and then faxed, printed, or sent electronically to the EHR—or in some facilities, all of the above.

7. The ordering physician, nurses, pharmacists, and other care providers read the results report and respond appropriately.

Not all tests are performed in the laboratory. Certain tests may be performed by handheld instruments at the patient's bedside or even the patient's home. This is called point-of-care testing. One example of such an instrument is a glucose monitor. The glucose monitor measures the amount of a type of sugar in a patient's blood. The results of this test can be electronically transferred from the glucose monitor device to the EHR. In a hospital, this is usually transferred through the LIS.

Medical laboratories are accredited by the College of American Pathologists (CAP). CAP accreditation is so thorough that it is accepted by the Joint Commission. In addition to the laboratory itself, CAP accreditation requires that nurses and other inpatient personnel who perform point-of-care tests at bedside be trained and certified to do so.

In addition to test orders and results, the LIS can be used to perform and keep track of non-patient-related duties. For example, it is necessary for the lab to calibrate the equipment periodically and to keep maintenance logs; the LIS system can do this.

The LIS provides management tools for maintaining records of the test equipment, certification of lab technicians who perform the tests, and nurses who perform point-of-care testing. Control tests are performed as required; serial or lot numbers of materials used for the tests are also tracked. These records are necessary for CAP audits and are, therefore, one of the most important benefits of the LIS.

### Stat Tests

*Stat,* from the term *statim,* means "without delay." It is used in the hospital to convey urgency in many instances of patient care. In the laboratory, stat orders are given the highest priority. Surgical pathology orders are sometimes ordered stat because the surgeon needs the results while the surgery is still going on. Nearly all orders from an emergency department are ordered stat, because the results are usually needed for the diagnosis or emergency care of patients.

---

**THE FIVE RIGHTS OF LABORATORY TESTING**[2]

1. Right patient
2. Right test
3. Right time
4. Right results
5. Right diagnosis

---

[2]Adapted from *Effective Diagnostic Decisions: The Five Rights of Laboratory Testing* (Tucson, AZ: Sunquest Information Systems, 2009), www.sunquestinfo.com.

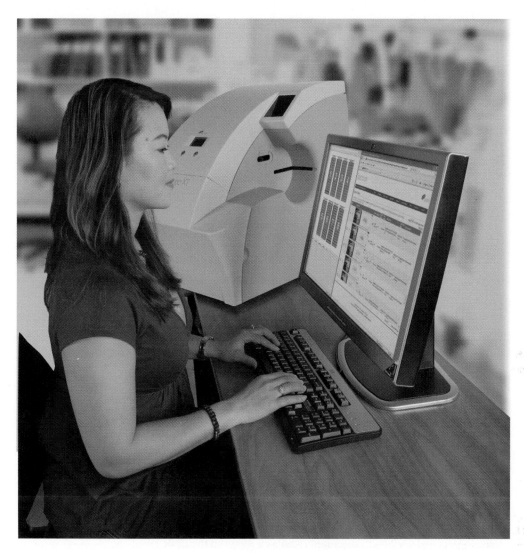

**FIGURE 8-6**

**A pathologist examines a specimen using digital pathology.**

(Courtesy of Aperio, Inc.)

## Digital Pathology

Digital pathology imaging systems work like a microscope, except that the image of the specimen slide is captured digitally. A computer monitor is used to display the image and allows the pathologist to digitally stain, zoom, or otherwise enhance the image. Computer software can also be used to recognize unusual patterns or cells in the image. A digital pathology system, the Aperio ScanScope XT™, is shown in Figure 8-6.

Recent developments can also use ranges of light beyond the visible spectrum, allowing pathologists to see what the human eye cannot. Another new breakthrough produces 3-D images of cells and proteins using a technology that works similar to a miniature MRI.

Digital pathology images can be stored in a PAC system. The advent of digital pathology has the potential to make the pathologist's workflow more like that of a radiologist.

# Radiology Department

Radiologists are physicians who specialize in interpreting diagnostic images of the patient, such as x-rays and CT scans. The information systems they use are specific to the needs of their department, not a standard function of a generalized EHR or HIS system. Radiology departments typically have a radiology information system (RIS), a picture archiving and communication system (PACS) for storing diagnostic images, and a dictation/transcription or voice recognition system.

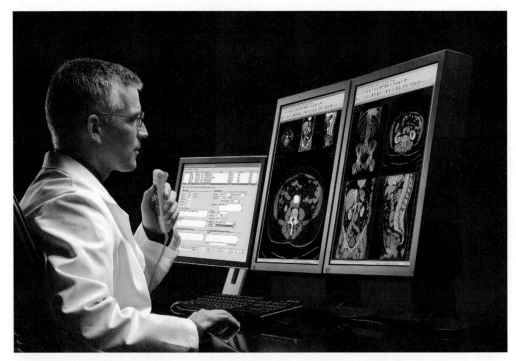

**FIGURE 8-7**    **Radiologist dictates report; monitors display RIS and PAC system.**

(Photo provided courtesy of Carestream Health, Inc.)

The radiology department will also have a large number of interfaces. Because the RIS is not typically a module of the HIS, interfaces to registration and billing will be necessary. Also, most of the imaging devices used in the department will transfer images directly to the PACS; the devices may also be capable of receiving order and patient data electronically from the RIS system. Patient data is then incorporated in the image when it is captured. Interfaces will be used to receive orders and send the transcribed radiology report to the EHR.

In Figure 8-7, a radiologist dictates the radiology report concerning the images displayed on the center and right monitors in the photo. The monitor on the left displays information from the RIS.

### Digital X-Ray Images

Traditional x-rays used to be taken on photographic film. To be stored in a PAC system, the film then had to be digitized using a scanner. Today, x-ray systems can record the image on a special plate that captures the image digitally, eliminating the steps of developing the film and then scanning it. Terminology from the days of film is still used though. For example, a set of related images interpreted by the radiologist is called a *study*; a *hanging* protocol refers to the number of images that simultaneously display on the radiologist's monitor. The term comes from the days when x-ray films were viewed by hanging them on light boxes.

---

**FLASH CARD**

Some x-rays are still taken with photographic film. When images are captured on film, a flash card is used. A flash card is a small card with the patient's name or ID on it that is photographed on the negative at the time the x-ray is exposed. This ensures that the x-ray is matched to the proper patient when the films are developed. Digital systems do not need a flash card; the patient information is stored in the DICOM file containing the image. DICOM stands for Digital Imaging and Communications in Medicine.

### CAT/CT, MRI, and PET Images

In addition to x-rays, other equipment used in the radiology department can capture images digitally and transfer them to a PAC system. These include:

- *Computerized axial tomography* (CAT) systems use x-rays to see into the patient's body and capture thousands of digital images. Using computer software, it then constructs a view of cross sections of the body from the digital images. In some facilities this is also referred to as CT or computed tomography.

- *Magnetic resonance imaging* (MRI) uses magnetic fields and pulses of energy to create images of organs and structures inside the body that cannot be seen by x-ray or CAT scan. Figure 8-8 shows an MRI device.

- *Positron emission tomography* (PET) combines CT and nuclear scanning using a radioactive substance called a tracer, which is injected into a patient's vein. A computer records the tracer as it collects in certain organs, then converts the data into 3-D images of the organ. PET can be used to detect or evaluate cancer.

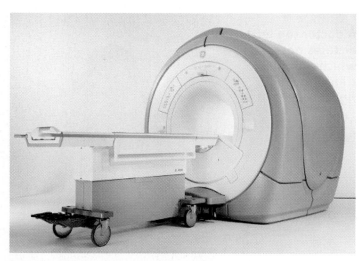

**FIGURE 8-8**
**Magnetic resonance imaging.**

(Used with permission of GE Healthcare.)

### High-Resolution Monitors

The radiologist must be able to see the smallest detail to ensure an accurate interpretation. To facilitate this, the computer monitor (screen) used by the radiologist has a higher resolution than a typical computer screen. *Resolution* refers to the size and number of pixels the screen can display. Radiology monitors have much smaller pixels, so they are capable of displaying a much larger quantity of them. This gives the radiologist a much better view of the image. The software radiologists use to view the image also has many features that allow the radiologist to enhance the digital image. Features include the ability to zoom in or out, change the contrast, and compare several images side by side.

## Dictation/Transcription Systems

Dictation systems are prevalent in healthcare. The clinician dictates his or her notes into a recording device. The dictation is subsequently transcribed (typed) by a professional called a medical transcriptionist. When completed, the transcribed document is returned to the clinician to review and approve.

The concept of dictating medical notes and having them transcribed has been around for many years. Transcribed documents provided a great improvement over illegible handwritten notes and reports. However, the process causes a significant delay between the time when patients are treated and when their charts are updated. It also does not produce a codified medical record and adds numerous steps to the workflow:

1. The doctor examines the patient.
2. The doctor dictates the note (usually from memory after leaving the exam room).
3. The recording of the dictation is sent to the transcriptionist.
4. The transcriptionist types the document as he or she listens to the recording.
5. The transcriptionist or a supervisor checks the document for accuracy.
6. The document is sent to the doctor for approval.
7. The doctor reads the document (usually without benefit of the original recording).
8. If there are errors, the doctor notes the necessary corrections and waits for the transcriptionist to make the changes.

**FIGURE 8-9**
**A doctor (on left) dictates notes which are then transcribed (on right).**

(Photos Courtesy Nuance, Inc.)

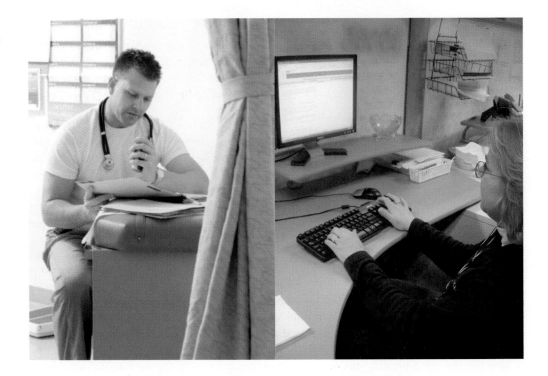

**9.** The doctor signs the completed document.

**10.** A file clerk pulls the patient chart from the filing system, inserts the document, and refiles the chart.

One of the benefits of an EHR is to eliminate the time delay and extra work inherent in using dictation/transcription for most medical specialties. The EHR improves the workflow because the note is finished when the exam is finished and does not require additional steps of transcribing, reviewing, and filing. There are, however, some specialties where dictation/transcription is likely to continue. Two of the specialties mentioned in this chapter, pathology and radiology, are examples.

Pathologists performing autopsies must dictate their findings because they cannot use a keyboard at that time. Similarly, radiologists use the computer to display and manipulate images, which keeps their hands busy, so they cannot easily type at the same time. Therefore, most radiologists dictate their observations as they are viewing them.

In both group practices and hospitals, there may also be some established physicians who are unwilling to stop dictating their exam notes or discharge summaries. In these cases, word-processed files of the transcribed documents can be imported into the EHR. This is preferable to scanning the typed document.

There are also costs associated with transcription. Transcription charges are based on number of lines or words that are transcribed. Line calculations are based on a 65-character line. A newer method proposed for calculating transcription charges is based on visible black characters (VBCs); in other words, characters you can see (not spaces or tabs).[3]

Dictation may be recorded on microcassette tapes, digital voice files, or even via telephone. Transcriptionists use special equipment that allows their hands to remain on the keyboard (Figure 8-9). A foot pedal controls the playback of the recording as the transcriptionist word processes the report.

---

[3]*A Standard Unit of Measure for Transcribed Reports,* AHIMA/MTIA Joint Task Force on Standards Development White Paper (Chicago: AHIMA, February 14, 2007), http://library.ahima.org/xpedio/groups/public/documents/ahima/bok1_034023.html.

## Speech Recognition Software

Speech recognition software translates the sounds of the human voice into text. In some places it is used to eliminate the dictation/transcription steps; elsewhere it is used to complement the process, by providing the transcriptionist with a text file to be reviewed and edited. Because radiologists rely heavily on dictation/transcription, they are leading the way in using voice recognition systems.

Having clinical dictation instantly and automatically transcribed by a computer reduces turnaround time and reduces or eliminates the cost of a transcription service. For some doctors, speech recognition systems can accurately recognize up to 99% of their words, but with most people, it seems to average about 95%. This means a full-length dictation will have one or more errors that must be corrected. The time spent backing up and making corrections slows down the overall rate of efficiency. This is one reason some practices using speech recognition software continue to use transcriptionists to edit and correct their documents.

Even though speech recognition systems make errors, they improve as they are used. Each time the speaker makes a correction, the system learns a little more about the speaker's voice patterns. Recognition is also improved by using special medical versions of the software that recognize medical terms that might not be used in a layperson's vocabulary.

Most often speech recognition is used to produce a text document, but it is possible to use speech recognition to produce a codified medical record. Ray Kurzweil, a scientist and inventor, brought the first commercial large vocabulary speech recognition systems to medicine in 1985. By 1990, his system was able to create structured medical records by voice recognition alone. Today at least one system, CliniTalk, enables a clinician to use speech recognition to record findings hands-free in the same EHR shown in Chapter 7, Figure 7-11.

**HOW SPEECH RECOGNITION SOFTWARE WORKS**   The words we speak are really made up of multiple sounds called *phonemes*. When you look up a word in the dictionary, you will find its pronunciation represented with symbols for its phonemes (for example, **phoneme**: fō´nĕm).

In English, there are about 16 vowel sounds and 24 consonants making about 50 phonemes. Computer scientists measuring electrical patterns of sound waves found that phonemes were represented by differing levels of energy across various frequency bands over a period of time.

The first step in speech recognition is to transform the sound of your voice into a digital file. A noise-canceling microphone discards background noise and sends your word sounds to the computer, which converts it into digital data.

Using mathematical calculations, the speech recognition software identifies the phonemes in the digital data. The phonemes are then compared to the "language model," which contains the rules of the speech recognition software.

Because certain sounds would be impossible to articulate, phonemes cannot appear in just any order. Therefore, the language model knows that only certain sequences of phonemes actually correspond to words or word syllables.

An average word has about six phonemes. Most people speak about three words per second. This means the computer must process about 18 phonemes per second. The software must not only identify the phonemes, it must also group them correctly into words. For example, the phonemes b + el instantly match "bell" while t + el match "tell." Though English has 10,000 possible syllables, these also will normally appear only in certain combinations and sequences.

One problem is that words such as *they're, their,* and *there* sound alike. To identify the correct word, the language model compares groups of three to four words called *trigrams* to common speech patterns to help it identify the correct word. For example, if you dictated: "There appears to be a blockage . . . ," the software would recognize that you didn't mean *their* or *they're* by the placement of the word *there* in the sentence.

Once the correct words are identified, they are displayed on the screen as though you had keyed them in. Usually there is a lag of a few seconds between the words you just spoke and the appearance of the text on your screen. If the software misidentifies a word, you can back up and correct it.

Each time the software misrecognizes a word and you correct it using the speech recognition software, the computer stores your pronunciation for the corrected word. The next time you dictate that word, it will then identify it correctly.

## A REAL-LIFE STORY

# Radiology in the Digital Age

*By Wesley McCann*

*Wesley McCann, BA, MA, RT-R, a Registered Technologist in Radiography and PACS clinical assistant at a large hospital in Michigan.*

---

Our radiologists work in a darkened room using multiple monitors, three to four in most cases. One monitor displays our RIS (radiology information system), while images associated with these charges are retrieved from the PACS (picture archiving and communication system) and displayed on two high-resolution monitors, normally 2 to 5 megapixels. A dual-monitor review station can cost $49,000, compared to a few hundred dollars for the normal CRT monitors used by the radiological technologists and most other personnel in the hospital. Our RIS is where we enter, store, and review all patient radiology charges.

Before PACS, every patient study was handled by numerous people before the radiologist. This goes back to the days when staff would have to hang films in a certain order on a large image viewing box, like that seen on the show *Scrubs*. Staff would have to find old relevant exams for that patient and hang them in a certain order according to the radiologist's preference. For example, if a person came in for a chest x-ray, the staff would find an old chest x-ray and hang it alongside the new exam in a certain order. This is called *hanging protocol*. The radiologist's hanging protocol and prior relevancy rules will determine how many studies are displayed and how the images are arranged on the screen. Each radiologist is very particular about how they want to review studies. With PACS, we can automate this entire process.

In general radiology we have what we call a study tree under which the exams are organized. Different parts of the anatomy are separated into different groups. If the technologist selects chest x-ray, everything that could be captured during a chest x-ray would be available for them. They can then choose ribs or chest within that subset. PACS puts the entire exam realm at their fingertips.

With film, the radiologist never had the capability to change the image contrast level, making it brighter or darker. You just had an image. If it wasn't perfect, you had to take it again. With a digital x-ray, radiologists can adjust the image any way they wish, which is good for the patient because it will reduce the radiation exposure caused by repeated studies due to inferior images.

We use both computed radiography (CR) and digital radiography (DR) systems for general radiology. The advantage of CR is that it uses the same x-ray equipment used for film-based x-rays, except

that a phosphor plate captures the image instead of film. However, the CR image plate must then be scanned and digitized using a CR reader, which converts the analog image to digital.

With digital radiography, no digital conversion is required. Images are captured digitally and displayed instantly, thereby decreasing the time technologists have to wait to review their study. If there is a disadvantage to DR, it is that it requires replacing existing equipment, and DR systems can cost up to four times as much as CR systems.

All of our radiology images are stored on our PACS archive in DICOM files. DICOM is a national standard that most vendors are now adhering to. DICOM files include data fields about the patient and the study. We no longer have to use flash cards to burn that information on the image; PACS takes care of that. Most everything is DICOM based, but we have to map it specifically for each machine. For example, our CR machine populates a field called "series description." But when we purchased a new DR from a different vendor, we had to program PACS so that it would populate the field, otherwise there was no data there and we would have had to manually type it in.

We also can import studies the patients bring with them on CD, or that we receive electronically over a high-speed network connection we have with the University of Michigan. However, our PACS is very strict; the patient, the medical record number, and the accession number have to match or else the system will not allow us to import the images correctly. To accomplish this, we create an order number and assign the imported images to it. When the doctor pulls the images up, it will clearly indicate that it is from an outside source, and is only for comparison, not interpretation.

We can also burn a CD for patients to take with them. We do this a lot for ER patients, so they can take copies of their x-rays back to their physician. Normally we can fit an entire study on a CD, but longer studies like angiograms may require two disks.

PACS has increased the availability of data to be exchanged from facility to facility, reduced patient exposure, and improved patient care. PACS has also allowed the healthcare community to make a patient health record portable in one form or another. No longer does a patient have to carry film jackets. With PACS, their entire record can be recorded on a few CDs.

---

Speech recognition software must also deal with the diversity of regional accents and the variety of ways that we pronounce words. Most programs start with a simple training session in which you read into the software a document that it already recognizes. It then compares your pronunciation of the words to its existing language model and adjusts accordingly. It continues to build a personal profile of your speech by learning from its mistakes.

Modern speech recognition software typically comes with a vocabulary of about 150,000 words, most of which you do not have to train the system to recognize. Medical versions of the software have language models with additional medical terminology. Healthcare facilities using speech recognition should purchase a medical version.

## Pharmacy Systems

All acute care hospitals have inpatient pharmacies. These pharmacies have one or more computer systems for tracking, ordering, and dispensing medications. These systems are interfaced with the registration, billing, CPOE, and EHR systems.

The hospital pharmacy receives and fills medication orders and delivers the drugs to the nursing units and other departments. Most hospitals will also store some drugs in the patient care areas where nurses can access them immediately, without waiting on the pharmacy. These drugs are usually locked in cabinets that dispense a prepackaged amount of the drug when an authorized person enters a medication order in the dispensing system computer. The pharmacy stocks these cabinets and reconciles the records of medications that have been given to patients from them.

Most of the drugs dispensed by hospital pharmacies today are manufactured by pharmaceutical companies and come in vials, tablets, capsules, or other standard forms. However, inpatient pharmacies also create medications by combining ingredients according to the doctor's order. In particular, the pharmacy prepares solutions for intravenous (IV) administration to patients.

Ever since the IOM report (discussed in Chapter 7) revealed that high numbers of deaths have occurred due to preventable medical errors, hospitals have increased their focus on patient safety. These efforts have included CPOE, computerizing the pharmacy, and using positive identification systems to correctly match the medication with the patient, thus ensuring the right patient receives the right medication.

---

### MEDICATION ADMINISTRATION—THE FIVE RIGHTS

1. Right patient
2. Right time and frequency
3. Right medication
4. Right dose
5. Right route of administration

---

When an order for medication is received in the pharmacy system, it is reviewed by a pharmacist and compared with information from the EHR. The pharmacist performs a drug utilization review (DUR), which you learned about in Chapter 7. DUR software in the pharmacy system may be used to automate this review.

If the DUR reveals any potential problems, the ordering doctor is notified. In some hospitals, the pharmacist has the authority to change the drug order. The pharmacist also serves as a consultant for the hospital doctors and may know of or suggest other drugs that would be more effective that the one originally prescribed. The pharmacist may also notify the hospital's dietary service if the effectiveness of the drug might be compromised by certain foods.

Filling the medication order may be a manual or automated process. Medication labels are printed, which include the patient location and identification. The labels may include barcodes. A small pharmacy may fill the order by manually counting the appropriate number of pills from a larger container and packaging and labeling them with the patient ID. Larger facilities use a more automated process.

Figure 8-10 shows a robotic Rx system in operation. The pharmacy has stored its drugs in individual packages labeled with barcodes that identify the drugs. A computerized dispensing

**FIGURE 8-10**

Electronic order
system. Guided Rx
robot fills
medication orders.

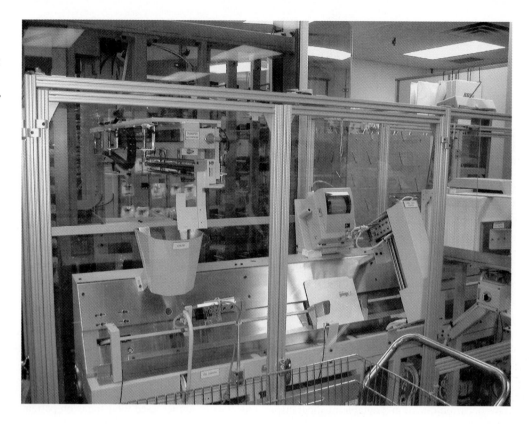

**FIGURE 8-11**

Rx robot restocks
prepackaged drugs
using barcode
reader.

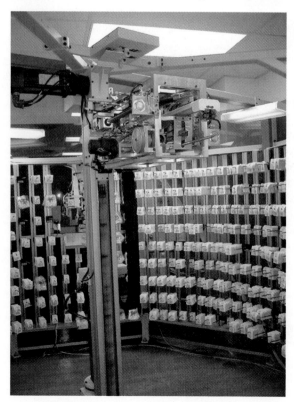

system receives the medication order data and directs the robotic arm to locate and retrieve the drugs on the order. These are then deposited into a container or bag for delivery to the nursing unit caring for the patient. The system is highly accurate. A barcode reader on the arm of the robot confirms the drug before selecting the package. When it is not being used for filling orders, the robot can also be used to restock the storeroom, as shown in Figure 8-11.

Once the orders have been filled, they are transported to the nursing unit, emergency department or other department. The pharmacy system also transfers charge information to the billing system.

A nurse, doctor, or other caregiver administers the medication and records the fact in the patient's chart. The patient wears a wristband that positively identifies the patient. The band may include a barcode, and in some facilities, a radio-frequency identification (RFID) device. The patient identity is compared to the patient ID on the medication and the medication is compared to the doctor's order. Only if everything matches is the drug administered to the patient.

Pharmacy systems also include decision support, patient medication administration reports, controlled substance tracking, and extensive intervention documentation.

Non-patient-related aspects of pharmacy systems include management functions for inventory control, pricing, purchasing, repackaging of large quantities into smaller units, and distribution from the central pharmacy to smaller units throughout the facility. These functions require additional interfaces to administrative systems such as accounts payable and to outside companies that supply the pharmacy.

# Emergency Department Systems

The emergency department (sometimes called ER for emergency room) is one of the busiest places in an acute care hospital. Patients arrive at the emergency department by ambulance or by presenting themselves for care. ER cases range from the most serious, life-threatening traumas to the common cold.

When a patient presents at the emergency department, the first step is to register. A registration clerk will search the master patient index (MPI) to determine if the patient has been previously registered at the hospital or an affiliated facility. If the patient's records are found, then the information is updated. If they are not found, the patient's demographic and insurance information will be entered in the registration system computer. In either case, the patient may be asked to sign routine forms required by the facility. Except for cases of serious injury, the patient will likely be directed to a waiting area until he or she can be seen.

When patients arrive by ambulance, they are immediately taken into the ER, bypassing the waiting room. The emergency medical technician (EMT) accompanying the patient will convey to the ER staff the presenting problem, vital signs, and patient information, which have been gathered during the drive to the hospital. In some cities, this information can be communicated to the ER while the ambulance is en route.

In emergency rooms, specially trained *triage nurses* are the first responders to patients. Their job is to quickly prioritize patient needs. Their review is often a simplified, organ-specific review of systems determined by the presenting complaint. Emergency room triage nurses help to decide how long treatment can be delayed without deterioration of the condition. Emergency department physicians use this screening to begin determining the diagnosis. In doing so, the nurse aids the physician assessment by presenting critical information to the physician for review.

Some issues concerning emergency departments:

- The ER may use a different software system than the rest of the hospital.
- The ER may not have access to the patient's records in the HIM department; the ER is not likely to have access to the patient's doctor's office records.
- ER patients who are victims of accidents or crimes may not be conscious and may have not yet been identified.
- Patient allergy or medical history information may not be known until a family member can be contacted.
- Patients without a primary care physician may treat the ER as a walk-in clinic, using emergency resources for ordinary conditions.

One of the principal challenges for the HIM department in terms of the emergency department concerns the patient who is unconscious and has not been identified. Patient records cannot be accessed without knowing who the patient is. Orders, medications, tests, and procedures require a medical record number. Typically, the patient is registered with minimal information as John or Jane Doe, and records begin to be created with this temporary ID. Once the patient is conscious or identified, then the records must be modified. If the patient already has a medical record number, then the records that were created under the temporary ID must be merged into the patient's actual chart.

Traditionally, emergency departments used white boards (similar to those found in classrooms) to track the patients in their care. Today, emergency departments rely on computer software to provide real-time updated information. For example:

- ER census and capacity
- Staffing assignments
- Patient wait times
- Patient location
- Patient chief complaint
- Patient acuity status

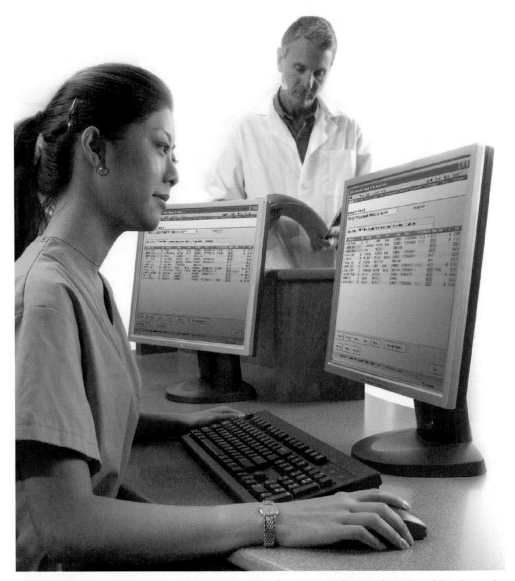

**FIGURE 8-12    Emergency department software replaces the ER white board.**

(Courtesy of GE Healthcare.)

- Order status
- Pending consults.

This information is important because the ER relies on other departments, such as radiology and laboratory, to perform diagnostic testing and on specialists to consult with ER physicians in specific cases. Waiting for results and consults from these other departments can force emergency departments to keep patients for a prolonged time. Staying current with the status of many patients can be a challenge. Emergency department software, such as that shown in Figure 8-12, improves emergency department workflow, patient care, and satisfaction.

Once the patient has been examined and diagnosed by the ER physician, the patient is either treated and sent home or admitted to the hospital. If the patient is admitted, then the ER records need to become part of the inpatient record for the current stay. If the patient is treated and sent home, charge data must be transferred to the billing system. However, if the patient is sent home, but then admitted to the hospital within 72 hours of the ER visit, the billing for the emergency room visit will be canceled and changed to inpatient billing.

# Biomedical Systems

A hospital's biomedical department is responsible for those devices that actually touch or attach to patients. Examples include instruments for measuring vital signs and cardiac and arterial blood gas monitors. Today, many of these devices have wired or wireless telemetry to transmit their information to nurses and into the EHR.

Although biomedical devices contribute a significant quantity of data to the EHR, in many facilities the biomedical department is separate from the IT department and does not report to the CIO. The devices themselves may require special software or interfaces for the EHR to be able to receive the data. The best outcome for the patients requires cooperation and effective communication between the biomedical and other departments.

# Surgical Department Systems

Hospital surgical departments not only provide restorative and lifesaving procedures, but are also a significant source of patients and revenue. As such, surgery departments wield great influence in the selection of perioperative software, even when their choice is different from the other hospital information systems.

The term *perioperative* refers to the entire surgical event from surgery scheduling, the arrival of the patient in the presurgery holding area, the actual surgery in the OR suite, and the immediate recovery in the postanesthesia area. Perioperative software includes nonpatient functions, such as management and scheduling of the operating rooms, surgical supplies, equipment, and personnel. It may also include software for the anesthesiologist.

## Operative Reports

The surgeon and anesthesiologist create preoperative notes prior to the surgery. Nurses' notes document preoperative preparation of the patient. The surgical procedure itself is recorded in its entirety. Records are kept of the anesthesia during the operation and postanesthesia recovery. The anesthesia report includes the preanesthesia evaluation. The operative report includes:

- Preoperative and postoperative diagnosis
- Surgeons' and their assistants' names
- Date, time, and duration of surgery
- Descriptive name of the surgery
- Type of anesthesia used
- Estimated blood loss
- Detailed record of the procedures performed
- Any unique or unusual events that occurred during the surgery
- Number of ligatures, sutures, packs, drains, and sponges used
- Description of all organs explored and all normal and abnormal findings.

If tissue is removed and sent to pathology, the pathologist's report is also included with the operative reports. As mentioned in Chapter 5, informed consent documents for the operation signed by the patient are also filed with the operative reports.

Prior to, during, and following the surgery, various biomedical devices are attached to patients for monitoring purposes. Following surgery, the patients are moved into a special area called the recovery room where they will continue to be monitored. The recovery room report documents patients' postanesthesia recovery, nurses' notes, vital signs, and administration of intravenous fluids and medications. Patients remain in the recovery area until the effects of the anesthesia have worn off and they are sufficiently stable to move to another location.

Surgery requires a great deal of record keeping. Electronic surgical record systems can store data from the patient monitors and record the nurses' and surgeons' notes.

**FIGURE 8-13**

**Anesthesiologist using a GE Centricity perioperative system.**

(Courtesy of GE Healthcare.)

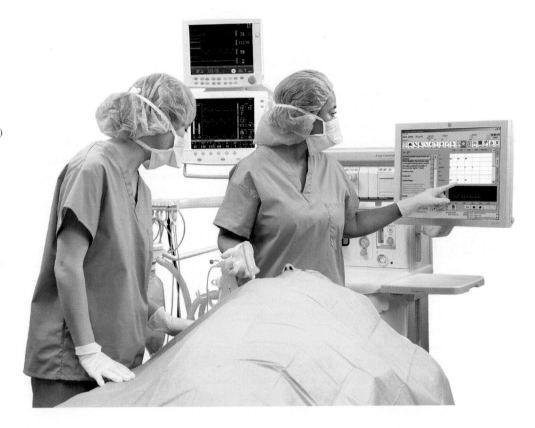

Figure 8-13 shows a perioperative anesthesia system for documenting and tracking standard care elements with device level data capture. Perioperative software is also used for scheduling and planning for the needs of the surgery. For example, surgeon *preference cards* specify the equipment and supplies the surgeons will need on hand for different types of surgeries. Instruments must be tracked through assembly, sterilization, storage, and use. Consumable supplies must be purchased and managed. Surgical case scheduling software, which replaces the traditional white board, can be accessed via the Internet by surgeons to find times when an OR is available.

## Implant Registry

Another record system that is a direct result of surgery is the implant registry. An implant is a device or substance intentionally put into the body to serve a particular purpose. Common implants include heart valves, pacemakers, breast implants, and artificial joints. Implant registries allow patients to be identified in the event of safety issues regarding a particular type of implant. For example, in the 1990s silicone breast implants received much negative publicity and were removed and replaced with saline implants, which were considered safer.

Implant registry data also facilitates the study of the performance and longevity of implants. Adverse events involving medical devices must be reported. To facilitate reporting, implant registry data includes:

- Patient demographic data
- Facility
- Implant manufacturer (name and address)
- Generic name of the implant and the manufacturer's brand name
- Model, serial, catalog, and lot numbers
- Description of the adverse event
- Who the adverse event was reported to (the FDA, implant distributor or the manufacturer).

## Transplant Registry

Whereas implants are substances or devices, transplants are tissues or organs. Most but not all transplanted organs come from organ donors who have died as a result of an accident. However, some types of transplants, such as bone marrow, are transplanted from living donors. Like implants, all transplants are carefully tracked and monitored.

To be successful, a transplant organ or tissue must come from a biologically compatible donor. Transplant registries are used to keep track of potential recipients and to communicate with international registries to locate the best match. The most prominent of these registries is the United Network for Organ Sharing (UNOS), and for bone marrow transplants, the National Marrow Donor Program (NMDP). Patients with the greatest need for a transplant are given the highest priority; therefore, the registry includes clinical data about patient status and condition.

In addition to the recipient data, transplant registries maintain information on the donor as well. This includes the cause of death, organ donor medical history, medications the donor was taking, the procurement process, and consent of the donor or family to donate the organs.

Post-transplant records are kept on the recipient, and in the case of living donors, on the donor as well. Post-transplant information on the recipient includes orders for immunosuppressive drugs, survival rate, functional status, graft status, and one-year and five-year follow-ups.

# Research and Clinical Trials

Both inpatient and ambulatory facilities participate in clinical trials of new drugs and devices. Clinical trials are authorized by the FDA to ensure the safety and efficacy of new drugs by testing them on small groups of patients in controlled studies, tracking the results and any adverse side effects.

The FDA divides clinical trials into four phases; each phase is considered a separate clinical trial. Though a drug may have been tested in the laboratory or on animals, the first phase of testing on human subjects is usually to see if the drug is safe and tolerated by a healthy person. Very small groups of subjects are tested in a controlled setting.

Phase II testing is performed on patients for whom the treatment is intended. Phase II focuses on finding the right dosage levels and proving the drug works. Once the drug has been shown to be safe and promises to be effective, phase III testing begins. Phase III uses larger groups of patients, and typically some are given the new drug or device being tested, while others are given a placebo. Phase III clinical trials may continue while FDA approval is pending. Phase IV trials occur after the drug has been approved and is on the market. Phase IV trials are used to survey its interaction once it is in general use.

Clinical trials are conducted according to designed protocols. Clinical trials may require the use of special software or tracking of data not normally in the facility's EHR. One problem clinical trials pose for HIM is that they sometimes require separate entry of the same data in two different systems: the normal EHR and a special system provided by the organization conducting the clinical trial. In cases where the normal EHR system can be used, care must be taken that data given to the research company is confined to just the clinical trial patients, in order to comply with HIPAA's "minimum necessary" rule. Clinical trial software is discussed further in Chapter 11.

# Chapter 8 Summary

### Departmental Information Systems

Data for health records flow into the EHR from many different systems. An acute care hospital may have 60 to 400 different software applications. Many of these are departmental systems, such as those used by the laboratory, radiology, or surgery departments. Others are software provided by a vendor to operate a particular instrument or device, but which are capable of exchanging data with the EHR or HIS systems. Doctor's medical practices tend to have fewer systems.

### Patient Registration

The core system for a hospital is called the health information system (HIS). The principal system for a medical office is the practice management system. One important function of these systems is patient registration. In hospitals, the patient registration system is sometimes referred to as the ADT system.

A master patient index is a list of all the patients who have previously been registered. In a large healthcare organization with multiple facilities, the MPI will be a special database that contains records of patients registered at all related facilities. In a healthcare organization with only a single facility, the MPI may be the same as the patient registration database. The purpose of the MPI is to prevent duplicate entry of the same patient and to provide a quick universal lookup of patients for all systems interfaced to the HIS. In paper-based systems, the MPI is necessary to locate the patient's medical record number.

A Soundex field may be included in the MPI system to allow surnames to be found based on how they sound phonetically when the user is unsure of the name's spelling.

## Laboratory Systems

A laboratory information system (LIS) receives orders and sends results of medical tests performed by the lab. The laboratory services include:

- Hematology
- Chemistry
- Immunology
- Blood bank (donor and transfusion)
- Pathology
- Surgical pathology
- Cytology
- Microbiology
- Flow cytometry.

The laboratory is supervised by a pathologist. There are two branches of pathology:

- Clinical pathology uses chemistry, microbiology, hematology and molecular pathology to analyze blood, urine, and other body fluids.
- Anatomic pathology performs gross, microscopic, and molecular examination of organs and tissues and autopsies of whole bodies. Surgical pathology performs gross and microscopic examination of tissue removed from a patient by surgery or biopsy.

Many of the clinical pathology tests can be performed using automated instruments that receive orders from the LIS and send results back to the LIS.

Results of anatomic pathology findings (and clinical pathology tests that are not performed on automated analyzers) are entered in to the LIS system manually. Pathology reports are sometimes dictated and transcribed.

When the LIS has received the test results data or pathology reports, it generates a lab report. These maybe printed or faxed reports. If the LIS is interfaced with the EHR, the lab report data is sent to the EHR as well.

Digital pathology captures specimen images digitally and displays them for the pathologist on a computer monitor.

The images can be stored on a PAC system. Digital pathology has the potential to allow the pathologist to see cells in a way that an ordinary microscope cannot.

Medical laboratories are accredited by the College of American Pathologists (CAP). The laboratory, equipment, supplies used for testing, and all personnel must meet certain CAP criteria regarding polices, procedures, and training to remain certified.

## Radiology Department

A radiology information system (RIS) is used to manage the workflow in radiology departments, communicate with PAC systems, schedule and track radiologic studies and post charges. RIS systems communicate with other systems such as HIS, EHR, and billing.

Radiologists are specialists who interpret x-rays and CT, MRI, and PET scans and other diagnostic tests. A *hanging protocol* is used to automatically display a number of images in the order the radiologist prefers.

Today most of the images the radiologist studies are digital. Traditionally, x-rays were taken with photographic film and then developed. Computed radiography (CR) replaces the film with a phosphor plate that can be processed by a computer to yield a digital x-ray image. Digital radiography (DR) captures the image directly and does not require processing.

Digital radiology images are stored in a Picture Archiving and Communication System (PACS) using a standard file format called DICOM, which stands for Digital Imaging and Communications in Medicine. The DICOM file includes fielded data about the patient and the study, eliminating the need for flash cards. Flash cards were used to add patient ID information when film x-rays were exposed.

High-resolution monitors allow the radiologist to see the smallest detail. *Resolution* refers to the size and number of pixels a screen can display. Radiology monitors have much smaller pixels, so they are capable of displaying a much larger quantity of them. Software used to view the images allows the radiologist to change the contrast, intensity, zoom in, zoom out, and otherwise enhance the image. The radiologist's interpretation of the study is produced in a radiology report.

## Dictation/Transcription Systems

Radiologists and many other medical specialists often dictate their reports and patient notes and either have the report transcribed or use speech recognition software. Though necessary in some situations, dictation/transcription does not produce a codified medical record, adds steps to the workflow, and takes longer to produce the final note or report.

Speech recognition software interprets the sound of the human voice and converts it into text. The results are not perfect and require some editing or correction. However, over time the computer learns the speaker's diction and recognizes more words, which reduces the error rate.

## Pharmacy Systems

All acute care hospitals have inpatient pharmacies. A hospital pharmacy receives and fills medication orders and delivers the drugs to the nursing units and other departments. Most of the drugs are in pill, vial, or capsule form and are manufactured by pharmaceutical companies; but some hospital pharmacies also create medications by combining ingredients into solutions for intravenous (IV) administration to patients.

Hospital pharmacies have one or more computer systems for tracking, ordering, and dispensing medications. These systems are interfaced with the registration, billing, CPOE, and EHR systems. Generally, medication orders are filled by the pharmacy and delivered to the nursing units on the floors. The nurses then administer the medications to the patient.

Hospital pharmacists act as consultants to doctors, performing drug utilization reviews (DURs) on medication orders and suggesting therapeutic alternatives where appropriate. Hospital pharmacists are also responsible for purchasing and managing pharmacy inventory.

## Emergency Department Systems

The emergency department or emergency room (ER) is one of the busiest places in an acute care hospital. Patients are seen in the ER for problems that range from the common cold to the most life-threatening injuries. Patients who come to the ER on their own begin with patient registration. Patients who arrive by ambulance are taken directly into the ER.

A specially trained triage nurse sees the patient first. The triage nurse's job is to quickly decide which patients need priority and to help decide how long treatment can be delayed without deterioration of the patient's condition.

The situation is especially complicated when an injured person arrives unconscious and without identification. Because the emergency department physicians need a medical record number to order tests or medications, a temporary chart is created. Once the patient is identified, these records must be merged into the patient's actual health records.

Emergency room treatment is often dependent on laboratory, radiology, and consultation reports. With a high volume of patients and many urgent activities occurring simultaneously, emergency room software is used to monitor and track the status of each patient.

After being treated by the emergency department, patients are either sent home or admitted to the hospital as inpatients.

Important issues concerning emergency departments include these:

- The ER may use a different software system than the rest of the hospital.
- The ER may not have access to the patient's records in the HIM department; the ER is not likely to have access to the patient's doctor's office records.
- ER patients who are victims of accidents or crimes may not be conscious and may have not yet been identified.
- Patient allergy or medical history information may not be known until a family member can be contacted.
- Patients without a primary care physician may treat the ER as a walk-in clinic, using emergency resources for ordinary conditions.

## Biomedical Systems

Prior to, during, and following the surgery, various biomedical devices are attached to the patient for monitoring purposes. The biomedical department is responsible for any systems that are attached to or come in contact with the patient. Modern biomedical monitoring devices transmit data to the EHR.

## Surgical Department Systems

Surgical departments provide restorative and lifesaving procedures, but are also a significant source of patients and revenue for the hospital.

The entire surgical event from surgery scheduling, the arrival of the patient in the presurgery holding area, the actual surgery in the OR suite, and the immediate recovery in the postanesthesia area is encompassed by the term *perioperative*.

Perioperative software records all aspects of presurgery, surgery, and postsurgical recovery. It also includes nonpatient functions, such as management and scheduling of the operating rooms, surgical supplies, equipment, and personnel. It may also include software for the anesthesiologist.

The operative report is a combination of reports from the surgeon, assistant surgeon, nurses, anesthesiologist, and pathologist. The patients' informed consent documents are filed with the other operative reports.

During some operations, patients receive an implant or transplant. An implant is a device or substance intentionally put into the body to serve a particular purpose. Common implants include heart valves, pacemakers, breast implants, and artificial joints.

A transplant operation replaces some part of the patient's body with an organ or tissue from a human donor. Some examples of transplanted organs include the kidney, heart, or liver. Bone marrow replacement is also considered a transplant.

Implant registries and transplant registries are separate. They are used to track what was put in the patient (recipient) and where it came from, how well it worked, and what the patient's functional status was as a result. Transplant registries also track donors.

## Research and Clinical Trials

Clinical trials are authorized by the FDA to ensure the safety and efficacy of new drugs and medical devices by testing them on small groups of patients in controlled studies, tracking the results and any adverse side effects. Large and small healthcare organizations alike participate in clinical trials. There are four phases of clinical trials on humans:

Phase I    Very small groups of subjects are tested in a controlled setting to see if the drug is safe and tolerated by a healthy person.

Phase II    Testing is performed on patients for whom the treatment is intended and focuses on finding the right dosage levels and proving the drug works.

Phase III    In this phase, larger groups of patients undergo controlled studies, in which some patients are given the new drug or device being tested and others are given a placebo.

Phase IV.    This phase surveys the drug's interaction in general use once the drug has been approved and is on the market.

Clinical trials follow designed protocols and sometimes require duplicate entry of patient exam data in special software used by the researcher. In cases where the normal EHR system can be used, care must be that data given to the research company is confined to the clinical trial project to comply with the HIPAA "minimum necessary" rule.

## Critical Thinking Exercises

1. Using Figure 8-3 determine the Soundex code for your surname.
2. Many medical errors occur when patients are given medications. How do the "five rights" prevent these errors? How does a CPOE system contribute to patient safety?

## Testing Your Knowledge of Chapter 8

1. What does the acronym PACS stand for?

2. What does the acronym MRI stand for?

3. What does the acronym DUR stand for?

4. Name at least four things checked for in a DUR.

5. What is an MPI? What is its purpose?

6. Which branch of pathology is concerned with blood: anatomical or clinical?

7. What is a *hanging protocol*?

8. What organization audits and certifies medical laboratories?

9. Where is a patient taken after surgery?

10. What is the difference between an implant and a transplant?

11. Which devices are the biomedical department responsible for?

12. What does it mean when an order is "stat"?

13. What is the standard file format for diagnostic radiology images?

14. Name three problem areas related to health records for emergency departments.

15. *True or false?:* Clinical trials violate the HIPAA privacy rule.

# Comprehensive Evaluation of Chapters 5-8

This comprehensive evaluation will enable you and your instructor to determine your understanding of the material covered so far.

1. Health records are classed as primary or secondary records. Which of the following is a primary record?
   a. insurance claim
   b. quality improvement report
   c. aggregate admissions data
   d. patient history and physical

2. Health records are classed as primary or secondary records. Which of the following is a secondary record?
   a. admission report
   b. operative report
   c. insurance claim
   d. discharge summary

3. What is an E-visit?
   a. emergency room visit
   b. emergency department visit
   c. electronic visit
   d. extended visit

*A patient health record is comprised of administrative and demographic data and clinical data. For each of the following indicate whether the data is administrative or clinical:*

4. HIPAA Consent to Use and Disclose PHI form
   a. administrative data
   b. clinical data

5. Doctor's orders
   a. administrative data
   b. clinical data

6. Consult referral
   a. administrative data
   b. clinical data

7. How many pages are in the average inpatient paper chart?
   a. 10
   b. 20
   c. 50
   d. 100

8. Using terminal digit filing, which section of the file room would chart 46-78-01 be found?
   a. section 01
   b. section 04
   c. section 46
   d. section 78

9. When paper charts are filed alphabetically the file system must be reorganized periodically. Why is this necessary?
   a. Paper charts wear out.
   b. Charts get misfiled.
   c. Some charts are thicker than others.
   d. More surnames start with certain letters.

10. A group medical practice adds 100 patients per month. The average thickness of a new patient's chart is 1/4 inch. If each file room shelving unit can hold 368 inches of files, how many new shelving units must be added per year just to accommodate new patient charts?
    a. 1
    b. 5
    c. 10
    d. more than 10

11. What is a nomenclature?
    a. an EHR coding system
    b. a PHI encryption system
    c. a network protocol
    d. a medical protocol

12. Which of the following is a nomenclature?
    a. DICOM
    b. PACMED
    c. SNOMED
    d. HL7

*The tabs on an EHR screen are used to logically group findings. The tabs have medical abbreviations. Write the meaning of each of the following acronyms:*

13. Sx _____

14. Hx _____

15. Px _____

16. What does *stat* mean on a test order?
    a. statistical analysis timed
    b. send to administration
    c. double-blind test
    d. without delay

17. Which branch of pathology analyzes body fluids?
    a. anatomical
    b. surgical
    c. clinical
    d. hydraulic

18. A biomedical device is
    a. a lab instrument
    b. a medical chemistry analyzer
    c. a device attached to a patient
    d. none of the above

19. Where is the patient taken after surgery during post-anesthesia?
    a. operating room
    b. recovery room
    c. patient's room
    d. admission, transfer and discharge

20. What is the standard file format for diagnostic radiology images?
    a. ACORN
    b. RIS
    c. DICOM
    d. RADCOM

21. Which of the following emergency department problems affects the HIM department?
    a. Patients without physicians who use the ER as a walk-in clinic
    b. Patients who arrive by ambulance
    c. Patients who arrive without their insurance cards
    d. Patients who are unconscious and do not have identification

22. Which of the following is not checked during a DUR?
    a. dosage
    b. diagnosis
    c. expiration
    d. interaction with other medications

23. Clinical trials are permitted by the HIPAA privacy rule.
    T. true
    F. false

24. Patient health records serve as the primary communication document between various providers who might care for the patient at different times in different departments.
    T. true
    F. false

25. Filing by reverse chronological order puts the newest documents at the front.
    T. true
    F. false

26. Having patients entering their own symptoms and history poses a security risk for the EHR.
    T. true
    F. false

27. The minimum record retention period for adult health records is age 65 or five years after the last encounter.
    T. true
    F. false

28. Terminal digit filing is not used where medical record numbers exceed six digits.
    T. true
    F. false

29. A deficiency report indicates items that are incomplete or missing from a chart.
    T. true
    F. false

30. HIM policies and procedures help ensure quality patient records.
    T. true
    F. false

31. Doctors and nurses do not have to follow HIM policies and procedures because they do not report to the health information manager.
    T. true
    F. false

32. The patient record provides the basis for all billing and reimbursement.
    T. true
    F. false

# Healthcare Coding and Reimbursement

9

## LEARNING OUTCOMES

After completing this chapter, you should be able to:

- Identify patient and insurance billing terms
- Name the coding standards used for billing
- Discuss reimbursement methodologies
- Explain managed care
- Compare prospective payment systems for hospitals
- Describe how a DRG is determined for billing purposes
- Explain the outpatient prospective payment system
- Discuss situations of healthcare fraud and abuse

## ACRONYMS USED IN CHAPTER 9

Acronyms are used extensively in both medicine and computers. The following acronyms are used in this chapter.

| | | | |
|---|---|---|---|
| **ABC** | Alternative Billing Codes | **HAC** | Hospital-Acquired Condition |
| **AMA** | American Medical Association | **HCPCS** | Healthcare Common Procedure Coding System |
| **APC** | Ambulatory Payment Classification | **HHA** | Home Health Agency |
| **CC** | Complication/Comorbidity Code | **HHRG** | Home Health Resource Group |
| **CF** | Conversion Factor | **HHS** | U.S. Department of Health and Human Services |
| **CHAMPVA** | Civilian Health and Medical Program–Veterans Affairs | **HIPAA** | Health Insurance Portability and Accountability Act |
| **CMS** | Centers for Medicare and Medicaid Services | **HMO** | Health Maintenance Organization |
| **CPT-4®** | Current Procedural Terminology, Fourth Edition | **ICD-9-CM** | International Classification of Diseases, Ninth Revision, Clinical Modification |
| **DME** | Durable Medical Equipment | **ICD-10** | International Classification of Diseases, Tenth Revision |
| **DRG** | Diagnosis-Related Group | **ICD-10-PCS** | International Classification of Diseases, Tenth Revision, Procedure Coding System |
| **EHR** | Electronic Health Record | | |
| **EOB** | Explanation of Benefits | | |
| **FECA** | Federal Employee Compensation Act | **IDN** | Integrated Delivery Network |
| **GPCI** | Geographic Practice Cost Indices | **IHS** | Indian Health Service |

| | | | |
|---|---|---|---|
| **IPA** | Independent Practice Association | **PPO** | Preferred Provider Organization |
| **IPF** | Inpatient Psychiatric Facility | **PPS** | Prospective Payment System |
| **IPPS** | Inpatient Prospective Payment System | **RAI** | Resident Assessment Instrument |
| **LOS** | Length of Stay | **RBRVS** | Resource-Based Relative Value Scale |
| **LTCH** | Long-Term Care Hospital | **RUG, RUG-III** | Resource Utilization Group; Resource Utilization Group, Third Version |
| **MCC** | Major Complication/Comorbidity | | |
| **MDC** | Major Diagnostic Category | **RVU** | Relative Value Unit |
| **MDS** | Minimum Data Set | **RW** | Relative Weight |
| **MS-DRG** | Medicare Severity–Diagnosis-Related Group | **SNF** | Skilled Nursing Facility |
| | | **UHDDS** | Uniform Hospital Discharge Data Set |
| **OASIS** | Outcome and Assessment Information Set | | |
| **OIG** | Office of Inspector General | **UR** | Utilization Review (Renamed Utilization Management) |
| **OPPS** | Outpatient Prospective Payment System | **VA** | U.S. Department of Veteran Affairs; also Veterans Administration |
| **OR** | Operating Room | | |
| **PCP** | Primary Care Physician | **WC** | Workers' Compensation |
| **POA** | Present on Admission | **WHO** | World Health Organization |

## Healthcare Business

There is no question that healthcare providers must be paid for their services, but the method of determining what that payment will be has changed over the years. Efforts to control spiraling healthcare costs have resulted in numerous and complex methodologies of reimbursement, which are the subject of this chapter.

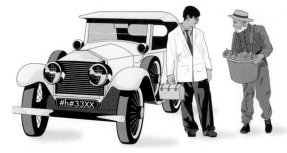

Up until the 1930s, usually only two entities were involved in a healthcare transaction: the guarantor and the provider. Patients or their family paid the doctor or hospital directly for medical services. Though it seems a cliché, country doctors did on occasion accept goods from patients in exchange for their services (as shown in Figure 9-1.)

As health insurance became more prevalent, a *third party* became involved in the payment for medical services: the insurance plan. Today about 85% of patients have some form of health plan. The various health plans and reimbursement schemes used by these plans are complex. We will discuss these plans in more detail once we have covered a few basic concepts.

**FIGURE 9-1**

**Doctors did not always receive money for services.**

## Patient Accounts and Registration

Chapter 8 discussed patient registration with emphasis on demographic information and the master patient index. The patient registration process also gathers information that will be necessary to obtain payment for the services rendered. This includes guarantor and insurance information. The *guarantor* is the person responsible for the patient's portion of the bill. For example, when the patient is a child, the parent is the guarantor.

Suffice it to say, the registration process must capture all of the information necessary for billing. The screen in Figure 9-2 has tabs across the top for accessing guarantor and payor information.

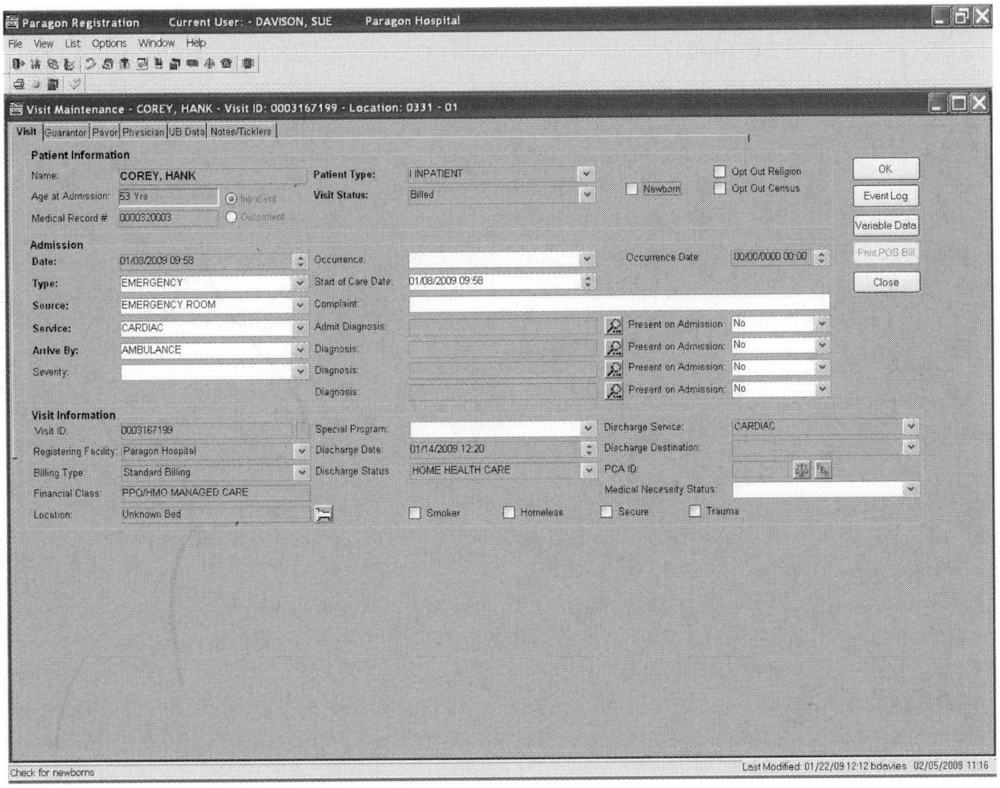

**FIGURE 9-2**

**Patient registration for inpatient admission from emergency department.**

(Courtesy of McKesson Corporation.)

## Patient and Insurance Billing Terms

Adding to the complexity of dealing with third-party payers is the fact that health plans use different terms for the same or similar concepts. The following list explains some of the terms that are used during the registration process:

- *Patient account:* Acute care hospitals create a new account for each episode of care, that is, for each new admission or emergency department visit. Medical practices create a new account on the first visit and use the same account for the life of the patient (except for family accounts, which may change when the children have grown up or marry.)

- *Guarantor:* The person responsible for paying amounts not covered by insurance is called the *guarantor* of the account. In many cases the guarantor is the patient. In other cases, the guarantor may be a parent or spouse. When the patient is not the guarantor, the name, address, and phone numbers of the guarantor must be recorded so they can be used for account billing later.

- *Health plan or payer:* A health plan may be a for-profit or not-for-profit insurance company, an employer self-insurance fund, or a government program such as Medicare. Government programs are not technically health plans, but are set up in the registration computer system the same way. CMS programs contract with various companies to process claims and disburse payments on their behalf. These companies are called *fiscal Intermediaries.*

    Health plans are sometimes also referred to as *payers.* Generally, the billing address and other information necessary to file claims are in a master file. The registration clerk usually just has to select the plan from a list and the address fields are automatically completed. One company may offer numerous plans, each with a different billing address. If one company offers multiple plans, the registration clerk must match the information displayed with that printed on the patient's insurance card.

- *Subscriber:* The primary person who is named on the health insurance card is referred to as the *subscriber, insured party, enrollee, member,* or *beneficiary.* That person's insurance ID is used to determine eligibility and during claims processing to determine which dependents and services are covered.

- *Beneficiary:* The beneficiary is a person who is entitled to receive benefits from the plan. Plan coverage is not limited to the subscriber and frequently includes spouses and children. In some systems these are called *dependents*.

- *Member number:* A unique ID is assigned by a health plan to each policy or by a government program to each participant. This is called the *member number*, *policy number*, or sometimes *insurance ID*. Some plans assign a unique member number to each dependent as well. Keeping accurate records of these IDs is vital to getting paid by the health plan.

- *Group number:* In many cases health insurance is obtained through an employer who has negotiated special rates and coverage. In such cases, the insurance card may include a group number. This number is used to further identify the policy and the benefits to which the patient is entitled.

If the patient has multiple insurance plans, the preceding insurance information is gathered for each plan.

## Additional Insurance Billing Terms

You should also be familiar with these additional insurance billing terms:

- *Claims:* The bill to insurance for healthcare services or supplies is called a *claim*. Claims are submitted electronically or on paper to the health plan or fiscal intermediary using standardized forms or in an electronic format specified by HIPAA.

- *Assignment of benefits:* Today, nearly all medical claims are filed by the provider, not the patient. The patient, during registration, signs a document authorizing the plan to pay the doctor directly. This is called *assignment of benefits*.

- *Adjudication:* The processing of the claim by the health plan is called *adjudication*. The coded information in the claim is processed by a computer, which compares the information to a set of coding rules called *claim edits* and a list of benefits covered by the patient's policy. If the claim does not meet the computer criteria, it is denied or suspended. If certain items are not covered by the policy or are not considered medically necessary, they are not paid. All items on the claim that pass the adjudication process are paid according to provisions of the policy and the provider's contract with the plan.

- *Explanation of benefits or remittance advice:* Explanation of the items and the amounts being paid are communicated to the provider as a remittance advice or explanation of benefits (EOB). An EOB is also sent to the patient.

- *Allowed amount:* Providers enter into contractual agreements with health plans that establish the amount the provider will receive from all parties for each service. This is called the *allowed amount*. It is usually less than the provider's usual customary charge for the service.

- *Remittance or reimbursement:* The remittance is the amount the provider receives from the insurance plan. It is sometimes called *reimbursement,* a term dating back to a time when patients filed their own claims and were subsequently reimbursed by the plan.

- *Adjustments:* Providers who have contractually agreed to participate in a health plan have agreed not to collect more than the allowed amount. An entry is made in the patient accounting system to reduce the original charge to the allowed amount. This is called a *contractual adjustment* or a *write-down adjustment*.

- *Coordination of benefits:* When a patient is covered by more than one insurance plan, one plan will be considered *primary* and the other *secondary*. The primary plan will adjudicate the claim first and determine the allowed amount for the services billed. The secondary claim will include information about what the primary plan allowed, paid, and denied.

  There are many reasons why a patient might have secondary insurance. When both parents work, children may be covered by both parents' plans. Adult patients may be covered by more than one employer. Medicare patients may purchase Medicare supplemental insurance that pays for the amounts not covered by Medicare. Indigent elderly patients may have both Medicaid and Medicare.

Coordination of benefits is the process by which two or more health plans determine which plan pays first and how much the other plans pay. As mentioned earlier, some plans electronically forward claims to the second plan, eliminating the need for the provider to file the second claim. These are called *crossover* or *piggyback claims.*

■ *Copay:* Most health plans require the patient to pay a portion of the charges. This amount may be referred to as the *copay* or *coinsurance* amount. The copay is usually a fixed amount per visit. The amount is often printed on the patient's insurance card and is collected at the time of the visit.

■ *Coinsurance:* Coinsurance is usually a percentage of the allowed amount. Because the exact amount is often not known until the health plan has adjudicated the claim, the patient may be billed at a later date for the coinsurance amount. For example, the patient due portion or coinsurance for many services is 20% of the allowed amount.

■ *Deductible:* Health plans often have a deductible amount. This is a fixed minimum that the patient must pay before the plan begins paying. Some plans have several deductibles, for example, one amount for doctor visits and another deductible for hospital stays. The deductible is usually for one year, and starts over each calendar year.

Claims are submitted and adjudicated as described above, but the provider is not paid; instead, the remittance advice will indicate that all or part of the allowed amount is "patient due" because of the deductible. Until the deductible is met, it is up to the provider to collect from the patient.

The plan keeps track of the amounts that have been credited toward the deductible and will begin paying providers once the patient has met the deductible. Because the patient may see several different doctors, sometimes providers have difficulty determining if the deductible has been met.

■ *Patient billing:* Amounts that are determined to be the responsibility of the patient are billed to the patient. A bill and a statement are not the same thing. A bill is akin to an invoice you might receive for a purchase. A statement is a list of charges, payments, and adjustments posted to the account during the period covered by the statement. Most healthcare facilities send patient statements, though some may call them patient bills. These will be discussed in more detail in Chapter 10.

# Codes for Billing

The first step in preparing a health insurance claim is to assign procedure codes for the services rendered and the supplies used, and diagnosis codes representing the disease or medical condition treated. Procedure and diagnosis codes are derived from the documentation in the patient's health record. Procedures and supplies are coded using the HCPCS/CPT-4 codes. Diagnoses are coded using the ICD-9-CM codes. Health plans and providers have been using procedure and diagnosis codes to communicate claim information on standard forms for 40 years; however, HIPAA made specific code sets mandatory.

## HIPAA Transaction Coding Standards

As you learned in Chapter 3, HIPAA not only established privacy and security rules, but also mandated specific standards for electronic transactions and required the use of standardized codes in those transactions. Here is a bit of background on HIPAA codes used for billing and reimbursement.

**CPT-4** CPT stands for Current Procedural Terminology. The number "4" represents the fourth edition of the coding system. CPT-4 codes are standardized codes for reporting medical services, procedures, and treatments performed for patients by the medical staff. CPT was created in 1968 by the American Medical Association (AMA) to provide a uniform nomenclature that accurately identified medical, surgical, and diagnostic services. Though originally shorter, the codes today are numeric, five digits in length. An example of several different groups of CPT-4 codes is shown in Figure 9-3.

**FIGURE 9-3**

**Small sample of CPT-4 codes.**

| CPT-4® Codes | |
|---|---|
| **Code** | **Description** |
| **Evaluation and Management Codes** | |
| 99212 | Outpatient visit, established patient, problem focused history/exam; straightforward medical decision making. |
| 99213 | Outpatient visit, established patient, expanded problem focused history/exam; medical decision making. |
| 99214 | Outpatient visit, established patient, detailed history/exam; medical decision making of moderate complexity. |
| 99215 | Outpatient visit, established patient, comprehensive history/exam; medical decision making of high complexity. |
| **Eye Surgery Codes** | |
| 66850 | Removal of lens material with aspiration. |
| 66940 | Removal of lens material; extra capsular |
| 66984 | Extra capsular cataract removal with insertion of intraocular lens prosthesis |
| **Psychological Services Codes** | |
| 90804 | Psychotherapy 20–30 minutes |
| 90806 | Psychotherapy 45–50 minutes |
| 90857 | Psychotherapy interactive group therapy |

**HCPCS** In 1983, CPT-4 codes were adopted by the government as part of the Healthcare Common Procedure Coding System (HCPCS) and became standard for private insurance and Medicare and Medicaid claims. CPT-4 expanded to include generic codes that covered almost any service that needed to be billed, but it did not include codes for billable supplies. Therefore, HCPCS II codes were created for billing supplies, injectable medications, and blood products.

Subsequently, various state Medicaid programs as well as private insurance companies were allowed to add codes (designated HCPCS III) that were not part of CPT-4. These were often "local codes" used by only one plan or in one region. This created nonstandardization in the HCPCS code set. Today local codes have been eliminated from HCPCS and differences between state Medicaid codes have been resolved primarily because of HIPAA legislation that required the adoption of national standards. HCPCS and CPT-4 became designated code sets under HIPAA. Figure 9-4 shows a sample of some HCPCS codes

**PROCEDURE MODIFIER CODES** Procedure modifiers are a set of two-digit codes used in conjunction with HCPCS/CPT-4 codes for billing purposes. For example, when two surgeons are billing for the same surgery, a modifier is used to indicate the assistant surgeon. Figure 9-5 shows a list of procedure modifier codes.

**ABC** ABC codes are alternative medicine billing codes created to meet the need for codes to document and bill for alternative types of care that are not addressed by other coding standards. Providers such as acupuncturists, ayurvedic doctors, behavioral healthcare workers, chiropractors, homeopaths, body workers, massage therapists, midwives, naturopaths, nurses, nutritionists, Oriental medicine practitioners, social workers, and somatic educators did not have sufficient codes to adequately describe their services.

ABC codes are similar in structure to CPT-4 codes but are not part of the CPT or HCPCS code sets. The codes are alphanumeric, five characters in length and allow a two-character modifier. ABC codes are accepted as billing codes only by some payers.

| HCPCS Codes | |
|---|---|
| **Code** | **Description** |
| **HCPCS Supply Codes** | |
| A4206 | Syringe With Needle, Sterile 1cc, Each |
| A4207 | Syringe With Needle, Sterile 2cc, Each |
| A4208 | Syringe With Needle, Sterile 3cc, Each |
| A4209 | Syringe With Needle, Sterile 5cc Or Greater, Each |
| A4210 | Needle-Free Injection Device, Each |
| A4211 | Supplies For Self-Administered Injections |
| **HCPCS Administration Codes** | |
| J0128 | Injection, Abarelix, 10 Mg |
| J0132 | Injection, Acetylcysteine, 100 Mg |
| J0133 | Injection, Acyclovir, 5 Mg |
| J0135 | Injection, Adalimumab, 20 Mg |
| J0180 | Injection, Agalsidase Beta, 1 Mg |

**ICD-9-CM**    ICD stands for International Classification of Diseases, which is a system of standardized codes developed collaboratively between the World Health Organization (WHO) and 10 international centers. Today's coding system evolved from the International List of Causes of Death, which was used by physicians, medical examiners, and coroners to facilitate standardized mortality studies. In 1948, WHO expanded and renamed the system to make it useful for coding patient medical conditions as well.

The number "9" represents the ninth revision of the coding system, which has been revised about every 10 years from 1900 to 1979. By the time the ninth revision was published, the U.S. National Center for Health Statistics began to modify the statistical study with clinical information.

The letters "CM" stand for Clinical Modification. Clinical modifications provided a way to code the clinical information about the health of a patient beyond that needed for statistical reports. In daily usage, the full acronym ICD-9-CM is often just referred to as ICD-9.

With the addition of clinical modifications, the codes became useful for indexing medical records, medical case reviews, and communicating a patient's condition more precisely. However, they took on even greater importance in 1989 when Congress made them mandatory on Part B Medicare claims. Other insurance programs followed suit, and ICD-9-CM codes became required by insurance carriers to process claims.

| Procedure Modifiers | |
|---|---|
| **Code** | **Description** |
| 51 | Multiple procedures (within an operative session) |
| 53 | Discontinued procedure (due to extenuating circumstances) |
| 80 | Assistant surgeon |
| 91 | Repeat clinical diagnostic laboratory test |
| 99 | Multiple modifiers |

**FIGURE 9-5**    **Small sample of procedure modifier codes.**

**FIGURE 9-6**

**Small sample of ICD-9-CM codes.**

| ICD-9-CM Codes (Diagnosis) | |
|---|---|
| **Code** | **Description** |
| **Diseases of Other Endocrine Glands** | |
| 250 | Diabetes mellitus |
| 250.0 | Diabetes mellitus without mention of complication (NOS) |
| 250.00 | Diabetes mellitus type II, not stated as uncontrolled |
| 250.01 | Diabetes mellitus type I (juvenile) not stated as uncontrolled |
| 250.02 | Diabetes mellitus type II, uncontrolled |
| 250.03 | Diabetes mellitus type I, (juvenile) uncontrolled |
| 250.1 | Diabetes with ketoacidosis |
| 250.2 | Diabetes with hyperosmolarity |
| 250.3 | Diabetes with other coma |
| **V Codes (circumstances other than disease or injury)** | |
| V22.0 | Supervision of normal first pregnancy |
| V22.1 | Supervision of other normal pregnancy |
| V70.0 | Routine general medical examination (health checkup) |
| V72.1 | Examination of ears and hearing |
| V72.1 | Encounter for hearing following a failed hearing screening |
| **E Codes (Classification of external causes of injury or poisoning)** | |
| E813.0 | Driver in a motor vehicle accident involving collision with other vehicle |
| E813.1 | Passenger in a motor vehicle accident involving collision with other vehicle |
| E813.3 | Motorcyclist in a motor vehicle accident involving collision with other vehicle |

ICD-9-CM is currently published in three volumes. The first two volumes provide a listing and an index of diagnosis codes; the third volume lists codes for hospital inpatient procedures. Figure 9-6 shows a sample list of codes from volumes 1 and 2.

The diagnosis codes are three characters, followed by a decimal point and up to two numerals. The first three characters of an ICD-9-CM code identify the primary diagnosis; the two digits to the right of the decimal point further refine the diagnosis specificity.

Insurance billing allows for the use of multiple ICD-9-CM codes for a single procedure, indicating one code as the primary diagnosis and additional codes as secondary conditions for which the treatment was done. Today insurance reimbursement is tied to the proper use of ICD-9-CM codes, in the proper order (of primary, secondary, etc.), and at the right level of specificity (number of decimal places.)

The historical intent of the ICD was to classify similar causes of mortality and disease conditions into statistical reportable data. When it became required for insurance billing, the code set had to be further modified. The problem was that if an ICD-9-CM code was required for an insurance claim, but the patient was perfectly healthy, what code should be used? To solve this problem, ICD-9-CM added a section of codes that start with the letter "V"; these V codes indicate nonillness conditions that can be used for billing. For example, when a child has a regular pediatric checkup, the visit would be coded as "V20.2 Well-Child Check-Up."

Volume 1 also includes "E" codes (listed at the bottom of Figure 9-6). These are not used for diagnosis, but to classify the cause of an injury or poisoning. For example, the billing diagnosis 823.0 indicates the patient had a closed fracture of the tibia. The code E813.1 provides

**FIGURE 9-7**

**Comparison of a small sample of DRG and MS-DRG codes.**

| DRG Codes | | |
|---|---|---|
| **MDC** | **DRG** | **Description** |
| | | **Surgical DRGs** |
| 01 | 529 | Ventricular shunt procedures with CC |
| 01 | 530 | Ventricular shunt procedures without CC |
| | | **Medical DRGs** |
| 04 | 79 | Respiratory infections & inflammations age > 17 with CC |
| 04 | 80 | Respiratory infections & inflammations age > 17 without CC |
| 04 | 81 | Respiratory infections & inflammations age 0–17 |
| 04 | 82 | Respiratory neoplasms |

| MS-DRG Codes | | |
|---|---|---|
| **MDC** | **MS-DRG** | **Description** |
| | | **Surgical MS-DRGs** |
| 01 | 031 | Ventricular shunt procedures w MCC |
| 01 | 032 | Ventricular shunt procedures w CC |
| 01 | 033 | Ventricular shunt procedures w/o CC/MCC |
| 01 | 034 | Carotid artery stent procedure w MCC |
| 01 | 035 | Carotid artery stent procedure w CC |
| 01 | 036 | Carotid artery stent procedure w/o CC/MCC |
| | | **Medical MS-DRGs** |
| 04 | 177 | Respiratory infections & inflammations w MCC |
| 04 | 178 | Respiratory infections & inflammations w CC |
| 04 | 179 | Respiratory infections & inflammations w/o CC/MCC |
| 04 | 180 | Respiratory neoplasms w MCC |
| 04 | 181 | Respiratory neoplasms w CC |
| 04 | 182 | Respiratory neoplasms w/o CC/MCC |

further detail that the broken leg is the result of an auto accident in which the patient was a passenger.

**DRG** DRG stands for diagnosis-related group. Over the past three decades, Medicare and other insurance plans began to reimburse hospitals based on the DRG. They found that certain diagnoses required about the same length of stay (LOS) and consumed the same amount of resources. Researchers at Yale University found that they could predict the reimbursement for inpatient hospital stays by categorizing the thousands of ICD-9-CM codes into 25 major diagnostic categories (MDCs) comprising 538 DRG codes. In 2008, Medicare expanded the DRG system to account for medical severity. The new MS-DRG system has 745 codes. Figure 9-7 compares a small sample of DRG codes to the new MS-DRG codes.

By analyzing the procedures performed and the principal diagnosis and secondary diagnoses of comorbidity or complication (if any), a computer program arrives at a DRG code, which is then used to determine how much the hospital should be paid for services rendered related to this DRG. Further details about how payments based on DRGs are calculated are given later in the discussions about prospective payment systems.

**FIGURE 9-8**

A comparison of ICD-10 codes and ICD-9-CM codes.

| Comparison of ICD-10 and ICD-9-CM codes | | | | |
|---|---|---|---|---|
| **ICD-10** | **Description** | **ICD-9-CM** | **Description** | |
| R31.0 | Gross hematuria | 599.7 | Hematuria | |
| R31.1 | Benign essential microscopic hematuria | 599.7 | Hematuria | |
| R31.2 | Other microscopic hematuria | 599.7 | Hematuria | |
| R31.9 | Hematuria, unspecified | 599.7 | Hematuria | |
| N36.41 | Hypermobility of urethra | 599.81 | Urethral hypermobility | |
| N36.42 | Intrinsic sphincter deficiency | 599.82 | Intrinsic sphincter deficiency | |
| N36.43 | Combined hypermobility of urethra and intrinsic sphincter deficiency | | | |
| N364.4 | Muscular disorders of urethra | | | |
| N36.8 | Other specified disorders of urethra | 599.83 | Urethral instability | |
| N36.8 | Other specified disorders of urethra | 599.84 | Other specified disorders of urethra | |

**FUTURE DEVELOPMENTS: ICD-10**   ICD-10 is the latest revision to the International Classification of Diseases. It was released by WHO in 1992 and is used broadly in Europe and Canada. ICD-10 contains about twice as many categories as ICD-9 and uses more alphanumeric codes. Effective January 1, 1999, ICD-10 was officially implemented in the United States for reporting the cause of death on death certificates. It has not been implemented for billing, and should not be used in place of ICD-9-CM for reporting diagnoses on insurance claims. The U.S. Department of Health and Human Services (HHS) has proposed that the ICD-10 code sets be used for billing effective October 1, 2013.

Just as clinical modifications were added to the ICD-9 codes to create ICD-9-CM, work is now under way to add clinical modifications to ICD-10 to produce ICD-10-CM. However, even when the work is completed, industry-wide transition to revision 10 will require considerable time and effort. In the 20 years since the creation of ICD-9-CM, nearly all medical practices and insurance plans have become computerized. Their systems contain coding and claim adjudication rules based on ICD-9-CM that will have to be modified before ICD-10 can be implemented as a standard. The clinical modifications in ICD-10-CM will include only volumes 1 and 2 (the diagnosis codes). Figure 9-8 compares several ICD-9-CM and ICD-10 codes.

**ICD-10-PCS**   Hospitals use volume 3 of ICD-9-CM for coding inpatient procedures. It has been proposed that the volume 3 procedure codes be replaced by a new procedure coding system called ICD-10-PCS. These procedure codes are not technically part of, nor derived in any way from, ICD-10; only the name is similar. These codes were created by 3M Health Information Systems under a contract with Medicare. The ICD-10-PCS codes are seven-digit alphanumeric codes and are intended to provide better codification of any underlying issues associated with a procedure performed.

There is some resistance to adopting the ICD-10-PCS codes partly because the adoption would have the same impact on computerized billing and claim systems as just discussed: Computer systems would require numerous modifications. However, the AMA is also concerned that ICD-10-PCS would replace the CPT-4 codes, becoming the single coding standard for all inpatient and outpatient procedures.

### Billing Codes Differ from EHR Nomenclatures

Having read the previous chapters, you might wonder why there are so many coding systems. Why, if ICD-9-CM is already an international standard that codifies most known medical conditions, wouldn't it make a satisfactory system for use with an electronic health record? The answer is the granularity of information represented by the code.

The insurance claim format does not have a place for (nor would the claim processor want) all the detailed findings that are found in the health record. For example, a pediatrician might use the ICD-9-CM code "V20.2 Well-Child Check-up" when submitting a claim for a child's exam. Obviously that code does not communicate anything about the child's size, growth rate, disposition, or demeanor—conversely, those types of details about the child's size and so on would not communicate to the claims processing system the purpose of the visit.

When coding medical information for statistical analysis or billing, ICD-9-CM classifications are sufficient, but they do not have enough detail to code the nuances of EHR findings.

Similarly, the CPT-4 code 99212 conveys to the health plan the fact, duration, and complexity of the patient visit. It does not, however, provide any clues as to what was discussed or observed during the visit, nor is that necessary for the claim. Thus, when recording medical findings about a patient, EHR data should be meaningfully specific; when reporting claims data, it is merely necessary for a code to represent the service and the justifying medical condition for that service.

# Reimbursement Methodologies

Being familiar with the coding standards used in healthcare transactions is a necessary first step because they are used in most reimbursement methodologies. By reimbursement methodology, we mean how the provider payment is determined.

Because the methods of reimbursement for professional services and hospital services are so different, we will discuss professional and institutional reimbursement separately, beginning with doctors.

### Fee for Service

Physicians and other medical professionals set their own fees for the services they provide. These fees are the amount they charge every patient. However, rarely are they paid the full amount of the charge by a third-party payer. The reason for this is that they have contractually agreed to provide services to beneficiaries of certain health plans at a discounted rate.

### Allowed Amount

Discounted fees are usually listed on the EOB as the allowed amount. The provider has multiple fee schedules: the amounts that they charge for the service rendered and the amounts that they have contractually agreed to accept from patients of certain health plans. The difference between these two amounts is posted as an accounting adjustment called a *write-down*.

The providers who enter into these contracts are called *participating providers*. Participating providers agree not to collect more for a service than the amount allowed by the contract, even if part of the fee is to be paid by the patient or a second insurance plan. In exchange for discounting their fees, the physicians hope to gain more patients. In areas where most patients have health insurance, not participating with a plan could cost the doctor patients.

Even though the doctor has agreed to accept the allowed amount, many plans do not pay the entire allowed amount, requiring the provider to collect a copay or coinsurance amount from the patient. For example:

| | |
|---|---|
| Physician's fee | $120.00 |
| Write-down adjustment | –$ 20.00 |
| Allowed amount | $100.00 |
| Insurance payment | $ 80.00 |
| Patient coinsurance | $ 20.00 |

The physician's usual fee is written down to the amount allowed by the insurance plan. The insurance pays 80% (of the allowed amount, not the original charge). The doctor must collect the remaining 20% from the patient. In the above example, the original charge is written down to $100. The insurance payment of 80% is $80 and the patient coinsurance is 20% or $20.

## Managed Care

Even though contractual agreements for discounted fees allowed third-party payers to limit the amounts paid for services, the utilization of those services has increased. This caused a rise in overall healthcare costs. New methodologies termed *managed care* were developed to control patients' use of services. There are several variations of managed care. We will discuss each.

Primary care physicians (PCPs) are physicians practicing family care, internal medicine, pediatrics, general practice, and sometimes gynecology. These are the types of physicians that patients often go to first when a health problem arises.

In a pure managed care scenario, primary care physicians serve as gatekeepers. Patients must choose a PCP from a list of plan doctors, even if it means changing from their regular doctor. Patients who need to see a specialist or have a diagnostic test must first see their PCP, who will refer the patients to a specialist or diagnostic center that is also under contract to the managed care plan.

Health maintenance organizations (HMOs) were authorized by congress in 1973. An HMO acts as both the insurer and the provider. HMO patients must use the HMO for all services, except medical emergencies. Several types of HMOs exist:

**Staff Model:**

- HMO owns the facilities and employs the doctors.

**Group Practice Model:**

- HMO contracts with facilities and physicians to provide the services.

**Independent Practice Association (IPA) Model:**

- A number of independent physicians form a business arrangement (IPA) for the purpose of contracting with the HMO. The IPA receives payment from the HMO and distributes it among the IPA physicians.

**Integrated Delivery Network (IDN) Model:**

- Facilities and physicians form a business arrangement (IDN) for the purpose of contracting with the HMO to provide both hospital and physician services.

HMO plans control patient access to as much of the healthcare delivery system as possible, requiring preapproval for all services except visits to the PCP, and refusing to pay for services received out of network (i.e., from non-HMO facilities or providers.)

Kaiser Permanente, discussed in Chapter 1, is an example of a very successful staff model HMO. Kaiser Permanente owns hospitals and clinics. The doctors are salaried employees. Other HMO plans where the physicians are not employed directly by the HMO (IPA, IDN, and group practice) sometimes reimburse the doctors using a capitation model.

## Capitation

*Capitation* (meaning "head count") is a payment based on the number of members who select a certain PCP or participating group as their HMO provider (see Figure 9-9). The PCP, IPA, or IDN

**FIGURE 9-9**

**Number of members per month determines PCP capitation payments.**

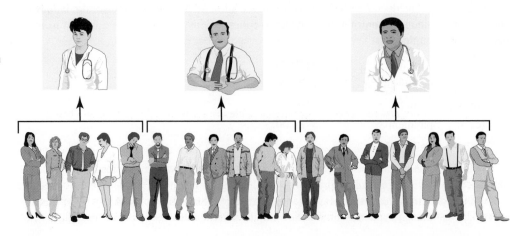

is paid a flat rate per member per month by the HMO, whether a provider sees the patient or not. The PCP sees patients of the plan, but does not get paid per visit. The PCP is also responsible for controlling patients' access to specialists and expensive procedures, acting as the gatekeeper to those services.

The capitation model succeeds when the group of HMO patients is large enough that the costs of treating members who need services and those who never see the doctor average out. Similarly, the HMO contracts with employer groups in the hope that with a large enough group of enrollees the number of patients needing little or no care will balance out those who need a lot.

Most provider HMO contracts have a provision to reimburse the provider differently for very ill patients whose care will require significantly more resources than the normal HMO member. These cases are considered exceptions and can be reimbursed beyond the capitation. The term for these cases is *outliers*.

## Preferred Provider Organizations

One problem with the managed care reimbursement methodology that became apparent early on was that different plans contracted with different PCPs. Hence, when an employer changed plans or a patient changed employment, that person was often forced to change family doctors as well. Also, patients and doctors felt they were giving medical decision making over to the insurance company. To address these problems, a modified form of managed care was created called the preferred provider organization (PPO) model.

The PPO model gives more choices to the patient. Doctors are contracted by the health plan as participating physicians, and patients are encouraged to use the PPO physicians. However, patients have the option of using other physicians or facilities; but when doing so, the patient must pay a higher coinsurance. The PPO tries to encourage members to make choices that save the plan money; but if the patient chooses to go outside the network the plan is protected, because the patient pays a larger share of the cost.

PPO plans may also use copay instead of coinsurance for primary care visits. Remember, a copay is a flat amount per visit, whereas coinsurance is a percentage. Copays encourage patients to use PPO doctors because patients pay only a small fee regardless of the complexity of the visit. If they see a non-PPO doctor they typically must pay 20% to 30% of the charge for the visit.

None of this discussion should be construed to infer that managed care plans are bad. Kaiser Permanente and others found that by emphasizing quality care, health maintenance, and preventive screenings, patients stayed healthier, which resulted in reduced health costs. When a managed care plan helps patients stay healthy, it is good for the patient and good for the plan.

## Government-Funded Health Plans

Plans that pay for healthcare services and that are funded by federal or state governments are not technically health insurance plans. They are the result of legislation and are legally called *entitlements*. They are not corporations or not-for-profit organizations like other insurance plans. However, in many other respects they are similar: They contract with providers and (through fiscal intermediaries) process and pay claims. Government-funded plans include the following:

- *CHAMPVA (Civilian Health and Medical Program–Veterans Affairs)* covers dependents and survivors of military veterans with disabilities and those killed in the line of duty.
- The *VA (Veterans Administration)* provides hospitals and healthcare services to military veterans.
- *TRICARE* provides healthcare for active duty military personnel, military retirees, and their dependents.
- The *IHS (Indian Health Services)* provides healthcare for Native Americans and Native Alaskans.
- *FECA (Federal Employee Compensation Act)* provides healthcare costs and lost income from work-related injuries for federal employees.
- *WC (workers' compensation)* provides healthcare costs and lost income from work-related injuries for employees in most types of businesses. Employers pay premiums into a state worker compensation fund in most states. States that do not operate worker compensation

funds require employers to purchase worker compensation coverage through self-insurance funds or commercial insurance companies.

■ *Medicaid* provides medical assistance for low-income patients with limited financial resources. Medicaid programs are state programs that receive federal funding.

■ *Medicare* is a health insurance program for:

• People age 65 or older

• People under age 65 with certain disabilities

• People of any age with end-stage renal disease (permanent kidney failure requiring dialysis or a kidney transplant).

The largest and most significant government program is Medicare. Medicare is not only the largest payer in America, but its polices, procedures, and reimbursement models serve as templates for commercial and nonprofit health plans. Simply put, many plans will not cover a service that Medicare does not, and will not pay more for a service than Medicare allows. Medicare and Medicaid are the responsibility of CMS, as described in earlier chapters. There are four types of Medicare coverage, Part A, Part B, Part C, and Part D:

■ *Medicare Part A (hospital insurance)* helps cover inpatient care in hospitals and skilled nursing facilities, but not custodial or long-term care. It also helps cover hospice care and some home healthcare. For most people, the premium for Part A was paid through their payroll taxes during the years they were working.

■ *Medicare Part B (medical insurance)* helps cover doctors' services and outpatient care. It also covers some other medical services that Part A doesn't cover, such as some physical and occupational therapy services, and some home healthcare. Part B helps pay for these covered services and supplies when they are medically necessary. Most people pay a monthly premium for Part B. Part B requires most patients to pay a deductible and coinsurance (usually 20% of the Medicare *allowed amount* for the service).

■ *Medicare Part C (Medicare Advantage Plans)* are health plans that are approved by Medicare but run by private companies. These plans are referred to as Medicare Part C. When a patient joins a Medicare Advantage Plan, they are still in Medicare. However, the plans operate like an HMO or PPO and often requires patients to use doctors and facilities in their network. The Medicare Advantage Plan provides all of the Part A and Part B coverage. Some plans also include Part D coverage. The patient pays a premium, but their overall costs may be less than what they would pay for Part B premiums and coinsurance.

■ *Medicare Part D (prescription drug coverage)* is insurance provided by private companies to Medicare patients. Everyone with Medicare can get this coverage, which may help lower prescription drug costs and help protect against higher costs in the future. Beneficiaries select a drug plan and pay a monthly premium.

■ *Medigap (Medicare supplemental insurance)* refers to health insurance policies sold by private insurance companies to fill "gaps" in Medicare plan coverage. Patients who have Medicare Advantage Plans (Part C) do not need a Medigap plan. For others, Medigap plans generally pay the portions of the medical expenses not paid by Medicare due to deductible or coinsurance. They do not necessarily pay for a service that is not covered by Medicare. Medigap is not part of Medicare and patients must purchase it separately in addition to paying their Medicare B premiums.

In terms of reimbursement methodologies, Medicare B uses a discounted fee-for-service model, which we will discuss in more detail in the next section. Medicare C uses any of the several HMO models we have just covered. Medicare A reimburses hospitals and other institutions using a prospective payment system (PPS) model, which will be explained later in the chapter.

## Medicare Part B Reimbursement

Medicare Part B is important not only because it is the largest payer, but also because by understanding its methods you will understand how other health insurance companies determine what to pay providers.

As stated earlier in this chapter, providers use HCPCS/CPT-4 codes to bill for professional services and supplies. A file called a *charge master* or *procedure code* file contains all of the HCPCS codes regularly used by the medical practice. Each code has a dollar amount that represents the doctor's fee for that service or supply. This represents the doctor's *fee schedule*. The file also contains a description and numerous other fields that contain numbers and values used for accounting, sorting, and reporting. One or more of those fields may be used for the *relative value units* (RVUs), as discussed next.

## Resource-Based Relative Value Scale

Relative value units were created to measure the value of one procedure compared to other procedures. It should be apparent that a complex surgery takes longer, has more risk, and requires greater skill than a simple one. However, several other factors need to be considered such as location, costs, and insurance. In 1985, Harvard University conducted a national study and created a Resource-Based Relative Value Scale (RBRVS). The RBRVS for each code is determined using three separate factors:

**Physician Work:**

■ the physician's time, mental effort, technical skill, judgment, stress, and the physician's education

**Practice Expense:**

■ direct expenses related to supplies and nonphysician labor used in providing the service, the pro rata cost of the equipment used, and an amount included for the indirect expenses

**Malpractice Expense:**

■ rates for malpractice insurance vary greatly by specialty.

In 1989, Medicare adopted RBRVS for determining its payment schedule, which became effective January 1, 1992. Medicare realized that there were regional differences in what it costs to provide medical services, so geographic practice cost indices (GPCI) values are also included in the payment calculation. The three GPCI values reflect cost variances by geographic setting. The geographically adjusted relative value is calculated using the following formula:

$$(\text{work} \times \text{GPCI work}) + (\text{expense} \times \text{GPCI expense})$$
$$+ (\text{malpractice} \times \text{GPCI malpractice})$$

The formula result is multiplied times a fixed dollar amount called the national conversion factor (CF) to calculate the Medicare fee (allowed amount). Compare, for example, the standard relative value units for an outpatient office visit in 2009 when the GPCI is calculated for different cities:

|  | RVU | Payment Amount |
| --- | --- | --- |
| Standard office visit, established patient | 1.72 | $62.03 |
| Adjusted for Atlanta, Georgia | 1.71 | $61.81 |
| Adjusted for New York City | 1.98 | $71.51 |

The result of the geographic adjustment is that a New York doctor will receive approximately $10.00 more for the same type of visit because his or her costs are higher.

Each year a committee led by the AMA adds new procedure codes and delete obsolete codes. A separate committee determines and assigns the RBRVS units to the codes. Once every five years, the committee reevaluates the values of all codes.

Each year, CMS updates the Medicare payment schedule for all procedure codes. There are actually two Medicare schedules. The first, a fee schedule, is used to calculate how much a participating provider is paid by Medicare and the patient (allowed amount). The second schedule is called the limiting charge. Providers are not required to participate with Medicare or accept assignment of benefits; but if they do not participate, they are prohibited by law from collecting more from Medicare patients for covered services than the limiting charge.

*(A)* Notifier(s):

*(B)* Patient Name:                   *(C)* Identification Number:

# ADVANCE BENEFICIARY NOTICE OF NONCOVERAGE (ABN)

<u>NOTE</u>: If Medicare doesn't pay for *(D)*_____ below, you may have to pay.

Medicare does not pay for everything, even some care that you or your health care provider have good reason to think you need. We expect Medicare may not pay for the *(D)*_____ below.

| *(D)*_____ | *(E)* Reason Medicare May Not Pay: | *(F)* Estimated Cost: |
|---|---|---|
|  |  |  |

## WHAT YOU NEED TO DO NOW:

- Read this notice, so you can make an informed decision about your care.
- Ask us any questions that you may have after you finish reading.
- Choose an option below about whether to receive the *(D)*_____ listed above.
    **Note:** If you choose Option 1 or 2, we may help you to use any other insurance that you might have, but Medicare cannot require us to do this.

| *(G)* OPTIONS:       Check only one box. We cannot choose a box for you. |
|---|

❑ **OPTION 1.** I want the *(D)*_____ listed above. You may ask to be paid now, but I also want Medicare billed for an official decision on payment, which is sent to me on a Medicare Summary Notice (MSN). I understand that if Medicare doesn't pay, I am responsible for payment, but **I can appeal to Medicare** by following the directions on the MSN. If Medicare does pay, you will refund any payments I made to you, less co-pays or deductibles.

❑ **OPTION 2.** I want the *(D)*_____ listed above, but do not bill Medicare. You may ask to be paid now as I am responsible for payment. **I cannot appeal if Medicare is not billed.**

❑ **OPTION 3.** I don't want the *(D)*_____ listed above. I understand with this choice I am **not** responsible for payment, and **I cannot appeal to see if Medicare would pay.**

*(H)* Additional Information:

**This notice gives our opinion, not an official Medicare decision.** If you have other questions on this notice or Medicare billing, call **1-800-MEDICARE** (1-800-633-4227/**TTY**: 1-877-486-2048).

Signing below means that you have received and understand this notice. You also receive a copy.

| *(I)* Signature: | *(J)* Date: |
|---|---|
|  |  |

Form CMS-R-131 (03/08)                      Form Approved OMB No. 0938-0566

**FIGURE 9-10**   **Medicare Advance Beneficiary Notice of Noncoverage form.**

Both participating and nonparticipating providers must tell a Medicare patient in advance if the patient will have to pay for a test or service because it is not covered by Medicare. If the patient agrees to the service, he or she must sign an Advance Beneficiary Notice of Noncoverage (ABN) form (shown in Figure 9-10.)

Federal and state laws require doctors to charge all patients the same fee for the same service. That means a doctor cannot charge a PPO patient less than a Medicare patient, even though he or she may be contractually required to accept less. Therefore providers' standard fee schedules tend to be substantially higher than the amount they will eventually collect. The amount of the original charge is subsequently reduced to the amount they are allowed to collect through an accounting entry called a contractual *adjustment* or contractual *write-down*.

The amount of a contractual adjustment or write-down is never recouped by the physician; it is just considered a cost of doing business. Just as a store might sell goods cheaper by the case than by the item, so the medical group hopes that contractually agreeing to participate with a health plan will bring them more patients.

Following the Medicare B example, many health insurance plans reimburse professional services based a discounted fee schedule. Like Medicare, these amounts are usually based on a multiplier of the RBRVS unit.

# Prospective Payment System Reimbursement

Hospitals do not bill insurance plans in the same way as physicians nor are reimbursements calculated the same way. Hospitals use a UB-04 claim form (shown in Chapter 10, Figure 10-6) that looks very different from the CMS-1500 claim form used for professional claims that is shown in Chapter 10, Figure 10-4.

Both types of claims begin with posting HCPCS and ICD-9-CM codes in a billing system. Once coded, a professional claim is ready to be sent. Hospital claim coders have to also identify the principal diagnosis and associate revenue codes with the procedures. The reason for these additional coding steps has to do with the method by which reimbursement is calculated, called a prospective payment system (PPS) or inpatient prospective payment system (IPPS). One way to understand prospective payments is to use Medicare Part A as an example.

## Medicare Part A and MS-DRGs

Medicare Part A is important not only because it is the largest payer, but also because Blue Cross and other health plans employ its policies and method to hospital reimbursements. Though the DRG method of reimbursement was first used by the New Jersey Department of Health, Medicare Part A was the first large payer to use it as a prospective payment system nationwide. Blue Cross and other plans followed.

Inpatient acute care hospitals are reimbursed a single total payment for each patient discharge based on a DRG code. The DRG model assumes that patients with the same sort of diagnoses require about the same length of stay and consume a similar amount of resources. Therefore, it is reasonable to pay the hospital a flat rate per hospital stay based on the type of case. This payment is considered full payment for all costs incurred by the hospital in treating the patient, other than physician services, which are billed separately by the physician.

Of course, medical complications could cause one patient to need more care than another. To allow for this, the DRG code is not determined from the principal diagnosis alone, but factors in whether the patient had more than one condition when admitted to the hospital. This is called *comorbidity*. Similarly, the DRG can be changed if a patient developed a complication (additional condition) while staying in the hospital. In 2008, Medicare revised the DRG system to allow for the medical severity of the illness in determining Medicare payments. The new system is called MS-DRG.[1]

---

[1]*Medicare Severity DRGs (MS-DRGs), Fiscal Year 2008 Inpatient Prospective Payment System,* CMS Transmittal 1374 (Baltimore, MD: Centers for Medicare and Medicaid Services, November 7, 2007).

When the claim is submitted, special software called the DRG Grouper determines the DRG (or MS-DRG) code. Reimbursement is calculated based on two factors, the relative weight and the hospital IPPS rate (operating + capital base rates).

**RELATIVE WEIGHT** Each DRG code is assigned a numerical value called a *relative weight* (RW) that reflects the average relative costliness of cases in that group compared with the costliness for the average Medicare case. The MS-DRG weights are recalibrated annually, based on standardized charges and costs for all inpatient PPS cases in each MS-DRG. The charges are reduced to costs by using national average ratios of hospital costs to charges for 15 different hospital departments. Unlike the RBRVS units discussed earlier, DRG relative weights do not vary by location; that is, the RW for a DRG code is the same nationwide. For example, consider the relative weights of the following two DRG codes. Though the length of stay is the same for both DRGs, the RW reflects the complexity of the surgery and costs to the hospital:

| MS-DRG | Description | Relative Weight |
|--------|-------------|-----------------|
| 134 | Tonsillectomy (other ear, nose, mouth, and throat OR procedures w/o CC/MCC ) | 0.82133378 |
| 508 | Major shoulder or elbow joint procedures w/o CC/MCC | 1.114330567 |

## Acute Inpatient Prospective Payment System
### Operating Base Payment Rate

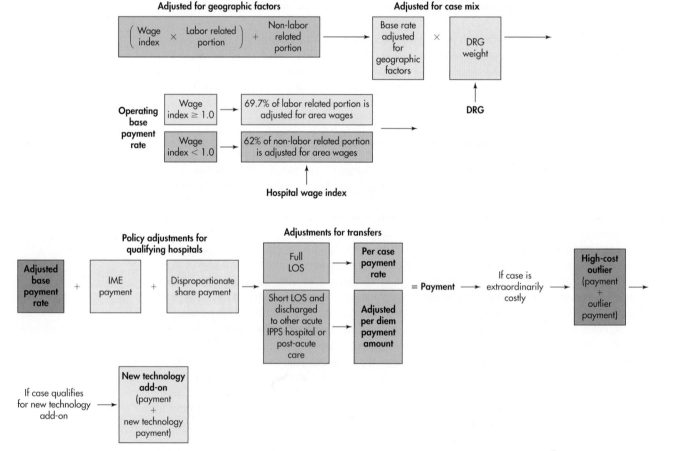

**FIGURE 9-11** **Determining the hospital's operating base rate.**[2]

---

[2]*Source: Acute Inpatient Prospective Payment System Fact Sheet,* Medicare Learning Network (Baltimore, MD: Centers for Medicare and Medicaid Services, 2007).

**PPS RATE**    The second factor is called the hospital's inpatient PPS rate. The IPPS rate is a dollar amount determined by the hospital's operating costs (labor and nonlabor) and whether it is located in an urban area with a population of more than 1 million.

IPPS payments are derived through a series of adjustments applied to separate operating and capital base rates. Operating payments cover labor and supply costs. Capital payments cover costs for depreciation, interest, rent, and property-related insurance and taxes. Figure 9-11 and Figure 9-12 show how each of these rates is determined. (*Note:* The concept of *case mix* shown in Figure 9-12 is explained in Chapter 11.)

The payment to which the hospital is entitled is calculated by multiplying the hospital's PPS rate (operating and capital base rate) times the RW of the DRG code. The following example shows the payment calculations for a hospital with a PPS rate of $6,000 (assuming there were no complications to the case):

Tonsillectomy          $0.82133378 \times \$6,000 = \$4,928.00$

Shoulder operation    $1.114330567 \times \$6,000 = \$6,685.98$

Payments are increased if the hospital serves a disproportionate number of low-income patients and are also increased for teaching hospitals. Additional amounts are paid for outlier cases in which the hospital's costs significantly exceeded the typical costs for the DRG.

## Acute Inpatient Prospective Payment System
### Capital Base Payment Rate

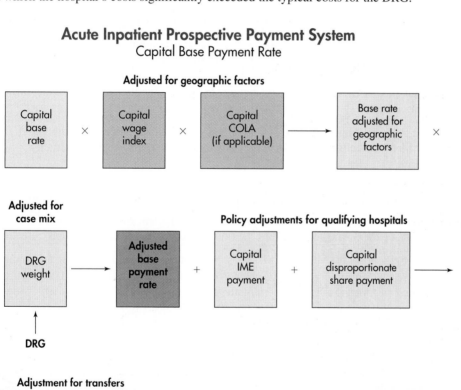

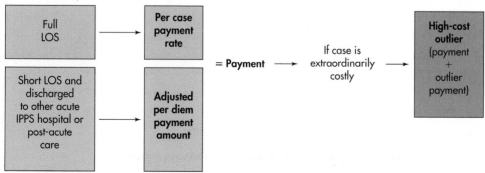

**FIGURE 9-12**
**Determining the hospital's capital base rate.[3]**

[3]Ibid.

Under the prospective payment system, the amount a hospital receives from Medicare A for a particular case may be less than the hospital's actual cost. The hospital must absorb this loss, but payments for other cases with the same DRG may be in excess of the hospital's costs; in that case, the hospital gets to keep the profit. The assumption of the prospective payment model is that over the course of the year the reimbursement for similar cases will balance out.

## Hospitals Excluded from Inpatient PPS

Certain hospitals' reimbursements are not based on PPS. These types of hospitals are paid based on reasonable costs (subject to maximum limits per discharge). These include children's hospitals, cancer hospitals, and critical access hospitals.

Alternative prospective payment systems are used to reimburse long-term care hospitals, skill nursing facilities, home health programs, and psychiatric and rehabilitation hospitals.

## Determining the DRG

An inpatient claim should encompass all of the charges for one stay. Though there are provisions for filing a corrected or supplemental claim, hospitals may lose revenue if they file incomplete or late claims. To prevent this, a bill-hold period is used by hospitals to delay billing to ensure that all charges are posted and therefore included in the claim.

The information on an institutional claim is used to determine the DRG. There is only one DRG for each claim, and it is assumed that the claim represents the entire case.

The determination of the DRG code is a complex algorithm that requires a software program called a DRG Grouper. The DRG Grouper software analyzes each case, assigning a DRG on the basis of the diagnoses, procedures, medical severity, and the patient's age, sex, and discharge status.

When preparing a claim, hospital coding specialists identify the principal diagnosis and any secondary diagnoses that represent complications or comorbidities:

- The principal diagnosis is the reason, after study, that the patient was admitted to the hospital. Medicare calls this the discharge diagnosis. It is a required element in the Uniform Hospital Discharge Data Set (UHDDS).

- Comorbidity is any condition that was present at admission but not inherent to the principal diagnosis. For example, a patient with pneumonia who also has a heart condition.

- Complications are conditions that arose while the patient was hospitalized. For example, a surgical patient who acquired a postsurgical *Staphylococcus aureus* (staph) infection.

There about 14,000 ICD-9-CM codes. This number would make for an unmanageable prospective payment system. So, DRG categorizes the thousands of ICD-9-CM codes into 25 major diagnostic categories (MDCs). Generally, the categories are based on the various body systems, though some MDCs can include multiple body or organ systems; for example, MDC 22—Burns.

The DRG Grouper software begins with the principal diagnosis, factors in secondary diagnoses of comorbidity or complication, analyzes the procedures performed, and takes into account the patient's age. Once the MDC is identified, the software follows a logical path called a decision tree. The DRG Grouper looks at the complication/comorbidity code (CC) list. If a secondary diagnosis on the claim is in the CC list and is not an inherent part of the principal diagnosis, the result may be a different DRG code with a higher reimbursement.

Prior to MS-DRGs, many claims resolved to one of two DRG codes with nearly identical descriptions. These are called *DRG pairs*. For example:

- *Surgical DRG pairs* were one code "without complications" and another code "with CC"

- *Medical DRG pairs* used one code for patients "under 17 years old" another code for patients "over 17."

MS-DRG replaced pairs with three levels of medical severity:

- *MCC (major complication/comorbidity):* the highest level of severity

- *CC (complication/comorbidity):* the next level of severity

- *Non-CC:* complication/comorbidity that does not significantly affect severity of illness and resource use.

## Appendectomy
### Major Diagnostic Category 6

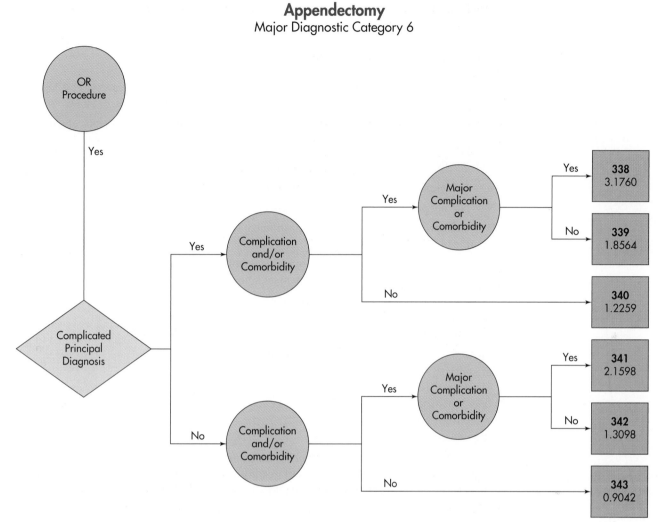

**FIGURE 9-13**   **Flow of MS-DRG Grouper logic.**[4]

The DRG Grouper generally selects the highest severity level of any secondary diagnosis. No additional consideration is given to the presence of multiple CCs. However, claims with certain high cost devices such as pacemakers an cardiac defibrillator implants are assigned a CC severity level if there is not one.[5] Figure 9-13 shows a flow sheet for the logic DRG Grouper uses.

### Exceptions

A higher DRG is not applicable if the secondary diagnosis (CC) is a hospital-acquired condition (HAC) that could have been prevented through the application of evidence-based guidelines. There are 10 categories of HACs:

1. Foreign object retained after surgery
2. Air embolism
3. Blood incompatibility
4. Stage III and IV pressure ulcers

[4]Ibid.

[5]Barbara O. Wynn and Molly Scott, *Evaluation of Severity-Adjusted DRG Systems: Addendum to the Interim Report* (Santa Monica, CA: RAND Health, May 2008).

5. Falls and trauma

6. Manifestations of poor glycemic control

7. Catheter-associated urinary tract infection

8. Vascular catheter-associated infection

9. Surgical site infection following a coronary artery bypass graft, gastroenterostomy, laparoscopic gastric surgery, or orthopedic surgery to the spine, neck, shoulder, or elbow

10. Deep vein thrombosis/pulmonary embolism following a total knee or hip replacement.

A present on admission (POA) indicator code is associated with each primary and secondary diagnosis code on the claim. HAC is determined from this code. The codes are:

Y = Yes, present at the time of inpatient admission

N = No, not present at the time of inpatient admission

U = Unknown, the documentation is insufficient to determine if the condition was present at the time of inpatient admission

W = Clinically undetermined; the provider is unable to clinically determine whether the condition was present at the time of inpatient admission or not

1 = Unreported/not used or exempt from POA reporting.

A few exceptional cases are directly assigned a DRG code without being assigned to an MDC. One example is heart transplants. Another is an extensive OR procedure unrelated to the principal diagnosis where, for example, something unexpected and unrelated is discovered and repaired during surgery.

There are also several DRG codes that are the result of coding errors. When the DRG Grouper reports these codes, the claim must be recoded or the hospital will not be paid.

### Outlier Cases

Prospective payment systems pay hospitals based on the assumption that most cases for the same MS-DRG will average out. When the cost of treating a particular patient exceeds the payment for the MS-DRG by a certain threshold amount, Medicare will increase the payment.

## Other Medicare Prospective Payment Systems

In addition to acute care inpatient hospitals, Medicare uses a prospective payment system for other entities as well. CMS has established prospective payment systems for other types of hospitals as well as home health agencies. However, PPS payments could not be calculated based on the same logic used for acute care hospitals, so different methods were designed.

### Inpatient Psychiatric Hospital Prospective Payment System

Medicare payments to inpatient psychiatric facilities (IPFs) are based on a per diem (per day) rate. The per diem rate includes both facility-level and patient-level adjustments. The facility-level adjustment factors in wage index, geographic location, and whether the facility is a teaching facility. The payment for an individual patient is further adjusted for various factors, such as the DRG classification, age, length of stay, and the presence of specified comorbidities. Additional payments are provided for cost outlier cases, a qualifying emergency department, and certain psychiatric therapy treatments.

### Long-Term Care Hospital Prospective Payment System

The PPS for long-term care hospitals (LTCHs) classifies patients into distinct diagnostic groups based on clinical characteristics and expected resource needs. The patient classification system groupings are called LTC-DRGs, which are the same MS-DRG codes used for acute care hospitals except that the relative weights have been modified to reflect the resources required to treat patients with medically complex health problems in long-term care facilities.

Relative weights for the LTC-DRGs account for the variation in cost per discharge, because they reflect resource utilization for each diagnosis. The LTCH PPS is adjusted for differences in wages and a cost of living, but no rate adjustment is made for geographic location, number of low-income patients, or indirect medical education.

Individual claims are adjusted for short-stay cases, interrupted-stay cases, cases discharged and readmitted to colocated providers, and high-cost outlier cases.

## Skilled Nursing Facility Prospective Payment System

The skilled nursing facility (SNF) prospective payment system reimburses skilled nursing facilities on a per diem basis. Unlike long-term care facilities, the rate is not based on DRGs, but on resource utilization groups, third version (RUG-III). SNF PPS rates include an adjustment for geographic differences in wages.

When a patient is admitted (transferred) to a SNF, a nurse or other healthcare professional assesses the patient using a standard form called a Resident Assessment Instrument (RAI). A sample page from the form is shown in Figure 9-14. The data collected includes the Minimum Data Set (MDS) discussed in Chapter 5. The first assessment (known as the five-day assessment) must be recorded within eight days of admission. Medicare requires patient assessments to be repeated on the 14th, 30th, 60th, and 90th day of patient stays.

SNF per diem payments for each admission are case-mix adjusted by the RUG-III system, which uses MDS data from RAIs to assign patients to one of 53 RUGs. Patients' cognitive and medical conditions, ability to care for themselves, and their service needs are used to determine the case-mix adjustment.

## Home Health Prospective Payment System

Medicare pays home health agencies (HHAs) a predetermined base payment. The payment is adjusted for the health condition and care needs of the patient, called the case-mix adjustment. The base payment is also adjusted for the geographic differences in wages.

A physician prescription is required for home health services. A nurse or therapist from the HHA uses the Outcome and Assessment Information Set (OASIS) instrument to assess the patient's condition. The OASIS data is then used to classify the patient into one of 80 home health resource groups (HHRGs). The case-mix adjustment is determined from the HHRG.

The HHA is paid for a 60-day episode of care. The physician must renew the order for home health care every 60 days. Although payment for each episode is adjusted to reflect the beneficiary's health condition and needs, the number of episodes a beneficiary who remains eligible for home health benefits can receive is not limited.

As with other prospective payment systems, outlier cases can result in higher reimbursements. However, HHAs can also receive lower reimbursement for patients who require very few home visits. These are called low-utilization cases and are paid on a per diem basis instead of the whole episode of care.

## Outpatient Prospective Payment System

Outpatient services provided by hospitals are reimbursed using an outpatient prospective payment system (OPPS). Outpatient services provided in doctor's offices is reimbursed by Medicare B (as described earlier) and does not use OPPS. OPPS is used for hospital outpatient services and for a few nonoutpatient situations:

- Partial hospitalization services by community mental health centers
- Administration of certain vaccines, splints, casts, and antigens by home health agencies
- Certain Medicare B services provided to hospitalized patients who do not have Medicare A.

OPPS differs from acute care IPPS in that it does not use DRGs. Payment is determined by an Ambulatory Payment Classification (APC) system, which is based on procedure codes instead of diagnoses codes.

In most cases, the unit of payment under the OPPS is the individual service or procedure. Services are assigned to APCs based on similar clinical characteristics and similar costs.

Resident _____  Numeric Identifier _____

## MINIMUM DATA SET (MDS) — *VERSION 2.0*
## FOR NURSING HOME RESIDENT ASSESSMENT AND CARE SCREENING
### *FULL ASSESSMENT FORM*
(Status in last 7 days, unless other time frame indicated)

### SECTION A. IDENTIFICATION AND BACKGROUND INFORMATION

| 1. | RESIDENT NAME | |
|---|---|---|
| | | a. (First)   b. (Middle Initial)   c. (Last)   d. (Jr/Sr) |

**2. ROOM NUMBER** ☐☐☐☐☐

**3. ASSESSMENT REFERENCE DATE**
a. *Last day of MDS observation period*
☐☐ — ☐☐ — ☐☐☐☐
Month   Day   Year
b. Original (0) or corrected copy of form (enter number of correction)

**4a. DATE OF REENTRY** Date of reentry from most recent temporary discharge to a hospital in last 90 days (or since last assessment or admission if less than 90 days)
☐☐ — ☐☐ — ☐☐☐☐
Month   Day   Year

**5. MARITAL STATUS**
1. Never married   3. Widowed   5. Divorced
2. Married   4. Separated

**6. MEDICAL RECORD NO.** ☐☐☐☐☐☐☐☐☐☐

**7. CURRENT PAYMENT SOURCES FOR N.H. STAY**
(*Billing Office to indicate;* **check all that apply in last 30 days**)

| Medicaid per diem | a. | VA per diem | f. |
|---|---|---|---|
| Medicare per diem | b. | Self or family pays for full per diem | g. |
| Medicare ancillary part A | c. | Medicaid resident liability or Medicare co-payment | h. |
| Medicare ancillary part B | d. | Private insurance per diem (including co-payment) | i. |
| CHAMPUS per diem | e. | Other per diem | j. |

**8. REASONS FOR ASSESSMENT**
[Note—If this is a discharge or reentry assessment, only a limited subset of MDS items need be completed]

a. Primary reason for assessment
1. Admission assessment (required by day 14)
2. Annual assessment
3. Significant change in status assessment
4. Significant correction of prior full assessment
5. Quarterly review assessment
6. Discharged—return not anticipated
7. Discharged—return anticipated
8. Discharged prior to completing initial assessment
9. Reentry
10. Significant correction of prior quarterly assessment
0. *NONE OF ABOVE*

b. *Codes for assessments required for Medicare PPS or the State*
1. Medicare 5 day assessment
2. Medicare 30 day assessment
3. Medicare 60 day assessment
4. Medicare 90 day assessment
5. Medicare readmission/return assessment
6. Other state required assessment
7. Medicare 14 day assessment
8. Other Medicare required assessment

**9. RESPONSIBILITY/ LEGAL GUARDIAN** (*Check all that apply*)

| Legal guardian | a. | Durable power attorney/financial | d. |
|---|---|---|---|
| Other legal oversight | b. | Family member responsible | e. |
| Durable power of attorney/health care | c. | Patient responsible for self | f. |
| | | *NONE OF ABOVE* | g. |

**10. ADVANCED DIRECTIVES** (*For those items with supporting* **documentation** *in the medical record,* **check all that apply**)

| Living will | a. | Feeding restrictions | f. |
|---|---|---|---|
| Do not resuscitate | b. | Medication restrictions | g. |
| Do not hospitalize | c. | Other treatment restrictions | h. |
| Organ donation | d. | *NONE OF ABOVE* | i. |
| Autopsy request | e. | | |

### SECTION B. COGNITIVE PATTERNS

**1. COMATOSE** (*Persistent vegetative state/no discernible consciousness*)
0. No   1. Yes   (**If yes, skip to Section G**)

**2. MEMORY** (*Recall of what was learned or known*)
a. Short-term memory OK—seems/appears to recall after 5 minutes
0. Memory OK   1. Memory problem
b. Long-term memory OK—seems/appears to recall long past
0. Memory OK   1. Memory problem

**3. MEMORY/ RECALL ABILITY** (*Check all* that resident was **normally able to recall during** *last 7 days*)

| Current season | a. | That he/she is in a nursing home | d. |
|---|---|---|---|
| Location of own room | b. | | |
| Staff names/faces | c. | *NONE OF ABOVE* are recalled | e. |

**4. COGNITIVE SKILLS FOR DAILY DECISION-MAKING** (*Made decisions regarding tasks of daily life*)
0. *INDEPENDENT*—decisions consistent/reasonable
1. *MODIFIED INDEPENDENCE*—some difficulty in new situations only
2. *MODERATELY IMPAIRED*—decisions poor; cues/supervision required
3. *SEVERELY IMPAIRED*—never/rarely made decisions

**5. INDICATORS OF DELIRIUM— PERIODIC DISORDERED THINKING/ AWARENESS** (*Code for behavior in the* **last 7 days**.) [Note: Accurate assessment *requires conversations with staff and family who have direct knowledge* **of resident's behavior over this time**].
0. Behavior not present
1. Behavior present, not of recent onset
2. Behavior present, over last 7 days appears different from resident's usual functioning (e.g., new onset or worsening)

a. EASILY DISTRACTED—(e.g., difficulty paying attention; gets sidetracked)
b. PERIODS OF ALTERED PERCEPTION OR AWARENESS OF SURROUNDINGS—(e.g., moves lips or talks to someone not present; believes he/she is somewhere else; confuses night and day)
c. EPISODES OF DISORGANIZED SPEECH—(e.g., speech is incoherent, nonsensical, irrelevant, or rambling from subject to subject; loses train of thought)
d. PERIODS OF RESTLESSNESS—(e.g., fidgeting or picking at skin, clothing, napkins, etc; frequent position changes; repetitive physical movements or calling out)
e. PERIODS OF LETHARGY—(e.g., sluggishness; staring into space; difficult to arouse; little body movement)
f. MENTAL FUNCTION VARIES OVER THE COURSE OF THE DAY—(e.g., sometimes better, sometimes worse; behaviors sometimes present, sometimes not)

**6. CHANGE IN COGNITIVE STATUS** Resident's cognitive status, skills, or abilities have changed as compared to status of **90 days ago** (or since last assessment if less than 90 days)
0. No change   1. Improved   2. Deteriorated

### SECTION C. COMMUNICATION/HEARING PATTERNS

**1. HEARING** (*With hearing appliance, if used*)
0. *HEARS ADEQUATELY*—normal talk, TV, phone
1. *MINIMAL DIFFICULTY* when not in quiet setting
2. *HEARS IN SPECIAL SITUATIONS ONLY*—speaker has to adjust tonal quality and speak distinctly
3. *HIGHLY IMPAIRED*/absence of useful hearing

**2. COMMUNICATION DEVICES/ TECHNIQUES** (*Check all that apply* during last 7 days)

| Hearing aid, present and used | a. |
|---|---|
| Hearing aid, present and not used regularly | b. |
| Other receptive comm. techniques used (e.g., lip reading) | c. |
| *NONE OF ABOVE* | d. |

**3. MODES OF EXPRESSION** (*Check all used* by resident to make needs known)

| Speech | a. | Signs/gestures/sounds | d. |
|---|---|---|---|
| Writing messages to express or clarify needs | b. | Communication board | e. |
| American sign language or Braille | c. | Other | f. |
| | | *NONE OF ABOVE* | g. |

**4. MAKING SELF UNDERSTOOD** (*Expressing information content—however able*)
0. *UNDERSTOOD*
1. *USUALLY UNDERSTOOD*—difficulty finding words or finishing thoughts
2. *SOMETIMES UNDERSTOOD*—ability is limited to making concrete requests
3. *RARELY/NEVER UNDERSTOOD*

**5. SPEECH CLARITY** (*Code for speech in the* **last 7 days**)
0. *CLEAR SPEECH*—distinct, intelligible words
1. *UNCLEAR SPEECH*—slurred, mumbled words
2. *NO SPEECH*—absence of spoken words

**6. ABILITY TO UNDERSTAND OTHERS** (*Understanding verbal information content—however able*)
0. *UNDERSTANDS*
1. *USUALLY UNDERSTANDS*—may miss some part/intent of message
2. *SOMETIMES UNDERSTANDS*—responds adequately to simple, direct communication
3. *RARELY/NEVER UNDERSTANDS*

**7. CHANGE IN COMMUNICATION/ HEARING** Resident's ability to express, understand, or hear information has changed as compared to status of **90 days ago** (or since last assessment if less than 90 days)
0. No change   1. Improved   2. Deteriorated

☐ = When box blank, must enter number or letter   ☐a. = When letter in box, check if condition applies

MDS 2.0 September, 2000

**FIGURE 9-14   Sample page from Resident Assessment Instrument (MDS 2.0).**

## Payment Rates Under the Hospital Outpatient Prospective Payment System

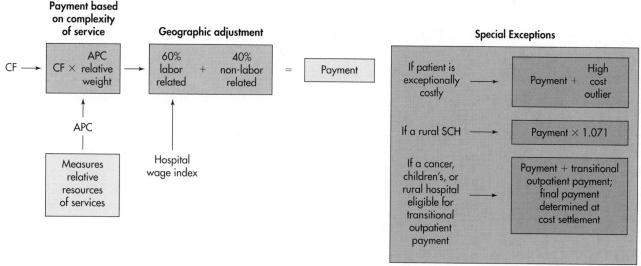

**FIGURE 9-15** **How an OPPS payment is calculated.**[6]

APCs have relative weights that represent the resource requirements of the service. The payment rates are determined by multiplying the APC's relative weight by a national conversion factor (dollar amount) to arrive at a national unadjusted payment rate for the APC. The payment rate is then further adjusted for geographic wage and price differences.

An important difference is that an outpatient claim can have multiple APCs, whereas an inpatient claim can have only one DRG. Most services are paid individually; the claim reimbursement is the sum of all the APC amounts added together. The exception is a service that is considered an integral part of another service on the claim. It is not paid under OPPS. Also, when multiple surgical procedures are performed in the same operation, the procedure with the highest APC is paid in full and other procedures performed at the same time are paid at 50%.

The APC is determined from the HCPC/CPT-4 codes on the claim. The ICD-9-CM diagnostic codes are reported but do not determine the payment (unless the diagnosis does not support the procedure performed). An additional code, called a *revenue code,* is reported on the claim. The revenue code indicates the provider's cost center (i.e., department that provided the service). It is used to map charges to costs for cost reporting. CMS does not instruct hospitals on the assignment of HCPCS/CPT-4 codes to revenue codes in the charge master since hospitals' assignments of costs vary.

Medicare beneficiaries must pay a coinsurance amount for outpatient services. Under OPPS, coinsurance due from the patient is generally 20% of the adjusted payment rate. The flowchart in Figure 9-15 shows how an OPPS payment is calculated.

## Non-Medicare Plans

Studying Medicare reimbursement methods is useful to understand how health plans reimburse doctors and hospitals. Though Blue Cross and other plans model reimbursement based on Medicare policies and methodologies, there are necessary differences. The average age of Medicare beneficiaries skews data toward services used by the elderly. Therefore, plans serving the general population must establish their own rates and determine reimbursements by factoring in the needs of their members and services of their participating providers, particularly with respect to pediatrics and obstetrics.

[6]*Source: Outpatient Prospective Payment System Fact Sheet,* Medicare Learning Network (Baltimore, MD: Centers for Medicare and Medicaid Services, 2007).

## A REAL-LIFE STORY

### Civil and Criminal Cases of Medical Billing Fraud

*From the files of the Office of Inspector General and the U.S. Attorney General.*

The following are real-life cases alleging medical billing fraud by corporations, employees, or medical professionals. These stories provide real-life examples of the results of some of the unethical and illegal fraudulent practices described in the following section.

The stories involve two types of cases, civil and criminal. Civil cases are settled with a civil monetary penalty in which the settling party has agreed to pay a fine without admitting any liability. In criminal cases, the corporation or individual has been prosecuted by the U.S. Attorney General and found guilty by a federal court.

### Billing the Wrong Code, Unnecessary Services, and Missing Signatures

The city of Chicago, Illinois, agreed to pay $6.9 million for allegedly submitting claims to Medicare for ambulance services that were not medically necessary, billing at the wrong level of service, and submitting claims without the patient's or other appropriate person's signature as required by CMS regulations.

### Billing Unnecessary Hospital Services

Sparks Health System, Sparks Medical Foundation, and Sparks Regional Medical Center agreed to pay $1,142,973 for allegedly billing Medicare for medically unnecessary hospital services.

### Reporting Fraudulent Hospital Costs

Sabine County Hospital District, Texas, agreed to pay $82,341, for allegedly fraudulently including physician recruiting fees on its cost report as a reimbursable expense.

### Charging Medicare Patients More than the Allowed Amount

A physician from Minneapolis, Minnesota, agreed to pay $53,400 to resolve his liability for allegedly violating his provider's assignment agreement. By accepting assignment for all covered services, a participating provider agrees that he or she will not collect from a Medicare beneficiary more than the applicable deductible and coinsurance for covered services.

The OIG alleged that the physician created a program whereby the physician's patients were asked to sign a yearly contract and pay a yearly fee for services that the physician characterized as "not covered" by Medicare. Because at least some of the services described in the contract were actually covered and reimbursable by Medicare, each contract presented to the Medicare patients constituted a request for payment other than the coinsurance and applicable deductible for covered services and was in violation of the terms of the physician's assignment agreement.

### Triple Billing of Medicare Visits

Temple Health Services, LLC, a medical clinic in New Haven, Connecticut, entered into a civil settlement agreement with the government in which it will pay $284,398 to resolve allegations that it violated the False Claims Act by billing Medicare for physical therapy services and physician's services that were not medically necessary or were not provided as billed.

Cardiologists would refer Medicare patients with certain cardiac conditions to Temple Health Services for cardiac rehabilitation. However, almost every time a Medicare patient went to the clinic for the cardiac rehabilitation services, Temple Health

## Fraud and Abuse

One aspect of HIPAA that wasn't discussed in Chapter 3 is that HIPAA also authorized the Office of Inspector General (OIG) to investigate cases of fraudulent healthcare practices. Currently, the OIG focuses on health claims paid through government programs, but HIPAA authorizes the OIG to investigate cases involving private health plans as well. The following are some examples of unethical and illegal fraudulent practices:

- Medically unnecessary services performed to increase reimbursement.
- Upcoding, the act of deliberately incorrectly coding a hospital claim so that the Grouper software will assign a DRG with a higher payment rate. This is also called maximizing.
- Unbundling, which consists of coding components of a comprehensive service as several HCPCS codes instead of the appropriate comprehensive code which encompassed the components. This is also called downcoding.

Services would bill Medicare for physical therapy services and a physician's office visit, in addition to the cardiac rehabilitation services. The physical therapy services and physician's services either were not medically necessary or were not provided as billed.

### Billing for Medical Equipment Never Provided

The owner of several durable medical equipment (DME) companies in Miami, Florida, was sentenced to 120 months in prison for his role in a multi-million-dollar healthcare fraud. The DME companies he owned collectively submitted more than $16,500,000 in false claims to Medicare for services and equipment that were never provided.

### Tampering with Lab Results and Health Records to Justify Billing

The owner and operator of two clinics, Medcore Group LLC and M&P Group of South Florida Inc., pleaded guilty to defrauding the Medicare program in connection with a $5.3 million HIV infusion fraud scheme. He and others used physicians, a physician's assistant, and phlebotomists to help facilitate the scheme.

Clinic employees intentionally manipulated patients' blood samples so that they would appear to need treatment, when in fact they did not. The owner/operator admitted that such tampering was done to make the medical files appear legitimate. Most patients were HIV positive or were given false diagnoses of cancer. The treatments for infused or injected drugs were not medically necessary, and he and others paid cash kickbacks to the patients for every visit to the clinic.

### Falsifying Utilization Review Documents

A registered nurse who managed, directed, and operated a business providing consulting services to skilled nursing facilities in Alabama and other states was sentenced by a federal court to serve 18 months in prison, two years of supervised release, and ordered to pay $600,000 in restitution to the Medicare program for intentionally creating documents that she knew were false and would mislead Medicare's fiscal intermediaries into believing that physicians working with her company were performing a larger portion of the utilization review (UR) services than they actually were, despite her knowledge that the physicians did not do so. She knew that the skilled nursing facilities would use these false statements to submit cost reports to Medicare fiscal intermediaries containing false information regarding the UR services.

Medicare guidelines state that only payments made to physicians for their services on UR committees are allowable as costs on a cost report for a skilled nursing facility. Nonphysician compensation associated with UR services are allowable only as part of the administrative costs of the skilled nursing facility and must be allocated as such.

### Necessary Infusions Billed, but Never Provided

The U.S. District Court in Savannah sentenced the owner of Longevity Care Services to 51 months imprisonment in connection with a scheme to defraud Medicare by billing for $3.4 million of phony infusion services that were never provided. Infusion services, when properly performed, are used to treat patients with immunocompromised conditions such as AIDS and cancer.

### OIG Case Involving Private Health Plans

Cannon Family Medicine, Inc., of Kannapolis, North Carolina, and its president plead guilty to four counts of healthcare fraud for submitting false claims to private health insurance companies as well Medicare, Department of Insurance, and the U.S. Office of Personnel Management.

- Billing for services not provided.
- Billing for levels of service that are not supported by documentation in the patient's health record.

## Corporate Compliance

The OIG outlined the minimum necessary elements for a comprehensive corporate compliance program. By following a compliance program encompassing these elements, an organization can fulfill its legal duty to ensure that it is not submitting false or inaccurate claims. Because the assignments of ICD-9-CM and HCPCS/CPT-4 codes determine how much is paid, a HIM compliance plan is integral to corporate compliance. The plan should include:

- A *code of conduct,* such as the AHIMA Standards of Ethical Coding, should be in place.
- *Policies and procedures,* such as a coding compliance manual that describes the organizations coding standards in writing, should be implemented.

■ *Education and training* sessions for coders should be provided monthly to ensure they are up to date on changes to ICD-9-CM and HCPCS/CPT-4 codes, the PPS, and coding guidelines.

■ *Effective communication* between managers and coding professionals and between coders and physicians is necessary when coding issues arise.

■ Ongoing *internal audits* should be conducted to ensure compliance with coding policies and issues and to identify problems that could result in sanctions and fines for the facility.

■ *Corrective action* should be taken to resolve problems and prevent similar problems in the future.

■ *Reporting* on compliance activities should be documented and reviewed by the corporate compliance officer.

# Chapter 9 Summary

## Healthcare Business

The business model for healthcare today involves at least three parties: the provider, the patient, and the health insurance plan, which is called the *third-party payer*. In most cases, the provider bills the insurance plan first. This is called an insurance claim. To know which plan to bill and to have the necessary data for billing, patient insurance information is recorded during registration and used when preparing the claim.

## Patient Accounts and Registration

A provider in a contractual relationship with the plan is called a *participating provider*. The participation agreement usually requires providers to accept an amount that is less than their usual fee, called the *allowed amount*.

• For professional and outpatient services, the allowed amounts are based on the procedures on the claim.

• For acute care hospitals, the payment is for the entire inpatient stay and is based on the *principal diagnosis* and the severity of any secondary diagnosis (*comorbidity* or *complication*).

Participating providers (both professional and institutional) must adjust the patient account for the difference between the original charges and the allowed amount. This is called an accounting adjustment or *write-down*.

A portion of each claim is usually the responsibility of the patient. This might be a flat rate per visit called a *copay*, or a percentage of the allowed amount called *coinsurance*. Patients may also have a *deductible* amount that must be paid by the patient each year. Patients and providers are sent explanations of benefits (EOBs) from the plan that list the procedures, allowed amount, insurance payment, and the portion for which the patient is responsible. The patient is sent a bill or statement by the provider showing the amount currently owed by the patient.

## Codes for Billing

Providers and payers are required to use standardized codes for healthcare transactions, such as insurance claims and remittance advice.

Billing for procedures, services, and supplies is done using the Healthcare Common Procedure Coding System (HCPCS), which includes the Current Procedural Terminology, Fourth Edition (CPT-4) codes.

Diagnoses codes are reported using the International Classification of Diseases, Ninth Revision, Clinical Modification (ICD-9-CM) codes. A tenth revision, ICD-10, has been created, but will not go into effect in the United States until at least 2013.

DRGs are used to classify ICD-9-CM codes into 25 major diagnostic categories (MDCs). The old DRG system had 538 codes; the newer MS-DRG system has 745 codes.

## Reimbursement Methodologies

Discounted fee-for-service plans attempt to control healthcare costs by controlling what the provider can charge.

Managed care plans attempt to control healthcare costs by controlling patients' utilization of services. There are several types of managed care plans:

■ *Staff Model:* HMO owns the facilities and employs the doctors.

■ *Group Practice Model:* HMO contracts with facilities and physicians to provide the services.

■ *Independent Practice Association (IPA) model:* A number of independent physicians form a business arrangement (IPA) for the purpose of contracting with the HMO. The IPA receives payment from the HMO and distributes it among the IPA physicians.

■ *Integrated Delivery Network (IDN) Model:* Facilities and physicians form a business arrangement (IDN) for the purpose of contracting with the HMO to provide both hospital and physician services.

The preferred provider organization (PPO) model allows patients to choose from PPO physicians and facilities, but also to use non-PPO providers. Patients are encouraged to stay within the PPO network because they must pay a higher share of the cost when they use a non-PPO provider.

Government programs, in particular Medicare and Medicaid, are the largest payers in the United States. As such, the policies and reimbursement models created by Medicare are adopted and emulated by many private payers.

Medicare Part A pays for inpatient hospital stays and skilled nursing facilities and reimburses hospitals per discharge based on a prospective payment system (PPS). Most Medicare Part A beneficiaries do not pay premiums because these were collected during their working years as Medicare taxes.

Medicare Part B pays for professional services and bases reimbursement on a discounted fee-for-service model. The amount allowed for each procedure is calculated by multiplying its relative value unit times a dollar amount conversion factor. The Resource-Based Relative Value Scale (RBRVS) varies the RVU by wage and geographic differences. Medicare B requires most patients to pay a premium.

Medicare C or Medicare Advantage Plans are HMO plans authorized by Medicare. The patient pays a premium to the HMO, which supplies all of the patient's Part A, Part B, Medigap, and sometimes Part D coverage.

Medicare Part D helps patients purchase prescription drugs at a lower cost. Patients pay a premium to private insurance plans for Medicare Part D coverage.

Medigap supplemental insurance is private insurance that pays the portion of Medicare claims and deductibles for which the patient is responsible.

## Prospective Payment System Reimbursement

Prospective payment systems use diagnosis-related groups (DRGs) to determine reimbursement for inpatient stays at all types of hospitals. Studies showed that patients with similar conditions had similar lengths of stay and used approximately the same amount of resources. The DRG is determined from the principal diagnosis and then a higher DRG is assigned if there are relevant diagnoses of comorbidities or complications (that are not the hospital's fault). Medicare improved the DRG system to better account for the medical severity of the health-related situations. This is called the MS-DRG or Medicare severity diagnosis-related groups.

The PPS adjusts the relative weight of the DRG for geographic and wage differences. Acute care hospitals are also reimbursed extra for serving low-income patients or acting as a teaching facility.

Outpatient services provided by hospitals are reimbursed using the outpatient prospective payment system (OPPS). This system does not use DRGs and does not apply to doctor's offices.

OPPS determines payment based on procedures instead of diagnosis groups. Procedures are assigned to an Ambulatory Payment Classification (APC), which has relative weights that represent the resource requirements of the service. Reimbursement is calculated from the relative weight of the APC times a national conversion factor, then adjusted for wage and geographic differences.

An important difference between inpatient prospective payment systems and OPPS is that an outpatient claim can have multiple APCs, whereas an inpatient claim can have only one DRG.

## Fraud and Abuse

It is both unethical and illegal to file false claims for unnecessary services, falsify medical records, violate participating provider agreements, or manipulate coding and billing. To prevent fraud and abuse, HIPAA authorized the Office of Inspector General (OIG) to investigate and prosecute cases of fraudulent healthcare billing to private insurance plans as well as government programs.

# Critical Thinking Exercises

1. Several reimbursement methodologies were described in this chapter. What incentive would a provider have to participate in each reimbursement type?
2. A clinic encourages Medicare patients to have tests that are not covered by Medicare. They always have the patient sign an Advance Beneficiary Notice. How do you feel about this policy?

# Testing Your Knowledge of Chapter 9

1. What is the difference between a diagnosis of comorbidity and complication?

2. Under what conditions will a complication not result in payment of a higher DRG?

3. Which Medicare plan pays for doctor's services—Part A or Part B?

4. Give an example of a type of hospital exempt from IPPS.

5. What is a standard method of calculating capitation payments?

6. What is the` difference between a staff model HMO and an IDN model HMO?

7. A participating provider's usual and customary fee for a service is $120, the Medicare allowed amount is $78. What is the amount of the write-down adjustment?

8. Two patients have the same insurance plan and the same DRG. Patient Jones's inpatient stay lasted 1 day. Patient Smith's inpatient stay lasted 2½ days. How much more will the PPS pay for Smith's claim?

*Write out the full name of the following acronyms:*

9. APC _____

10. DRG _____

11. EOB _____

12. PCP _____

13. RVU _____

14. When should you use the ICD-10 codes to code insurance claims?

15. What does it mean when a facility payment is calculated per diem?

# Healthcare Transactions and Billing

**10**

## LEARNING OUTCOMES

After completing this chapter, you should be able to:

- Describe the billing workflow
- Identify the eight types of HIPAA electronic transactions
- Compare the differences between hospital and professional claim forms
- Explain the functions of a clearinghouse
- Discuss the concepts of claim scrubbers, accounts receivable, and the payment floor
- Explain how electronic data interchange (EDI) transactions work

## ACRONYMS USED IN CHAPTER 10

Acronyms are used extensively in both medicine and computers. The following acronyms are used in this chapter.

| | | | |
|---|---|---|---|
| **ANSI** | American National Standards Institute | **EDI** | Electronic Data Interchange |
| **ANSI 837-D** | HIPAA-Compliant Dental Claim Format | **EFT** | Electronic Funds Transfer |
| | | **EHR** | Electronic Health Record |
| **ANSI 837-I** | HIPAA-Compliant Institutional Claim Format | **EMC** | Electronic Media Claims |
| | | **EOB** | Explanation of Benefits |
| **ANSI 837-P** | HIPAA-Compliant Professional Claim Format | **ER** | Emergency Room (Emergency Department) |
| **APC** | Ambulatory Payment Classification | **ERA** | Electronic Remittance Advice |
| **ASC** | Accredited Standards Committee | **FTE** | Full-Time Equivalent Employees |
| **CDA** | Clinical Document Architecture | **HCPCS** | Healthcare Common Procedure Coding System |
| **CMN** | Certificates of Medical Necessity | **HHS** | (U.S.) Department of Health and Human Services |
| **CMS** | Centers for Medicare and Medicaid Services | **HIPAA** | Health Insurance Portability and Accountability Act |
| **CMS-1500** | Paper Claim Form for Professional Services | **HIPPS** | Health Insurance Prospective Payment System Code Set |
| **COB** | Coordination of Benefits | **HIS** | Health Information Service |
| **CPT-4** | Current Procedural Terminology, Fourth Edition | **HMO** | Health Maintenance Organization |
| **DISA** | Data Interchange Standards Association | **ICD-9-CM** | International Classification of Diseases, Ninth Revision with Clinical Modifications |
| **DRG** | Diagnosis-Related Group | | |

| | | | |
|---|---|---|---|
| **IPPS** | Inpatient Prospective Payment System | **PPO** | Preferred Provider Organization |
| | | **PPS** | Prospective Payment System |
| **MS-DRG** | Medicare Severity—Diagnosis-Related Group | **RUG** | Resource Utilization Group |
| | | **SDO** | ANSI-Accredited Standards Development Organization |
| **NCCI** | National Correct Coding Initiative | | |
| **NCPDP** | National Council for Prescription Drug Programs (Pharmacy EDI Format) | **SNF** | Skilled Nursing Facility |
| | | **UB-04** | Universal Billing Claim Form for Institutional Billing (also known as CMS-1450) |
| **NPI** | National Provider ID | | |
| **OCR** | Optical Character Recognition | **WC** | Workers' Compensation |
| **OPPS** | Outpatient Prospective Payment System | **X12N** | ANSI Insurance Standards Committee Responsible for Developing and Maintaining HIPAA Transactions |
| **PCP** | Primary Care Physician | | |
| **PHI** | Protected Health Information (HIPAA) | | |

# Secondary Health Records and Business Processes

Chapter 5 described secondary health records as those that are created by abstracting relevant details from the primary records. The business or billing office is one of the main departments creating and using secondary health records. A principal example of secondary records is the health insurance claim.

This chapter will examine health insurance claims, billing, and other healthcare transactions. To put some of the terms from Chapter 9 into the context of business office processes, we begin with an overview of a general billing workflow. We then examine separately the business processes of medical professionals and of hospitals. Follow the workflow in Figure 10-1 as you read the following section.

### Billing Workflow

1. Providers of all types verify patient insurance eligibility with the health plan, either prior to or during the admission or visit. Medical offices collect and post copays at the visit.

2. The patient is treated and discharged or checked out.

3. As you learned in Chapter 9, the provider usually needs to bill a third party, the insurance plan, in order to receive payment. The insurance bill is called a *claim*. The first step in preparing the claim is to assign procedure codes for the services rendered and the supplies used and diagnosis codes representing the disease or medical condition.

4. Using these codes and the patient registration information, a computer program generates a paper or electronic claim to be sent to the insurance plan.

   Before the claim is sent to the insurance plan, an insurance or claim specialist reviews the claim to make sure there are no errors. Because of the volume of claims, a computer program is used to examine the claim data and identify problems. Once the claim is correct, it is sent to the insurance plan (usually electronically).

5. When the claim is received by the insurance plan, it is adjudicated. If the claim is correct, a payment is sent to the provider; this is called the *remittance*. A paper or electronic document is generated that explains the amounts that were paid. This is called the *remittance advice* or *explanation of benefits* (EOB).

6. When the remittance is received by the provider, the payment amount is recorded in the patient accounts system. Frequently, the amount billed does not equal the amount paid. This may be the result of a contractual agreement that stipulates that the provider will

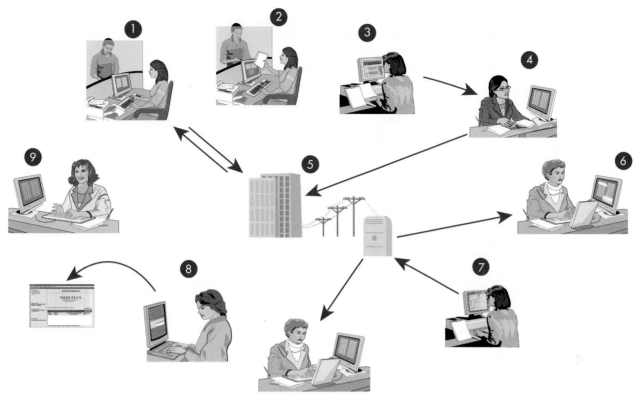

**FIGURE 10-1   Billing workflow.**

accept a discounted payment and/or that a portion of the charges is the patient's obligation. An accounting entry called a *write-down adjustment* is posted to adjust the charge.

7. If the patient has a secondary insurance plan, a claim is next sent to the second plan. In certain cases the first plan will automatically forward the claim to the second plan. This is called a "piggyback" claim or *coordination of benefit* (COB) claim. For example, when a Medicare patient has a supplemental insurance policy with the fiscal intermediary who processes the Medicare claims, the company will sometimes process the secondary claim automatically. This eliminates the need for the provider to file a second claim. These are also known as crossover claims.

8. Most health plans require the patient to pay a portion of the medical bill. These payments are referred to as the copay, coinsurance, and deductible amounts. The copay amount is usually stated on the patient's insurance card and collected during the patient visit. The coinsurance amount is usually a percentage of the allowed amount and is not known until the claim has been adjudicated. The EOB tells the provider what amount is the patient's responsibility.

   When all the patient's insurance plans have responded with remittance advice, a bill or statement is sent to the patient for any amounts due that are the patient's responsibility. The patient statement should clearly show the amounts paid or denied by the insurance plans, any adjustments to the charges required by the plan contract, and the amount due from the patient.

9. When patient payments are received by the medical office or hospital, they are posted to the patient's account. When the account balance is zero, no further statements will be sent.

## Patient Billing and Statements

Amounts that are determined to be "patient due" (i.e., the patient's responsibility to pay) are billed to the patient. A bill and a statement are not the same thing. A bill is akin to an invoice you might receive for a purchase. A statement is a list of charges, payments, and adjustments posted

Pay by check or credit card

If paying by credit card complete
reversed side

Rosa Garcia
1301 Paces Ferry Rd
Atlanta, GA 30339-1301

Patient ID 59301

Amount Due: 40.00
Due Date: June 10, 2010

**STATEMENT**
May 31, 2010

**Remit To:**
GOOD HEALTH ASSOCIATES
P.O. BOX 811
ATLANTA, GA 30305-0811

------------------------------- Detach and return top portion with your payment -------------------------------

| DATE | PROVIDER | DESCRIPTION | CHARGE | ADJ | INSUANCE PAID | PATIENT PAID | BALANCE DUE |
|------|----------|-------------|--------|-----|---------------|--------------|-------------|
| 04/07/2010 | C. Jones | Extended Office Visit | 70.00 | 16.51 | 33.49 | 20.00 | 0.00 |
| 04/07/2010 | C. Jones | CBC | 49.00 | 40.00 | 9.00 | 0.00 | 0.00 |
| 05/16/2010 | C. Jones | Extended Office Visit | 70.00 | | 0.00 | 0.00 | 70.00 |
| 05/23/2010 | M. Smith | Brief Office Visit | 45.00 | | 0.00 | 0.00 | 45.00 |

|  |  |
|--|--|
| **Subtotal** | 115.00 |
| **Billed to insurance** | 115.00 |
| **PATIENT due now** | 40.00 |

**PATIENT IS RESPONSIBLE FOR BALANCES NOT PAID**
**BY INSURANCE**

# GOOD HEALTH ASSOCIATES

P. O. Box 811
Atlanta, GA 30305-0811
PHONE (404) 555-2010

**STATEMENT**
May 31, 2010
Patient ID 59301
Amount Paid:

**FIGURE 10-2** **Example of an open item patient statement.**

to the account during the period covered by the statement. Most healthcare facilities send patient statements, though some may call them patient bills. Several types of patient statements are discussed next.

**BALANCE FORWARD PATIENT STATEMENT** A balance forward statement lists charges and payments for one period. Subsequent statements simply start with a line giving the balance from the previous statement, and then list any new payments, charges, or adjustments posted in the current period. A bank statement or credit card statement is an example of a balance forward statement. Balance forward statements work fine for banks. However, because healthcare reimbursement involves third-party payers and because it can take weeks or months for claims to be filed, adjudicated, and processed, balance forward statements confuse the patients. Payments listed on a balance forward statement may be for services provides several months ago, not services listed on the current statement; it is therefore not apparent to the patient to which charges the payments were applied.

**OPEN ITEM PATIENT STATEMENT**   An open item statement lists each charge, how much has been paid by the insurance plan, how much was written down by the provider, and how much is due from the patient. The charges for each visit are reprinted on subsequent statements until they are paid in full. The bottom of the open item statement clearly shows the amount pending with the insurance plan and the amount due from the patient. Figure 10-2 shows a sample of an open item statement.

**HOSPITALS BILLS OR STATEMENTS**   Patient bills from hospitals list charges for tests, services, and the inpatient stay, but do not usually detail every item that was used or charged. For example, a summary line may appear on the bill for use of the surgical suite and surgical supplies, but will not list in detail each of the supplies used, even though those items were recorded in the hospital's cost accounting system. (Note that the surgeon's and anesthesiologist's fees are not on the hospital bill; they are billed separately by the doctors.)

One reason hospitals summarize the details of charges is because hospitals are reimbursed under a prospective payment system (PPS), as discussed in Chapter 9, which is different from the way doctors and other healthcare providers are reimbursed. As mentioned earlier, hospitals start a new patient account for every stay. This method of accounting ensures that insurance payments are applied to the correct inpatient stay when a patient is hospitalized more than once. However, separate patient accounts mean that a patient who has been in the hospital several times will receive multiple bills and statements. This sometimes confuses patients.

# Electronic Data Interchange (EDI)

As discussed in Chapter 3, HIPAA mandated eight electronic transactions and required all but the smallest health plans to make them available to providers. The process of exchanging these transactions is called electronic data interchange or EDI.

Some forms of EDI, particularly the electronic media claim (EMC), had been in use for several years, but health plans used many different EMC formats and providers could not keep up. HIPAA standardized EDI formats by requiring specific transaction standards for eight types of electronic data interchange.

Seven of the eight transactions use standard formats developed by the American National Standards Institute (ANSI) Data Interchange Standards Association (DISA) Accredited Standards Committee (ASC) X12n. The ANSI X12 EDI standards have long alphanumeric designations, but they are often referred to in a shortened version (i.e., ASC X12 835 or ANSI 835). We will use the shorter ANSI designation throughout this text.

The eighth HIPAA-mandated transaction format, retail pharmacy claims, was not created by ANSI. It is instead a format maintained by the National Council for Prescription Drug Programs, Inc. (NCPDP), an ANSI-accredited SDO, but not part of the X12n committee.

To review, here are the eight transactions required by HIPAA and their ANSI and NCPDP format numbers:

1. Claims or equivalent encounters and coordination of benefits (ANSI 837). Due to differences in reimbursement methodologies, variations were made in this format to accommodate different providers. The formats are ANSI 837-P (professional claims), ANSI 837-I (institutional claims), and ANSI 837-D (dental claims)

2. Remittance and payment advice (ANSI 835, Health Care Claim Payment/Advice)

3. Claim status inquiry and response (ANSI 276, Health Care Claim Status Request; ANSI 277, Health Care Claim Status Response)

4. Eligibility benefit inquiry and response (ANSI 270, Health Care Eligibility Benefit Inquiry; ANSI 271, Health Care Eligibility Benefit Response).

5. Referral certification and authorization (ANSI 278, Health Care Services Request for Review and Response)

6. Health plan premium payments (ANSI 820, Payroll Deducted and Other Group Premium Payment for Insurance Products)

7. Enrollment and de-enrollment in a health plan (ANSI 834, Benefit Enrollment and Maintenance)

8. Retail drug claims, coordination of drug benefits and eligibility inquiry (NCPDP 5.1, Version D.0).

Transaction standards for two additional HIPAA transactions have not yet been finalized:

9. Health claims attachments (ANSI 275, Patient Information in Support of a Health Claim or Encounter; not final)

10. First report of injury for reporting workers' compensation incidents (not final).

Though transactions such as electronic insurance eligibility verification are important, the principal goal was to eliminate the work involved in producing and processing paper claims and paper remittance advice. Because those are the major components in healthcare business, we will examine them next. However, because the reimbursement models for healthcare professionals differ dramatically from those used for hospitals, their claims are different as well. Therefore, we will discuss these providers' claims separately.

## Professional Services

Medicare and other insurance plans use two different types of claims, one for professional billing and another for institutional billing. Physicians, chiropractors, osteopaths, therapists, and nearly all other medical professionals bill for their services using the professional claim ANSI 837-P or CMS-1500.

### Real-Time and Batch Posting

*Posting* is a term used for the act of putting charges and payments into the patient accounting system. In many medical offices, this is done in real time; that is, while the patient is still in the office. One advantage of real-time posting is that it allows for the collection of copay and sometimes coinsurance amounts due from the patient. Another is that it can shorten the revenue cycle, because at the end of the day the charge posting is complete and ready to be billed to insurance. *Charge posting* is also called *charge capture*.

Figure 10-3 shows an encounter form or superbill recommended by the American Academy of Family Practice for use in physician offices to communicate billing information about the visit. These are also known as charge tickets. The forms are numbered and identify the patient, provider, and date and time of the visit. They typically list the most common procedures and diagnosis codes used by the office. The doctor circles or checks the services and diagnosis. The person posting the charges enters the codes the doctor has marked on the form; the computer locates the item from the charge master and calculates the fee.

The process is essentially the same in batch posting, except that the superbills are not entered into the computer on the day of the visit. Instead they are gathered into a batch for the date and posted later. Some offices use a billing service to post charges, generate insurance claims, and send patient statements. The batch method is common when using a billing service.

With either method, superbills are numbered and missing numbers must be accounted for. A report of the payments and charges that have been posted is compared to the information on the superbills to ensure charges were posted correctly.

Some doctors do not see patients in the office. For example, anesthesiologists bill for their services, but do not have office visits. Many anesthesiologists use billing services. Other specialists such as radiologists and surgeons may see patients in their office, but also bill for

# Family Practice Management Superbill Template

From the American Academy of Family Practice (AAFP) Family Practice Management Toolkit
(http://www.aafp.org/fpm/20060900/43inse.html)

| | | |
|---|---|---|
| Date of service: | Waiver? ☐ | |
| Patient name: | Insurance: | |
| | Subscriber name: | |
| Address: | Group #: | Previous balance: |
| | Copay: | Today's charges: |
| Phone: | Account #: | Today's payment: check# |
| DOB:        Age:        Sex: | Physician name: | Balance due: |

| RANK | Office visit | New | Est |
|---|---|---|---|
| | Minimal | | 99211 |
| | Problem focused | 99201 | 99212 |
| | Expanded problem focused | 99202 | 99213 |
| | Detailed | 99203 | 99214 |
| | Comprehensive | 99204 | 99215 |
| | Comprehensive (new patient) | 99205 | |
| | Significant, separate service | -25 | -25 |
| | **Well visit** | **New** | **Est** |
| | < 1 y | 99381 | 99391 |
| | 1-4 y | 99382 | 99392 |
| | 5-11 y | 99383 | 99393 |
| | 12-17 y | 99384 | 99394 |
| | 18-39 y | 99385 | 99395 |
| | 40-64 y | 99386 | 99396 |
| | 65 y + | 99387 | 99397 |
| | **Medicare preventive services** | | |
| | Pap | | Q0091 |
| | Pelvic & breast | | G0101 |
| | Prostate/PSA | | G0103 |
| | Tobacco counseling/3-10 min | | 99406 |
| | Tobacco counseling/>10 min | | 99407 |
| | Welcome to Medicare exam | | G0344 |
| | ECG w/Welcome to Medicare exam | | G0366 |
| | Flexible sigmoidoscopy | | G0104 |
| | Hemoccult, guaiac | | G0107 |
| | Flu shot | | G0008 |
| | Pneumonia shot | | G0009 |
| | **Consultation/preop clearance** | | |
| | Expanded problem focused | | 99242 |
| | Detailed | | 99243 |
| | Comprehensive/mod complexity | | 99244 |
| | Comprehensive/high complexity | | 99245 |
| | **Other services** | | |
| | After posted hours | | 99050 |
| | Evening/weekend appointment | | 99051 |
| | Home health certification | | G0180 |
| | Home health recertification | | G0179 |
| | Post-op follow-up | | 99024 |
| | Prolonged/30-74 min | | 99354 |
| | Special reports/forms | | 99080 |
| | Disability/Workers comp | | 99455 |
| | **Radiology** | | |
| | | | |
| | | | |

| RANK | Office procedures | | |
|---|---|---|---|
| | Anoscopy | | 46600 |
| | Audiometry | | 92551 |
| | Cerumen removal | | 69210 |
| | Colposcopy | | 57452 |
| | Colposcopy w/biopsy | | 57455 |
| | ECG, w/interpretation | | 93000 |
| | ECG, rhythm strip | | 93040 |
| | Endometrial biopsy | | 58100 |
| | Flexible sigmoidoscopy | | 45330 |
| | Flexible sigmoidoscopy w/biopsy | | 45331 |
| | Fracture care, cast/splint | 29____ | |
| | Site: _____ | | |
| | Nebulizer | | 94640 |
| | Nebulizer demo | | 94664 |
| | Spirometry | | 94010 |
| | Spirometry, pre and post | | 94060 |
| | Tympanometry | | 92567 |
| | Vasectomy | | 55250 |
| | **Skin procedures** | | **Units** |
| | Burn care, initial | 16000 | |
| | Foreign body, skin, simple | 10120 | |
| | Foreign body, skin, complex | 10121 | |
| | I&D, abscess | 10060 | |
| | I&D, hematoma/seroma | 10140 | |
| | Laceration repair, simple | 120____ | |
| | Site: _____ Size: _____ | | |
| | Laceration repair, layered | 120____ | |
| | Site: _____ Size: _____ | | |
| | Lesion, biopsy, one | 11100 | |
| | Lesion, biopsy, each add'l | 11101 | |
| | Lesion, destruct., benign, 1-14 | 17110 | |
| | Lesion, destruct., premal., single | 17000 | |
| | Lesion, destruct., premal., ea. add'l | 17003 | |
| | Lesion, excision, benign | 114____ | |
| | Site: _____ Size: _____ | | |
| | Lesion, excision, malignant | 116____ | |
| | Site: _____ Size: _____ | | |
| | Lesion, paring/cutting, one | 11055 | |
| | Lesion, paring/cutting, 2-4 | 11056 | |
| | Lesion, shave | 113____ | |
| | Site: _____ Size: _____ | | |
| | Nail removal, partial | 11730 | |
| | Nail removal, w/matrix | 11750 | |
| | Skin tag, 1-15 | 11200 | |
| | **Medications** | | **Units** |
| | Ampicillin, up to 500mg | J0290 | |
| | B-12, up to 1,000 mcg | J3420 | |
| | Epinephrine, up to 1ml | J0170 | |
| | Kenalog, 10mg | J3301 | |
| | Lidocaine, 10mg | J2001 | |
| | Normal saline, 1000cc | J7030 | |
| | Phenergan, up to 50mg | J2550 | |
| | Progesterone, 150mg | J1055 | |
| | Rocephin, 250mg | J0696 | |
| | Testosterone, 200mg | J1080 | |
| | Tigan, up to 200 mg | J3250 | |
| | Toradol, 15mg | J1885 | |
| | **Miscellaneous services** | | |

| RANK | Laboratory | |
|---|---|---|
| | Venipuncture | 36415 |
| | Blood glucose, monitoring device | 82962 |
| | Blood glucose, visual dipstick | 82948 |
| | CBC, w/ auto differential | 85025 |
| | CBC, w/o auto differential | 85027 |
| | Cholesterol | 82465 |
| | Hemoccult, guaiac | 82270 |
| | Hemoccult, immunoassay | 82274 |
| | Hemoglobin A1C | 85018 |
| | Lipid panel | 80061 |
| | Liver panel | 80076 |
| | KOH prep (skin, hair, nails) | 87220 |
| | Metabolic panel, basic | 80048 |
| | Metabolic panel, comprehensive | 80053 |
| | Mononucleosis | 86308 |
| | Pregnancy, blood | 84703 |
| | Pregnancy, urine | 81025 |
| | Renal panel | 80069 |
| | Sedimentation rate | 85651 |
| | Strep, rapid | 86403 |
| | Strep culture | 87081 |
| | Strep A | 87880 |
| | TB | 86580 |
| | UA, complete, non-automated | 81000 |
| | UA, w/o micro, non-automated | 81002 |
| | UA, w/ micro, non-automated | 81003 |
| | Urine colony count | 87086 |
| | Urine culture, presumptive | 87088 |
| | Wet mount/KOH | 87210 |
| | **Vaccines** | |
| | DT, <7 y | 90702 |
| | DTP | 90701 |
| | DtaP, <7 y | 90700 |
| | Flu, 6-35 months | 90657 |
| | Flu, 3 y + | 90658 |
| | Hep A, adult | 90632 |
| | Hep A, ped/adol, 2 dose | 90633 |
| | Hep B, adult | 90746 |
| | Hep B, ped/adol 3 dose | 90744 |
| | Hep B-Hib | 90748 |
| | Hib, 4 dose | 90645 |
| | HPV | 90649 |
| | IPV | 90713 |
| | MMR | 90707 |
| | Pneumonia, >2 y | 90732 |
| | Pneumonia conjugate, <5 y | 90669 |
| | Td, >7 y | 90718 |
| | Varicella | 90716 |

| | Immunizations & Injections | | Units |
|---|---|---|---|
| | Allergen, one | 95115 | |
| | Allergen, multiple | 95117 | |
| | Imm admin, one | 90471 | |
| | Imm admin, each add'l | 90472 | |
| | Imm admin, intranasal, one | 90473 | |
| | Imm admin, intranasal, each add'l | 90474 | |
| | Injection, joint, small | 20600 | |
| | Injection, joint, intermediate | 20605 | |
| | Injection, joint, major | 20610 | |
| | Injection, ther/proph/diag | 90772 | |
| | Injection, trigger point | 20552 | |
| | **Supplies** | | |

| | Diagnoses |
|---|---|
| 1 | |
| 2 | |
| 3 | |
| 4 | |

**Next office visit**

| Recheck | Prev | PRN | _____ | D | W | M | Y |
|---|---|---|---|---|---|---|---|

Instructions:

**Referral**

To:

Instructions:

**Physician signature**

X _____

**FIGURE 10-3   Encounter form (also known as a superbill or charge ticket).**

services performed at the hospital. For these services, they do not use a superbill; instead, the charges are posted from a list or report provided by the doctor or hospital. These charges are batch posted.

### Payments

Payments are posted both in batches and real time. Patient payments, especially copay payments, are usually posted while the patient is present so that a receipt can be provided. Some offices collect the copay upon arrival; other offices collect the copay after the visit when the patient checks out.

Payments from insurance plans are often posted in batches. These payments may be accompanied by paper explanation of benefit (EOB) reports or electronic remittance advice (ERA) files. Both paper and electronic remittances can span multiple patients' claims and are sometimes dozens of pages long.

## Professional Claims Billing

The professional claim is a standard form. The paper version is the CMS-1500. The electronic version is the ANSI 837-P transaction. Medicare now requires all but the smallest provider to submit claims electronically. The most recent Medicare performance data available reported 94.8 percent of all Medicare Part B physician claims were electronic.[1] Whether claims are electronic or paper, most medical offices use a computer to generate the claim.

Though the majority of claims are electronic, the CMS-1500 form can be useful to understand what information is reported, since essentially the same content is required in paper or electronic format. A sample CMS-1500 form is shown later in Figure 10-5.

The fields on the CMS-1500 form are numbered boxes called *form locators*. Figure 10-5 describes some of the fields on the CMS-1500 form. Medicare requires the blank form to be printed in a special color of red ink. The fields are filled in by the provider in black ink. The red form allows some Medicare intermediaries to extract data from the paper form electronically using optical character recognition (OCR) software. This eliminates data entry for the intermediary.

As you will recall from Chapter 9, professional claim reimbursement is based on the charges for the procedures, services, and supplies provided. Therefore, each item is listed on the claim with its HCPCS/CPT-4 code and associated with one or more diagnoses that justify its medical necessity. The charges for each item are typically the providers' usual and customary rate for the item, not the contractual allowed amount they expect to be paid.

The same information is reported in an electronic claim. The difference is that electronic claims are sent in a file called a batch. Within that file are many claims for the same provider and possibly multiple claims for one or more patients. Because each paper claim is a form, it is necessary to repeat all the provider and patient information; with electronic claims, duplicate information is eliminated.

Figure 10-4 shows the structure of the ANSI 837-P electronic claim format required by HIPAA. The file structure of the ANSI 837-P starts with information about a transaction and the entity submitting the batch and then uses several loops to eliminate redundant repetition. Each loop in Figure 10-4 that is indented can be repeated so long as the information above it remains the same. For example, the billing provider is sent once; subsequent patients for that provider do not need to repeat the billing provider. Similarly, if the subscriber/patient has more than one claim, subsequent claims do not repeat the subscriber/patient information until the patient changes.

---

[1]*Electronic Media Claims (EMC) Rates for Medicare Carriers for Calendar Year 2007* (the most recent year available), www.cms.hhs.gov.

**Header** (Indicates start of transaction; the type and version of transaction)

> **Submitter** (Name and ID of entity authorized to submit claims)
> **Receiver** (Name of entity for which claim data is intended)

> > **Provider Loop** (Billing provider name and NPI information similar to CMS-1500 box 33)

> > > **Subscriber Loop** (Insured's information similar to CMS-1500 boxes 1a, 4, 7 and 11)
> > > **Patient Loop** (Patient information similar to CMS-1500 boxes 2–3, 5–6, and 8)

> > > > **Claim Loop** (Most claim information above and below the service loop in the CMS-1500 form; for example, boxes 14–23 [including diagnosis codes] as well as claims totals similar to boxes 28–30)

> > > > > **Service Line Loop** (Procedure code, modifier, amount, quantity; and rendering provider; similar to CMS-1500 boxes 24a–j with the addition of information about payments per line from other insurance plans)
> > > > > **Service Line Loop**—*Repeated for each procedure up to 999 lines*

> > > > **Claim Loop**—*Next claim, same patient*

> > > > > **Service Line Loop**—*Repeated for each procedure up to 999 lines*

> > > **Subscriber Loop** *Next subscriber and patient*
> > > **Patient Loop**

> > > > **Claim Loop**—*New claim, for this patient*

> > > > > **Service Line Loop**—*Repeated for each procedure up to 999 lines*

**Trailer** (indicated end of transaction set)

**FIGURE 10-4**

**Loop structure of ANSI 837-P electronic media claims.**

Other space-saving efficiencies are realized as well. For example, if the subscriber and patient are the same, the patient information is not repeated. Additionally, the data are separated by special characters and therefore require little more file space than the actual fielded data. Figure 10-6, shown later, allows you to see the efficiency of EMC data.

## Institutional Claims Billing

Hospitals and other institutions use a different claim form, both for paper and electronic billing, than do professional providers. This is necessary because as you learned in Chapter 9, hospital reimbursement is based on the principal diagnosis and diagnosis related group. The paper UB-04 form and the ANSI 837-I electronic format differ substantially from their counterparts used for professional claims. There are also differences in how hospital charges are posted.

### Hospital Batch Posting

Inpatient facilities do not bill until the patient is discharged and all of the records have been completed. For this reason, many hospitals do not begin coding and charge capture until the HIM department has analyzed the record and sent it for coding. Review the workflow illustrated in Chapter 2, Figure 2-1.

Hospitals often hold billing for a number of days after discharge to ensure that all the charges have been collected and coded. This is called the *bill-hold period*. At that point, there are hundreds of charges to be coded and posted. However, as hospital departments become computerized, the lab, pharmacy, supplies, radiology, and other departments are beginning to automatically post charges as the supplies or services are used; thus, reducing the number of items that must be manually posted.

One of the reasons hospitals have a bill-hold period is because both the DRG Grouper software used to determine the DRG and the OPPS Pricer software used for APCs analyze the diagnosis and procedure codes for the entire episode. If important services or diagnoses are missing, the wrong DRG may be used or APC codes may be missing from the claim. Although it is possible to submit a corrected or supplemental claim, it may not be paid. Also, claims must be submitted within a certain time frame or they will not be paid.

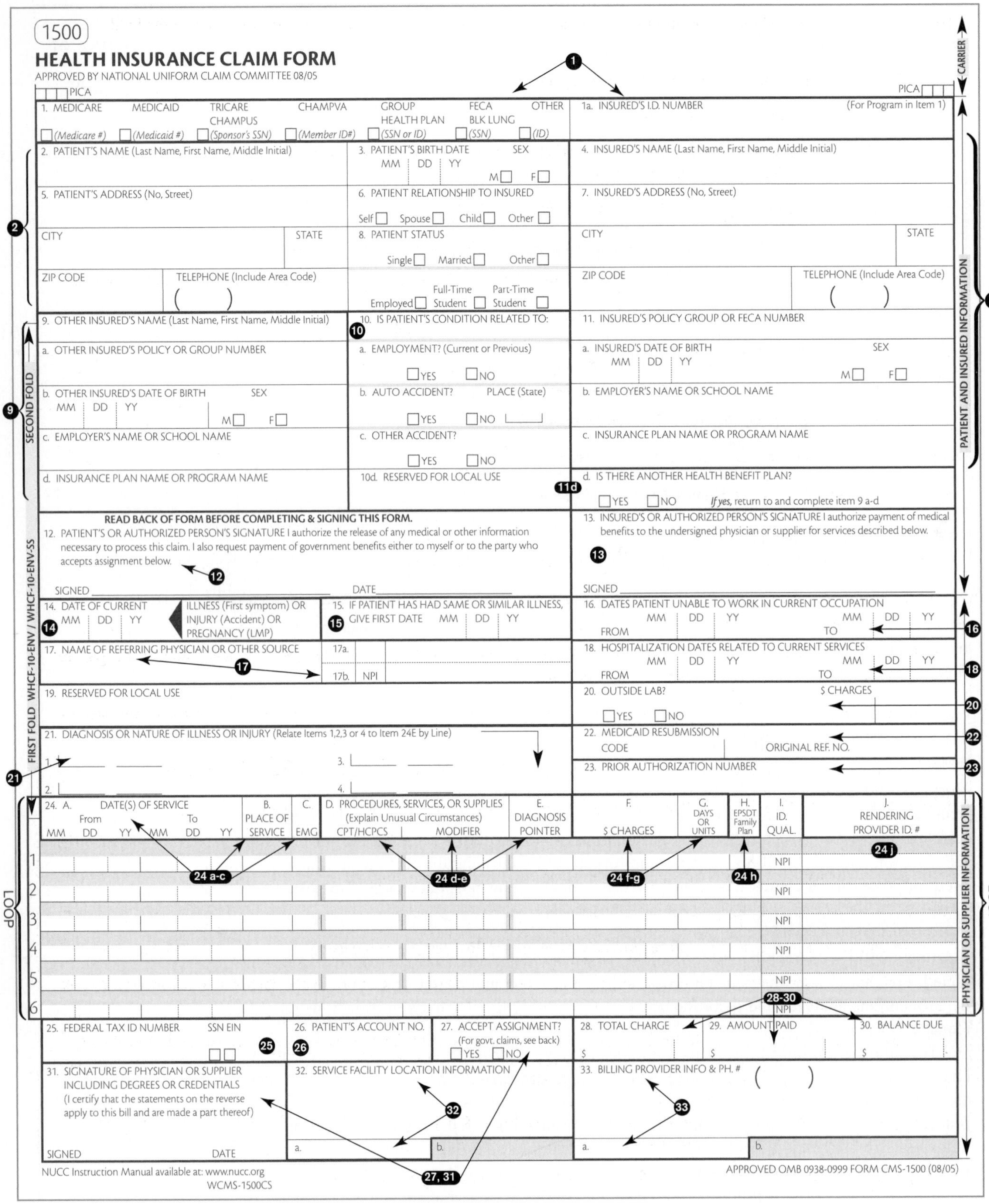

1500
HEALTH INSURANCE CLAIM FORM
APPROVED BY NATIONAL UNIFORM CLAIM COMMITTEE 08/05

PICA | PICA

1. MEDICARE (Medicare #) | MEDICAID (Medicaid #) | TRICARE CHAMPUS (Sponsor's SSN) | CHAMPVA (Member ID#) | GROUP HEALTH PLAN (SSN or ID) | FECA BLK LUNG (SSN) | OTHER (ID)

1a. INSURED'S I.D. NUMBER (For Program in Item 1)

2. PATIENT'S NAME (Last Name, First Name, Middle Initial)

3. PATIENT'S BIRTH DATE MM DD YY SEX M F

4. INSURED'S NAME (Last Name, First Name, Middle Initial)

5. PATIENT'S ADDRESS (No, Street)

6. PATIENT RELATIONSHIP TO INSURED Self Spouse Child Other

7. INSURED'S ADDRESS (No, Street)

CITY STATE

8. PATIENT STATUS Single Married Other

CITY STATE

ZIP CODE TELEPHONE (Include Area Code) ( )

Employed Full-Time Student Part-Time Student

ZIP CODE TELEPHONE (Include Area Code) ( )

9. OTHER INSURED'S NAME (Last Name, First Name, Middle Initial)

10. IS PATIENT'S CONDITION RELATED TO:

11. INSURED'S POLICY GROUP OR FECA NUMBER

a. OTHER INSURED'S POLICY OR GROUP NUMBER

a. EMPLOYMENT? (Current or Previous) YES NO

a. INSURED'S DATE OF BIRTH MM DD YY SEX M F

b. OTHER INSURED'S DATE OF BIRTH MM DD YY SEX M F

b. AUTO ACCIDENT? PLACE (State) YES NO

b. EMPLOYER'S NAME OR SCHOOL NAME

c. EMPLOYER'S NAME OR SCHOOL NAME

c. OTHER ACCIDENT? YES NO

c. INSURANCE PLAN NAME OR PROGRAM NAME

d. INSURANCE PLAN NAME OR PROGRAM NAME

10d. RESERVED FOR LOCAL USE

d. IS THERE ANOTHER HEALTH BENEFIT PLAN? YES NO *If yes,* return to and complete item 9 a-d

READ BACK OF FORM BEFORE COMPLETING & SIGNING THIS FORM.

12. PATIENT'S OR AUTHORIZED PERSON'S SIGNATURE I authorize the release of any medical or other information necessary to process this claim. I also request payment of government benefits either to myself or to the party who accepts assignment below.

SIGNED DATE

13. INSURED'S OR AUTHORIZED PERSON'S SIGNATURE I authorize payment of medical benefits to the undersigned physician or supplier for services described below.

SIGNED

14. DATE OF CURRENT MM DD YY — ILLNESS (First symptom) OR INJURY (Accident) OR PREGNANCY (LMP)

15. IF PATIENT HAS HAD SAME OR SIMILAR ILLNESS, GIVE FIRST DATE MM DD YY

16. DATES PATIENT UNABLE TO WORK IN CURRENT OCCUPATION FROM MM DD YY TO MM DD YY

17. NAME OF REFERRING PHYSICIAN OR OTHER SOURCE | 17a. | 17b. NPI

18. HOSPITALIZATION DATES RELATED TO CURRENT SERVICES FROM MM DD YY TO MM DD YY

19. RESERVED FOR LOCAL USE

20. OUTSIDE LAB? YES NO $ CHARGES

21. DIAGNOSIS OR NATURE OF ILLNESS OR INJURY (Relate Items 1,2,3 or 4 to Item 24E by Line)

1. 2. 3. 4.

22. MEDICAID RESUBMISSION CODE ORIGINAL REF. NO.

23. PRIOR AUTHORIZATION NUMBER

| 24. A. DATE(S) OF SERVICE From MM DD YY To MM DD YY | B. PLACE OF SERVICE | C. EMG | D. PROCEDURES, SERVICES, OR SUPPLIES (Explain Unusual Circumstances) CPT/HCPCS MODIFIER | E. DIAGNOSIS POINTER | F. $ CHARGES | G. DAYS OR UNITS | H. EPSDT Family Plan | I. ID. QUAL. | J. RENDERING PROVIDER ID. # |
|---|---|---|---|---|---|---|---|---|---|
| 1 | | | | | | | | NPI | |
| 2 | | | | | | | | NPI | |
| 3 | | | | | | | | NPI | |
| 4 | | | | | | | | NPI | |
| 5 | | | | | | | | NPI | |
| 6 | | | | | | | | NPI | |

25. FEDERAL TAX ID NUMBER SSN EIN

26. PATIENT'S ACCOUNT NO.

27. ACCEPT ASSIGNMENT? (For govt. claims, see back) YES NO

28. TOTAL CHARGE $

29. AMOUNT PAID $

30. BALANCE DUE $

31. SIGNATURE OF PHYSICIAN OR SUPPLIER INCLUDING DEGREES OR CREDENTIALS (I certify that the statements on the reverse apply to this bill and are made a part thereof)

SIGNED DATE

32. SERVICE FACILITY LOCATION INFORMATION a. b.

33. BILLING PROVIDER INFO & PH. # ( ) a. b.

NUCC Instruction Manual available at: www.nucc.org
WCMS-1500CS

APPROVED OMB 0938-0999 FORM CMS-1500 (08/05)



**FIGURE 10-5 CMS-1500 paper form for professional claims.**

**The fields on the CMS-1500 form are numbered boxes called form locators. The following describes some of the fields on the CMS-1500 form:**

**①** 1, 1a    Type of insurance plan, member ID or policy number.

**②** 2–3, 5–6, 8    Patient demographic information.

**④** 4, 7, 11a–c    Information about insured party; the primary person who is named on the health insurance card (also known as the subscriber, enrollee, member, or beneficiary).

**⑨** 9a–d, 11d    Information about secondary insurance, if any.

**⑩** 10    Is the condition the result of an accident? If so, auto or WC insurance may be responsible.

**⑫** 12    Patient signature to release PHI for claims processing; also for government programs, patient assigns benefits to provider.

**⑬** 13    Insured's signature to assign benefits to provider.

**⑭** 14    Date of onset of current illness or injury.

**⑮** 15    Date of previous occurrence of same or similar condition.

**⑯** 16    Dates patient is unable to work due to current condition.

**⑰** 17, 17b    Referring provider name and national provider ID number.

**⑱** 18    Hospitalization dates related to services on this claim.

**⑳** 20    If purchased lab services are included on claim, the name of lab and cost to provider are entered in this box.

**㉒** 22    If claim resubmitted to Medicaid, a reference number is entered in box.

**㉓** 23    If prior authorization required for services, an authorization number is entered in this box. For managed care plans, this is also called the referral number.

**㉑** 21    Diagnosis—up to four ICD-9-CM codes are entered in the numbered fields (called pointers). Later, in box 24e the pointer numbers will indicate the diagnoses for each procedure.

**Start Service Loop.**    Up to six procedures (related to four diagnoses) can be billed on the claim. Fields 24a–j are repeated for each procedure.

**24a–c** 24a–c    Dates of service, place of service (office, hospital, home, etc.), and whether visit was an emergency.

**24d–e** 24d–e    HCPCS/CPT-4 code, procedure modifier, and diagnoses codes pointers (from box 21).

**24f–g** 24f–g    Charge (dollar amount) and days or units; represent the fee for service. For example, $450 for 3 days of hospital visits.

**24h** 24h    Is service for Medicaid early periodic screening or family planning program.

**24j** 24j    National provider ID (NPI) of the provider who rendered the service.

**End service loop.**    When all the procedures have been printed, the charges are totaled.

**28–30** 28, 29, 30    Service loop totals; total of charges on claim, amount paid by primary plan (if this claim is secondary), and the balance due (charge minus payment),

**27,31** 27, 31    Provider accepts or declines assignment of benefits and certifies that the claim is accurate. (Most doctors do not sign every form; instead, they have signed a form permitting the facility to print "signature on file" on the claim. However, the doctor remains responsible for the accuracy of the claim.)

**25 26** 25, 26    Tax ID of the group practice, physician, or facility; the practice's internal account number for the patient, which is subsequently used to post payments to the correct patient account.

**32** 32, 32a    Facility where service was rendered and national provider ID (NPI) of facility.

**33** 33, 33a    Billing provider, address, and phone; national provider ID (NPI) of billing provider.

Once the codes for the services have been posted and checked by a coding or billing specialist, the claim is produced by a computer program (as described in Chapter 9). As with professional claims, institutional claims must be submitted electronically (with rare exceptions). The most recent Medicare performance data available reported 99.9 percent of all Medicare Part A hospital claims were electronic.[2] However, the UB-04 paper form can be useful to understand the information that is being sent in the ANSI 837-I electronic claim.

### UB-04 Claims

Figure 10-7 shows the UB-04 paper form used for institutional claims. The UB-04 is also known as Form CMS-1450. It is only accepted from institutional providers (hospitals, skilled nursing facilities, home health agencies, etc.) that are excluded from the mandatory electronic claims submission requirements.

The UB-04 form looks considerably different from the CMS-1500. Whereas the CMS-1500 has "yes/no" boxes for questions like "Accident," "Work-related," or "Student," the UB-04 does not. Because there are many more factors that could affect an inpatient claim "yes/no" check boxes and individual questions are replaced with coded fields. Special information affecting the claim is communicated through the use of condition codes, occurrence codes, and value codes. Also, because all of the charges for an inpatient stay might not fit on one piece of paper, the UB-04 claim is permitted to be nine pages long, which can accommodate 450 line items.

## Electronic Media Claims (EMCs)

HIPAA requires all but the smallest health plans to receive claims electronically in the ANSI 837 format and permits all types of providers to send them. Further, Medicare requires nearly all providers to submit claims electronically. As described earlier, there are variations in the content of the ANSI 837 to accommodate professional, institutional, and dental providers. However, the loop structure shown in Figure 10-4 remains consistent. EMC files are not usually a single claim, but batches of claims sent in one large file. The shaded portion of Figure 10-6 shows you what an ANSI 837-I transaction would look like if you could see inside the file. The numbered labels on the right side of Figure 10-6 help you identify the loops, but are not part of the transaction file.

### Clearinghouses

HIPAA defined a covered entity as a provider, health plan, or clearinghouse (see Chapter 3). A *clearinghouse* is generally thought of as an entity that acts as a transaction intermediary between the provider and the health plan. A clearinghouse receives claims from the provider, sends them to the plans, receives responses from the plans, and sends those responses to the provider. Technically, that function is called a *switch,* because HIPAA legally defines a clearinghouse as the specific function of converting data arriving in a noncompliant format into a HIPAA-compliant format.

Though clearinghouses do provide the conversion service defined by HIPAA, they serve a more practical purpose as well. A modern medical office may have 1,200 or more health plans defined in its computer system. In part, this is because different patients have different health plans. Another reason is that insurance companies offer many different plans. These plans may have different billing addresses and different fee structures; some of their plans may be fee-for-service, whereas others may be PPO or HMO; and so forth.

The result of this plethora of plans is that the billing department may be forced to deal with hundreds of EMC batches, one for each plan or unique carrier address. Imagine spending all week just transmitting files to all the different insurance carriers. So one service that clearinghouses provide is a single point of transmission.

---

[2]*Electronic Media Claims (EMC) Rates for Medicare Carriers for Calendar Year 2007* (the most recent year available), www.cms.hhs.gov.

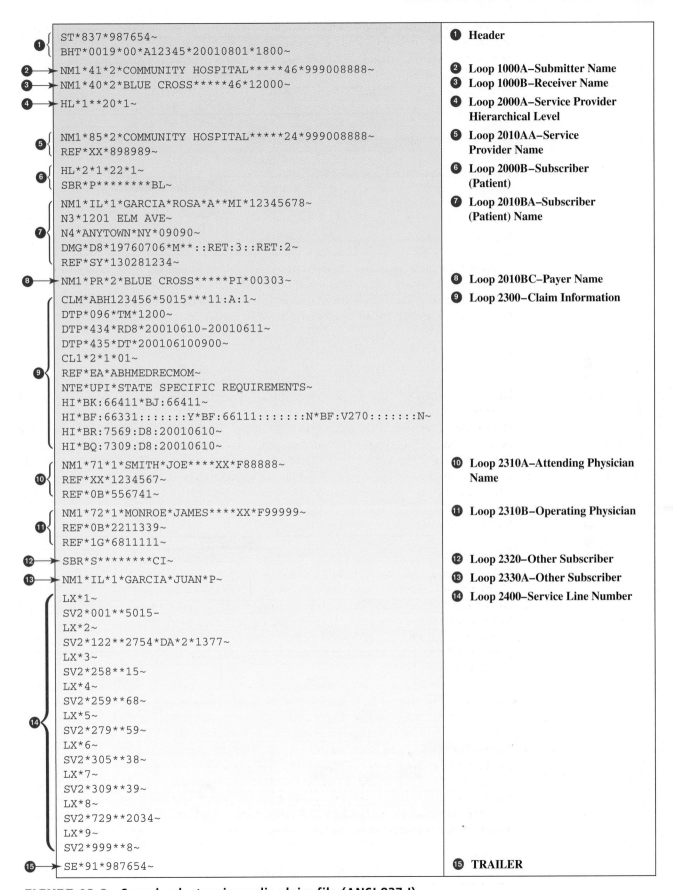

**FIGURE 10-6** Sample electronic media claim file (ANSI 837-I).

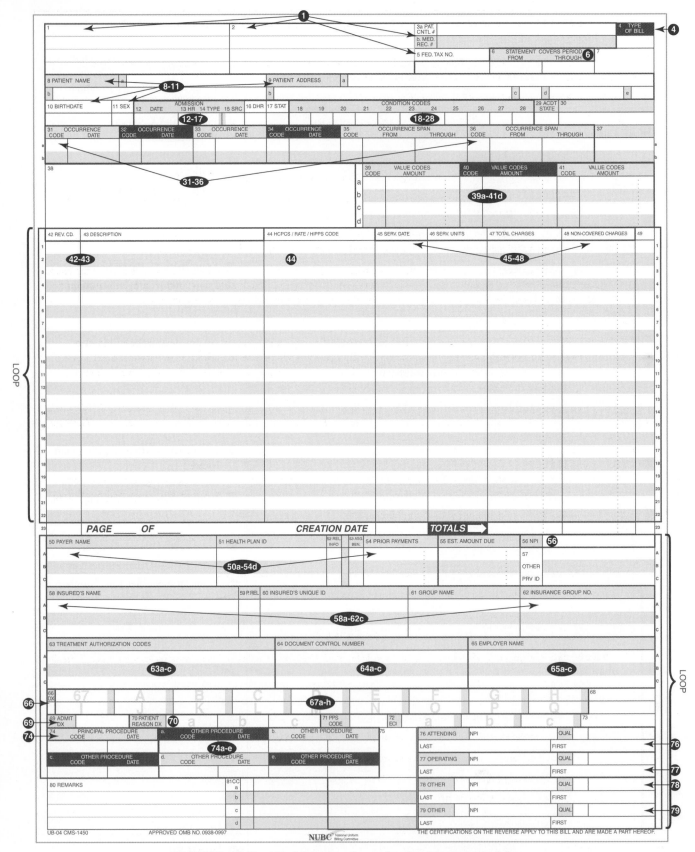

**FIGURE 10-7** UB-04 paper form for institutional claims.

**The fields on the UB-04 form are numbered boxes called form locators. The following describes some of the fields on the UB-04 form:**

**1**  1, 2, 3, 5   Name and address of (institution) provider, name and address to send payments, the facility's internal patient account and medical record numbers, and the facility's tax number.

**4**  4   Bill type 3 digit code indicating type of facility, type of care, and type of claim (admit-discharge, interim, replacement claim, etc.).

**6**  6   Dates covered on claim.

**8–11**  8–11   Patient demographic information.

**12–17**  12–17   Date, hour, type, and source of admission; discharge hour and status (sent home, transferred to SNF, etc.).

**18–28**  18–28   Condition codes are used to provide information relevant to the claim such as "condition related to work," "admission unrelated to discharge," or "neither patient nor spouse employed."

**31–36**  31–36   Occurrence codes and dates are used to provide information on a wide range of issues that affect the claim (examples: the date of an accident, date of last menstrual period for pregnancy claims, date of retirement).

**39a–41d**  39a–41d   Value codes followed by an amount are used to report numeric data that might affect adjudication of the claim. In most cases, these are monetary, such as the patient's Medicare coinsurance; but in some instances, the value codes are used to report a quantity, such as number of units of blood or number of passengers in an ambulance.

**Start Service Loop**   (repeated up to 450 times)

**42–43**  42–43, 45–48   Revenue code and description, date of service for outpatient claims or date of assessment for inpatient
**45–48**  claims, units, total charge, total noncovered charge. The lines are normally sorted and printed in revenue code order. A special revenue code 0001 is used to report the sum of all the charges and all the noncovered charges on paper claims; electronic claims have fields for these totals in a segment of the structure.

**44**  44   HCPCS or accommodation rate or HIPPS code, depending on the type of claim. Outpatient claims report the HCPCS code for the service or supply. Inpatient claims report the accommodation rate. Home health care, SNF, and long-term care facilities report the RUG code followed by an assessment code.

**End Service Loop**

**50a–54d**  50a–54d   Name and ID of health plans the patient has as well as indicators that the patient has signed a release of information and assignment of benefits. If the patient has paid a deductible or coinsurance amount, that is reported in 54a–54d.

**56**  56   Billing provider's national provider ID (NPI) number.

**58a–62c**  58a–62c   Insured party's name, patient's relationship to insured, insured's ID (member number), group name and number for each health plan listed in 50a–50c.

**63a–c**  63a–c   Treatment authorization or referral number (if one was issued for these services).

**64a–c**  64a–c   Document control (claim) number previously issued for this claim by a payer.

**65a–c**  65a–c   Employer name for workers' compensation claims.

**66**  66   Version number of ICD codes; currently always a 9 for ICD-9-CM codes.

**67A–H**  67A–H   The principal diagnosis code goes in field locator 67. Up to eight additional diagnoses codes are printed in fields 67A–H. Note fields 67I–Q are not used by Medicare.

**69**  69   Admitting diagnosis code.

**70**  70   Reason for visit code (for outpatient services).

**74**  74   Principal procedure code and date (used for inpatient claims where a procedure was performed).

**74a–e**  74a–e   Other procedures—codes and dates for other inpatient procedures.

**76**  76   Attending provider name and NPI.

**77**  77   Operating provider name and NPI (if surgical procedure).

**78 79**  78–79   Other providers (i.e., referring doctor) name and NPI.

When using a clearinghouse, the provider's computer produces the electronic claims file, but it can contain the claims for many different plans. The clearinghouse computer receives the larger file, separates the claims into individual files by payer, and retransmits the claims to the individual payers. (If the data is not in HIPAA format, the clearinghouse provides the conversion as well.)

When a plan receives a batch of claims, it returns a response file confirming it has received them. If the provider uses a clearinghouse, the clearinghouse gathers the responses from the various payers and produces a report for the provider. Clearinghouses may act as the conduit for the other HIPAA transactions as well.

Providers pay the clearinghouse for its services. The fee may be per transaction or a flat monthly rate. Health plans do not charge providers for EDI services.

### Claim Scrubbers

Claims that are incorrectly coded or have missing information will be rejected by the payer. In some cases, more than one claim will be rejected. For example, a missing patient's date of birth will result in all claims for that patient being rejected. Another example, a missing or incorrect provider ID could cause an entire batch of claims to be rejected.

With paper claims, a billing specialist could review the claim form before it was sent. With electronic claims, a prebilling report can be created that will allow the billing specialist to review information that is about to be assembled into the claim. This will allow corrections to be made before the claim is sent. However, there are hundreds of claims to be examined and many possible conditions that could cause a claim to be rejected. Modern offices and hospitals rely on computers to examine the data and prepare the claims.

To eliminate preventable billing errors and reduce rejected claims, providers use special software to analyze claims data prior to submission. This software is sometimes called a *claim scrubber,* because it produces "clean" or correct claims. The software may be a component of the billing system, in which case it may have the ability to prevent claims from being created until errors are corrected. In other cases the claim scrubbing software may examine a batch of claims and report if there are any errors before they are sent.

Payers use a list of rules called *claim edits* to examine received claims prior to adjudicating them. Claim scrubbers try to follow the same logic as the payer's claim edits to identify problems in advance.

# Provider Payments

Both professional and institutional providers endure long delays in receiving payment for their services. In addition to the bill-hold period described earlier, once a clean claim is filed, Medicare intermediaries impose a delay, called the *payment floor,* on paying the claim. The delay is 14 days for electronic claims and 29 days for paper claims. Many other health plans also impose a payment floor. Once the primary insurance has paid, the provider must still bill any secondary insurance plan, and then finally the patient. The uncollected money owed during this period is called *accounts receivable*. It is not unusual for providers to have a 90- to 120-day accounts receivable. This means that more than 90 days will pass from the date the patient was seen until the account is paid off.

When payment is received, it must be posted to the patient's account in the accounting system. Secondary insurance claims require information about what the primary plan has paid; therefore, a claim cannot be sent to the secondary payer until the payment from the primary payer is posted.

The process of posting payments also involves posting the contractual write-down adjustments and writing off or rebilling any services that have been denied. Payment is denied for many reasons, including coding errors, services not covered by the patient's plan, or services that require additional documentation to justify the claim. Denied claims require special handling, such as recoding and rebilling the claim, appealing the claim denial, or submitting requested supporting documents.

### Electronic Remittance Advice (ERA)

For every claim that is filed, a provider can expect to receive a remittance advice (or EOB) and hopefully a payment. Large payers often group payments for hundreds of patient claims into one check and create remittance advice reports that are dozens of pages long. Each of these payments must be posted to the correct patient account along with any necessary contractual adjustments. Responsibility for any amount remaining due on the claim is then transferred to secondary insurance or the patient. If responsibility is transferred to secondary insurance, the billing system will automatically produce a claim the next time the insurance billing software is run.

A large medical practice or busy hospital can literally receive mail sacks filled with insurance checks and EOBs that must be posted. Electronic remittance advice (ERA) systems can receive the remittance information from the payer in an ANSI 835 transaction.

A patient account number sent by the provider with the claim is returned in the ERA so the correct patient is identified. The computer then uses the information in the file to automatically post the payments, post the adjustments, and transfer responsibility for each item that was adjudicated. This saves the practice or hospital time and effort.

Special segments within the ANSI 835 transaction carry codified information about how the claim was adjudicated and codes for any adjustments that were made to the payment. This information is saved in the database and reported in an electronic claim to the secondary payer.

The ERA system produces a report of what has been sent in the file and how it has been applied to the patient accounts. If payment has been paid by check, the checks are reconciled to totals on the report. If payment has been made by direct deposit, the amount of the deposit is verified with the reported payments. Direct deposit is called electronic funds transfer (EFT) by which money is sent electronically directly to the provider's bank account. The ERA file is not sent to the bank because it contains PHI.

Figure 10-8 shows a sample paper remittance advice generated from an ERA file. Providers can use software provided by Medicare that will print data from an ANSI 835 file in a report similar to that shown in Figure 10-8. Though health plans format their paper EOBs differently, they generally contain the information shown in Figure 10-8. Studying this figure will help you understand the data that is sent in the ANSI 835 transaction.

# Insurance Eligibility and Other Transactions

Though EMC and ERA eliminate a majority of the paper transactions, several other HIPAA transactions are useful to providers.

### Insurance Eligibility

Determining if a patient still has the insurance plan listed in the registration computer or if the patient is eligible for certain services is a time-consuming but necessary task for many providers. Consider these examples:

- Medicaid patients can be eligible for services one month and then not eligible the next. Medicaid also requires precertification (getting permission in advance) for certain services.

- Managed care patients may change PCPs. Providers may want to verify they are still the PCP before seeing a patient.

- Providers may want to make sure the insurance information on file is correct.

- Medical offices are too busy while seeing patients to call insurance plans to verify eligibility; however, the patient insurance coverage on file may be out of date.

- Hospitals and ambulatory surgery centers often verify covered services before scheduling or performing a surgery.

Determining electronic eligibility involves a pair of transactions. The provider sends an eligibility inquiry in the ANSI 270 format to inquire about the eligibility, coverage, or benefits associated with a health plan, employer, plan sponsor, subscriber, or a dependent under the subscriber's policy. The payer responds with the requested information using the ANSI 271

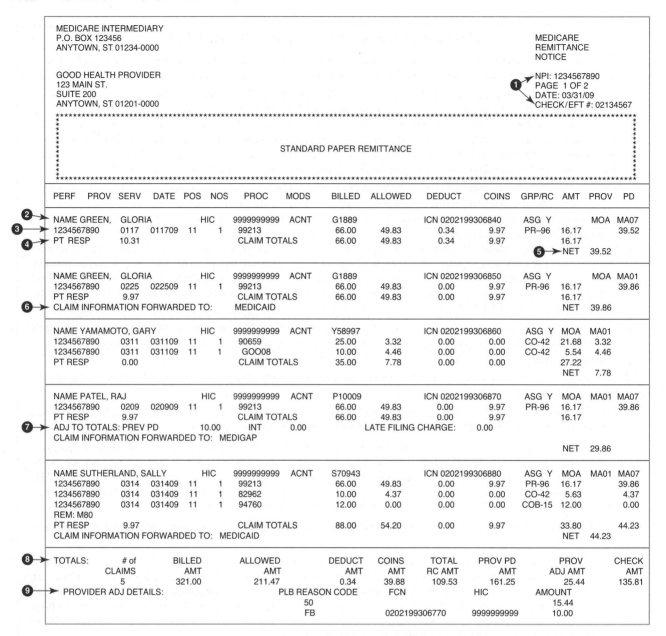

**FIGURE 10-8**   **Sample paper EOB remittance advice.**

transaction. The payer can also send ANSI 271 transactions to communicate information about, or changes to, eligibility, coverage, or benefits from payers to physicians, hospitals, and third-party administrators.

Though not as important as EMC and ERA in reducing paperwork for the health system at large, for hospitals that have full-time staff manually doing eligibility verification by phone, electronic eligibility verification offers a significant improvement. Additionally, providers of all sizes will reduce payment delays and rejected claims due to outdated records by verifying patients' insurance coverage before or during the patient encounter.

### Referrals and Authorizations

Some situations and health plans require providers to get prior authorization before performing certain services for patients of those plans. Historically, this has been a time-consuming process requiring that a high-level medical professional talk to the plan about the case. The ANSI 278 transaction, called the Health Care Services Request for Review and Response, can be used to

## Explanation of Numbered Points Shown in Figure 10-8

**1** The EOB header contains the addresses of the health plan and the provider. The NPI (national provider identifier) is that of the billing entity (group practice). The CHECK/EFT number is used to match the EOB with checks or electronic funds transfer deposits.

**2** This line contains a mix of information about the claim: NAME is the name of the beneficiary. HIC is the beneficiary's insurance number. ACNT is the medical practice's ID for the patient number; this might be the account, medical record, or a special number generated for this claim. ICN is an internal control number, a unique 13-digit number assigned to the claim by the plan during claims processing. ASG indicates whether the claim was assigned. MOA contains codes that correspond to remittance advice remarks. For example, MA01 is a standard remark advising providers that if they disagree with the approved amount they have the right to appeal the claim. The code MA07 indicates the claim has been forwarded to Medicaid.

**3** The claim details listed here correspond to the column labels at the top of this section: PERF PROV is the 10-digit national provider ID of the provider who provided the medical service. SERV DATE is the dates the service was performed. The dates can accommodate a range (from–to) and are listed in numeric format representing month, day, and year (in this example, January 17, 2009). POS is a 2-digit code for the place of service. NOS is the number of units of service or days. PROC is the HCPCS/CPT-4 code. MODS are up to four procedure code modifiers. BILLED is the amount the provider billed for the service. ALLOWED is the amount the provider is contractually allowed for the service. DEDUCT is the amount of deductible owed by the patient. COINS is the coinsurance amount owed by the patient. GRP/RC lists any group codes and claim adjustment reason codes associated with this service line. AMT is any adjustment amount related to the reason codes. PROV PD is the amount the provider is paid by the plan for this service. There will be a claim detail line for every procedure on the original claim.

**4** The claim totals line shows the totals of the details lines. PT RESP is the portion of the claim for which the patient is responsible (deductible plus coinsurance amounts). CLAIM TOTALS are the totals of all service-line-level amounts under each of the columns labeled BILLED, ALLOWED, DEDUCT, COINS, AMT, and PROV PD.

**5** NET is the amount actually being included in the check for this claim. Under certain circumstances this can be less than the PROV PD amount. An example of this is shown in the fourth claim on this EOB (see 7 below.)

**6** When a claim is automatically forwarded to the secondary payer, it is sometimes called a "piggyback" claim. A message on the EOB informs the provider that the claim has been forwarded to the beneficiary's second plan.

**7** An additional line can print on the EOB where there are additional adjustments to the amount paid for the claim. Often this occurs when a claim has been resubmitted. The line will begin with the label ADJ TO TOTALS. The data may include PREV PD, the amount previously paid for the services when the claim is an adjusted claim. INT is the interest amount (if any). LATE FILING CHARGE is the late filing charge (if any). Amounts in this line are added or subtracted from the PROV PD amount, which is the reason the NET amount can be different from the sum of the PROV PD for the items.

**8** After all the claims have been listed, a summary section totals the amounts for each of the columns and the amount of the check or EFT payment.

**9** Below the claim totals summary section, sometimes there is another section that lists provider-level adjustment details. These are adjustments that are not specific to a particular claim on this EOB. In most cases the plan is deducting money from the check for a previous claim it believes was paid in excess or in error. When this occurs a PLB REASON CODE is listed. The reason codes provide an explanation for the adjustment. In this example, code 50 is Late Filing Penalty, which is being deducted from this check for a claim on a previous EOB. The number listed under FCN is usually the ICN number from a previous EOB and the HIC number listed is the beneficiary number of the patient on that claim.

replace the phone call and conduct the referral certification and authorization process. Some examples where the ANSI 278 might be used include the following:

- Notifying the plan of an inpatient admission
- Precertification of planned inpatient admissions
- Precertification for transfer or admission to an SNF, rehabilitation services, or long-term care facility
- Prior approval for certain procedures
- Referrals for managed care patients.

In this transaction, the ANSI 278 is used to send the request for authorization and for the plan to return information about the authorization, certification, or referral to the provider. Even in cases where the response from the plan is an instruction to call a plan case manager, time is saved because the provider does not have to go through customer service or wait on hold.

## A REAL-LIFE STORY

## The Realities of Hospital Billing

*By Mary E. Bazan*

> *Mary Bazan is the director of billing and finance for a large multiple-facility regional healthcare system.*

**W**e have 45½ FTEs (full-time equivalent employees) in my department. There are 5 personnel who post payments, 28 billers, 7 collectors, and 5 management and administrative personnel. We also perform document scanning of financial documents, such as consent to pay, authorizations, correspondence, nonelectronic remittance advice, financial disclosures, uncompensated payers, and write-offs. The scanned document files are stored in the same system as our HIM department uses, but the document imaging management software keeps the financial documents separate from the clinical records.

In our organization, each revenue-generating department is responsible for entry of its particular charges. A great number of departments automate that process. For example, the surgery system sends us the surgery charges, as does the lab system, radiology, and pharmacy. There are still some departments that do manual posting, such as point-of-care testing, outpatient clinics, and our ER.

Our staff uses an online coding support system and has online access to CMS memos, the *Federal Register*, and payers' standards. We also have a compliance checker as part of our system that uses the National Correct Coding Initiative (NCCI) edits where they are required. NCCI is a Medicare standard for bundling and unbundling rules. For example, when you have certain procedures with fluoroscopy, you have to include the fluoroscopy in the procedure as opposed to billing separately for it.

Our hospital EHR enables our billers to access medical records right from the billing department, which can be very helpful in preparing claims. There are a number of claim elements that are situational in nature. So having ready access to the medical record is of great assistance to us.

We have two monitors on every desk, so a person can have a medical record displayed on one monitor and a coding reference on another, or a payment on one monitor and a claim record on the other.

About 97 percent of our claims go out electronically. For both inpatient and outpatient billing, we have a claim scrubber application that examines the claim data and applies the kinds of audits and standards that are required by different payers. One reason to have a claim scrubber is because no one can get a claim off their patient accounting system that will meet all the various payer standards. Despite the fact that HIPAA standardized transactions and code sets, it is still amazing to see the variety of ways plans process claims. For example, when you do multiple procedures on the same date, you are supposed to use the modifier on every line, yet I deal with one HMO whose system can't handle that. There are also substantial differences between Medicaid requirements and everyone else. With the commercial payers, Blue Cross is pretty particular about what revenue code they want and whether you use an HCPCS code or not. They don't do UB or transactions the way that Medicare would.

---

The authorization, certification, or referral number is subsequently reported on the claim so the plan will know the service was authorized and the claim will not be denied or suspended.

### Claim Status

Though a claim may pass the payer's edits, it may not be adjudicated. In certain cases the plan may ask for further information, supporting documentation, or test results relating to the case. These are called *suspended claims*. Sometimes providers lose track of these requests for additional information and so the claim goes unpaid. Even when the requested information has been supplied, the provider may not know what has happened to the payment.

Though providers have come to expect a built-in payment delay (called the *payment floor*), claims that have not been paid in a reasonable period of time must be investigated. The first step is to query the plan about the claim status. There are a number of ways to do this:

- Call the plan help lines and ask to speak to a customer service representative.
- Use an automated voice response phone system provided by the plan.
- Enter data on a web page provided by the plan.
- Send a Health Care Claim Status Request (ANSI 276 transaction) electronically and receive a Health Care Claim Status Response (ANSI 277 transaction) back from the plan.

Obviously, the EDI transaction is more efficient. The HIS computers can be programmed to automatically generate ANSI 276 requests for any claim that is not paid within a certain number

We send claims through a clearinghouse, rather than directly, because you basically have to do all the support of the setup and transmissions. So we have the clearinghouse expense for claims; but with the patient statements, I wish we could find a cheaper alternative. We pay the clearinghouse less than 10 cents a claim, but our patient billing has a pretty steep overhead. We aren't able to do guarantor level billing, so statements are sent at the account level, which generates a plethora of paper and is pretty confusing to the patients and costly to us. After the initial billing, we try to combine things into a single patient statement; however, for us this is a manual process.

There hasn't really been much progress improving patient billing in healthcare. Over the next few years, the industry should look at allowing patients to use the Internet to check on the status of their accounts, payments, and online statements. The banking, brokerage, telephone, and utility companies have succeeded in that area. We have had a fair number of people ask for online statements and payments.

The preponderance of our payers offer online access for claim status and eligibility. Medicaid, Medicare, and some others are transactional, but many other plans offer Internet-based lookup. Medicaid was the first program where we could do automatic generation of a 276 and get a 277 back. Probably the biggest issue is if we send those through our clearinghouse, they cost us a quarter each. We are trying to develop some kind of protocol that would only solicit those verifications when needed, because that is expensive, especially for programs like Medicaid where we are already not getting much money.

We receive electronic remittance transactions from Medicare, Medicaid, Blue Cross, and our biggest HMO. Those payers represent 75 to 80 percent of our volume. The electronic remittance transactions are coded with the data for secondary billing, allowing us to automate that as well.

None of the payers are doing electronic authorizations, and we have a fair number of Medicaid HMOs with fairly stiff authorization requirements that consume a lot of our time to do it with FTEs; so that transaction would be helpful.

None of our payers are working on electronic attachments. Right now they often want records that must be sent on paper. Another problem is that HIPAA requirements do not apply to workers' compensation (WC) and auto insurance plans. They are very work intensive for us because they require everything; they audit the entire record and are our slowest payers.

My advice is to automate as much as you can. Get as much out the door and back in electronically as possible. Also check that each step of the process happens as it should. It is possible for a large file of claims to get misrouted, lost, corrupted, or not get from the clearinghouse to the payer. Rather than wait for the payment floor, we are proactive about verification. We check the payer's website and the payer's system to validate that claim batches arrived and are showing on their system. We randomly select a number of claims each day and check the claim status. We can't afford to wait 14, 30, or 45 days to discover the claim didn't get there.

Another thing is to look at data relative to rejections and look at patterns for process improvements. Though it takes a fair amount of effort, I believe if you have statistically sound sampling you can find the cause of the problem. For example, suppose someone transposed two numbers in the charge master. Every time that code is posted it will be wrong and someone in billing has to correct that manually. By fixing the charge master, you eliminate the need to make corrections. I don't think there is any substitute for internal auditing. It takes time, but I have never found it to be anything but valuable.

of days. The ANSI 277 responses can be gathered and reported to a claims specialist at the hospital or medical office to determine what is holding up payment.

## Claim Attachments

Claim attachments are supplemental documents providing additional medical information to the claims processor that cannot be accommodated within the claim format. Common attachments are certificate of medical necessity (CMN), discharge summaries, and operative reports. They are sent to the health plan with the original claim or in response to a request from the plan. They are one of the main reasons claims are suspended (waiting the arrival of paper copies of the claim attachments).

HIPAA proposed to solve this problem by creating a transaction for the electronic transmission of claim attachments. The specification has been created by a joint effort of the ANSI ASC X12n work group and a HL7 workgroup assigned to create the format called the clinical document architecture (CDA). The CDA documents are both machine readable (they are easily parsed into data elements that can be processed electronically) and human readable (they can be easily viewed and read by a person.)

The HHS final rule to make the claim attachment standard official had not yet passed as of 2009, but a Notice of Proposed Rule Making defines six types of electronic claims attachments:

1. Clinical reports
2. Laboratory reports

3. Emergency department reports

4. Rehabilitative services (care plans)

5. Ambulance services

6. Medications (during treatment and upon discharge).

The ANSI X12n workgroup has defined the ANSI 275 transaction as "Additional Patient Information in Support of a Health Claim or Encounter." The ANSI 275 transaction can act like an envelope and carry the CDA data.

The X12n workgroup also proposed that the ANSI 277 claim status response act as a request to the provider to send the required attachment. Providers will also be allowed to submit the ANSI 275 with the ANSI 837 claim for cases they know will require an attachment, eliminating the need for the plan to request the attachment or suspend the claim.

---

## Chapter 10 Summary

### Electronic Data Interchange (EDI)

HIPAA standardized healthcare EDI by requiring the use of standard formats developed and maintained by ANSI. HIPAA mandated eight EDI transactions:

1. *Claims or equivalent encounters and coordination of benefits (ANSI 837):* Due to differences in the way doctors and hospitals bill, different implementations of this format were created:

   Healthcare professionals use ANSI 837-P, which is equivalent to the paper CMS-1500 form.
   Institutional providers use ANSI 837-I, which is equivalent to the paper UB-04 (also called the CMS-1450) form.
   Dentists use ANSI 837-D.

2. *Remittance and payment advice (ANSI 835):* Replaces the paper remittance advice or the provider's EOB. The transaction contains all the information necessary for a computer to automatically post payments to patient accounts and bill secondary insurance.

3. *Claim status inquiry (ANSI 276) and response (ANSI 277):* These two transactions permit providers to query a plan about the status of a claim and get a response. Claims are sometimes suspended in the payer's system awaiting further documentation. In the future, it may be possible for the ANSI 277 transaction to be used by plans to request claim attachments.

4. *Eligibility benefit inquiry (ANSI 270) and response (ANSI 271):* Eligibility benefit information may be requested by the provider to verify eligibility, coverage, benefits, employer, plan sponsor, subscriber, or dependents under the subscriber's policy. Plans may send ANSI 271 without an inquiry to inform providers and third-party administrators about changes in eligibility, coverage, or benefits.

5. *Referral certification and authorization (ANSI 278):* Some plans require prior authorization or precertification for certain procedures or treatments; for example, surgery, expensive diagnostic tests, inpatient admission, or transfer to a SNF. The ANSI 278 transaction, Health Care Services Request for Review and Response, is used. Managed care plans that require PCP referrals can also use this transaction.

6. *Health plan premium payments (ANSI 820):* The ANSI 820 transaction can be used to transmit health plan premium payments between employers and plans for employer group plans.

7. *Enrollment and de-enrollment in a health plan (ANSI 834):* The ANSI 834 Benefit Enrollment and Maintenance transaction is used by employers to enroll (and remove) employees from group health coverage.

8. *Retail drug claims, coordination of drug benefits and eligibility inquiry (NCPDP 5.1; Version D.0):* Retail pharmacies communicate with health plans using the NCPDP format.

Two additional healthcare transactions are being developed, but have not become official HIPAA transactions: Patient Information in Support of a Health Claim or Encounter (ANSI 275), which is used to send additional information necessary for processing certain claims, and the first report of injury transaction, which is used for reporting workers' compensation incidents.

### Posting, Billing and Payments

There are many steps involved in the accounting and billing departments for providers to be paid. Review the billing workflow shown in Figure 10-1 and the following information:

Entering procedure and diagnosis data for billing and the subsequent payments and adjustments into the patient accounts system is called *posting*. Posting is done in real time (while the patient is present) or in batches. Real-time posting is commonly used in medical offices; batch posting is commonly used by billing services and for hospital billing.

Hospitals delay billing for a designated period of time after discharge called the bill-hold period. This is done to ensure that all charges from the various hospital departments have been posted before producing the claim. Because inpatient prospective payment systems determine payment by analyzing all the codes on the claim, missed procedures or diagnoses could cause the hospital to be paid less.

Medicare and many other payers withhold payments for a period of time after the claim is adjudicated; for example, 14 days for electronic claims and 29 days for paper claims. This is called the payment floor.

In many cases if the patient has secondary insurance, the provider must wait until payment is received from the primary insurance before billing the secondary plan. In certain instances, payers will automatically forward the claim to the secondary plan. These are called piggyback, crossover, or COB claims.

Though providers can send EDI transactions directly to payers, many find that they have too many plans to send each batch separately. Clearinghouses can act like a switch, receiving a large batch of claims for many payers, repackaging the claims into individual batches, and forwarding them to each plan. Clearinghouses are one of the three covered entities defined by HIPAA; thus, they are permitted to process claim batches that contain PHI.

Because providers deal with so many plans with different rules, many providers use claim scrubbers (special software that examines claim data before it is sent to eliminate preventable billing errors).

When all of the plans have paid, any remaining balance that is patient responsibility must be collected from the guarantor or patient. From the date of the visit or admission to the date the account is finally paid off, the amount owed is called the accounts receivable.

Patient bills or statements are usually sent on a monthly or periodic basis to inform the patient about what insurance has paid and what is due. There are two types of patient statements:

- *Balance Forward*—begins with the previous month's balance and shows only charges or payments posted in the current period.
- *Open Item*—shows all unpaid items with payment, adjustments, and balance for each item.

## Critical Thinking Exercises

1. Locate the questions in Box 10 of the CMS-1500 insurance form shown in Figure 10-5. Why would a health plan want this information on its claim form?
2. What are some of the advantages of electronic media claims over paper claims?

## Testing Your Knowledge of Chapter 10

1. What is the name of the paper document explaining the insurance payment to the provider?

2. What is the name of the accounting entry posted to reduce the original charge to the allowed amount?

3. What does the acronym EMC stand for?

4. What does the acronym ERA stand for?

5. What does the acronym EDI stand for?

6. What is the name of the period of time hospitals delay billing?

7. What is meant by the term *payment floor*?

8. Name four of the eight EDI transactions required by HIPAA.

9. Name the two types of patient statements.

10. What are claim edits?

11. What is the difference between real-time and batch posting?

12. Which paper form was designed for professional claims?

*For each of the following statements circle true if it is correct, or false if the statement is not true:*

13. HIPAA requires all but the smallest health plans to receive claims electronically.
    *True        False*

14. A separate EMC file must be created for each claim.
    *True        False*

15. The first step in preparing a claim is to calculate the DRG.
    *True        False*

# 11

# Health Statistics, Research, and Quality Improvement

After completing this chapter, you should be able to:

- Explain why secondary health records are important
- Describe internal and external uses for secondary data
- Discuss different types of registries
- Compare the differences between an index and a registry
- Discuss HEDIS and the National Hospital Quality Measures
- Read an XML formatted file
- Explain data sampling
- Understand healthcare statistical terms and formulas
- Perform statistical calculations for *ratio*, *proportion*, *mean*, *median*, *mode*, and *range*
- Describe the relationship between hospital quality measures and pay-for-performance initiatives

## ACRONYMS USED IN CHAPTER 11

Acronyms are used extensively in both medicine and computers. The following acronyms are used in this chapter.

| | | | |
|---|---|---|---|
| **ACEI** | Angiotensin Converting Enzyme Inhibitor | **CMS** | Centers for Medicare and Medicaid Services |
| **AIS** | Abbreviated Injury Scale | **COB** | Coordination of Benefits |
| **AMI** | Acute Myocardial Infarction (Heart Attack) | **CTR** | Certified Tumor Registrar |
| | | **DRG** | Diagnosis-Related Group |
| **ANSI X12n** | ANSI Insurance Standards Committee Responsible for Developing and Maintaining HIPAA Transactions | **DNA** | Deoxyribonucleic Acid |
| | | **EHR** | Electronic Health Record |
| | | **FDA** | Food and Drug Administration |
| **ARB** | Angiotensin Receptor Blocker | **HBIPS** | Hospital-Based Inpatient Psychiatric Services |
| **CAC** | Children's Asthma Care | | |
| **CDC** | Centers for Disease Control and Prevention | **HEDIS** | Health Plan Employer Data and Information Set |
| **CMI** | Case Mix Index | **HF** | Heart Failure |

| | | | | |
|---|---|---|---|---|
| **HIPAA** | Health Insurance Portability and Accountability Act | **LVSD** | Left Ventricular Systolic Dysfunction |
| **HIS** | Health Information System | **NCQA** | National Committee for Quality Assurance |
| **HL7** | Health Level 7 | | |
| **HMO** | Health Maintenance Organization | **NHQM** | National Hospital Quality Measures |
| **HOP; HOP QDRP** | Hospital Outpatient Program; Hospital Outpatient Program–Quality Data Reporting Program | **P4P** | Pay for Performance |
| | | **PCI** | Percutaneous Coronary Intervention |
| **HX** | History | **PHI** | Protected Health Information (HIPAA) |
| **ICD-9-CM** | International Classification of Diseases, Ninth Revision, Clinical Modification | **PN** | Pneumonia |
| | | **PR** | Pregnancy and Related Conditions |
| **ICD-10-CM** | International Classification of Diseases, Tenth Revision, Clinical Modification | **SCIP** | Surgical Care Improvement Project |
| **IDSS** | Interactive Data Submission System | **TPO** | Treatment, Payment, and Operations (HIPAA) |
| **IRB** | Internal Review Board | **UM** | Utilization Management |
| **ISS** | Injury Severity Score | **VTE** | Venous Thromboembolism |
| **LBBB** | Left Bundle Branch Block | **XML** | eXtensible Markup Language |
| **LDL-c** | Low-Density Lipoprotein–Cholesterol | | |

# Secondary Health Records and Indexes

Chapter 5 introduced the concepts of primary and secondary health records. Chapter 10 described the creation of secondary health records as claims, which are used to obtain reimbursement. Claim data is also used for quality improvement purposes. For example, capitation managed care plans often require providers to file electronic or paper claims even though the claims will not be paid. These *claims equivalent encounters* are used by the HMO to collect and monitor data about the services provided.

Similarly, data from UB-04 and ANSI 837-I claims is used by CMS and state agencies to derive numerous healthcare statistics, including the hospital case mix index (described later). In addition to claims, providers submit data in several other forms. Some examples are the Uniform Hospital Discharge Data Set, HEDIS, and cancer and implant registries.

Providers also maintain indexes of the data within their patient health records for both internal and external reporting purposes and studies. When paper records were prevalent, these indexes were created by manually abstracting data from the patient chart and entering it into a special database. As health records became computerized, it was possible for the computer to perform this task automatically. For many EHR systems the data does not have to be extracted; it is simply indexed in place.

One example is the disease index. In manual systems, the HIM department would have to create an index of the patients and their discharge diagnosis ICD-9-CM code as part of discharge processing of the record before the chart was filed. This index could then be used by the facility to count the number of patients treated for certain conditions, as well as identify their medical record numbers if cases warranted further study.

Today the same index is created by simply programming the EHR computer to index the discharge diagnosis field in the database. Not only is it easier, but in most cases the data is more timely because the case is indexed as soon as the discharge record is entered. Medical records are also indexed by the attending physician, surgeon, procedures, discharge status, even the patient's age and zip code. One of the real benefits of coded, fielded data is the ability to automate the creation of an unlimited type and number of indexes.

## Internal and External Uses of Indexes

Indexes may be created to permit internal users of the healthcare organization to locate, count, or analyze the data for quality and process improvement of healthcare operations quickly. Indexes are also used to identify and sort records for external use, such as reporting to health plans or state or federal agencies quickly. Indexes may also be used to identify automatically any records to be abstracted for internal or external registries.

# Registries

Registries are different from indexes in that an index most often points to a medical record containing one or more fields to be reported or studied. A registry is a separate database into which certain data elements have been imported or manually entered.

For example, a hospital might maintain a trauma registry. The trauma registry entries might be built automatically by selecting cases with certain diagnosis codes. This would differ from the disease index, which includes all patients, because the trauma registry would only have patients with ICD-9-CM codes in the 800 to 959 range. In addition, the trauma registry might have additional fields that must be entered because they were not in the admission or discharge summary. For example, Abbreviated Injury Scale (AIS) and Injury Severity Score (ISS) might be manually entered by the registrar.

If the registry is used by the hospital to improve performance or processes or to satisfy accreditation requirements, the users are internal. If the registry is used to report data to, for instance, the National Trauma Data Bank, then the users are external.

An implant registry (discussed in Chapter 8) is another example of a registry created and maintained primarily for internal users, but essential for reporting in the case of an adverse event. The implant registry is necessary because it allows facilities to maintain information such as serial number, product number, and manufacturer of surgically implanted devices and materials. Because there is no longer a national implant registry, the implant registry is normally maintained for internal use (risk management). However, should an adverse event occur with an implant, the registry data will be necessary to make a report to the FDA. The implant registry may also be used to track follow-up data regarding the performance of the implant.

## Cancer Registries

One of the earliest types of registries is a cancer registry. Cancer registries date back to 1926; however, Congress did not begin funding the National Program of Cancer Registries until 1992. The facility-based cancer registrar enters data about cases by abstracting it from the health records of patients diagnosed with some form of cancer. These cases might be identified by using the disease index, discharge reports, or pathology reports or by gathering information for patients registered at outpatient cancer or radiation therapy centers.

Data collected in the facility-based registries is used internally for quality assessment of the facility, for research, and to measure the success of various treatment modalities. The registry data is also aggregated and reported to state and national cancer registries. These population-based registries are used to identify trends and changes in the incidence and survival rate for various types of cancers. Cancer registry data includes:

- Accession number (manually or automatically assigned to the case)
- Patient demographic information
- Occupational history of patient
- Date first diagnosed
- Type and site of the cancer
- Stage of the cancer (size and extent it has spread)
- Diagnostic methodologies
- Treatment methodologies
- Follow-up data (collected in subsequent years) determining cancer status and mortality.

Facilities report registry data to central cancer registries, which are part of the National Program of Cancer Registries. The Centers for Disease Control and Prevention (CDC) then collects and aggregates data from the state registries. A facility-based cancer registry is one of the requirements for certification of cancer programs by the American College of Surgeons. Registries are maintained by a trained cancer registrar, who may, by passing an examination, become a Certified Tumor Registrar (CTR).

# Processing and Maintaining Secondary Data

As we have seen from the previous examples, secondary data such as claims and registries can be created by simply pointing to relevant health records containing the desired cases (indexing), by exporting fielded data from patient records into a separate database, and by manually abstracting and entering the data. Often the process involves all three methods. This is true of the two types of secondary data we have studied so far, claims and registries.

Claims are created by processing a combination of charges automatically generated by departmental systems and charges posted by a coding technician or coding specialist who abstracts the patient health record. A coding or billing specialist then manually selects the principal diagnosis. The claim also includes patient demographics, insurance, provider, and COB payment information automatically retrieved from the HIS systems.

Similarly, registry data can be automatically populated from patient health records by using the disease index to select appropriate cases, but is supplemented by manual entry of data such as injury severity or stage of cancer.

### Data Quality

Errors in data not only affect its usefulness, but can have serious repercussions in decisions that are based on that data. Clinical data errors can harm patients. Coding and billing errors can result in financial losses, audits, or fines. Statistics based on erroneous data can result in false assumptions and incorrect decisions.

Automating the creation of secondary databases can reduce errors caused by manually rekeying existing data—if the primary data is correct. Several factors determine the quality of data:

- The *validity* or accuracy of the data is the foundation of everything else. Was the data entered properly, was the decimal in the right place, was the unit of measure correct (e.g., microgram or milligram)?

- The *reliability* and consistency of the data entry is important. Do all the records originate from a common nomenclature or are different terminologies being used? Do data dictionaries in different programs contributing to the database align?

- The *completeness* of the data is important. Missing data can skew results or cause false interpretations. Software can be programmed to require entry of all fields necessary to ensure complete records, but records that are completely missing are not so easily identified. Consider a patient medication list that is incomplete. How would the clinician know the patient is on the drug if it is not recorded?

- The *timeliness* of the data is important to ensure it is included when a claim, report, or study is generated. In situations where secondary data is created by exporting primary data, late-arriving data may never reach the secondary database or may require manual entry.

- The *security* of the data is paramount in healthcare. This not only means controlling access, but ensuring that the data is not lost, damaged, deleted, or modified. This is especially important where secondary data is not exported to a separate database, but reported directly from the primary data indexes.

### Data Confidentiality

HIPAA privacy rules govern data containing PHI. In some cases, such as claims, secondary data containing PHI is sent to external users (the payer) for the allowed purposes of treatment, payment, and operations (TPO). Similarly, data from the implant registry including PHI may be sent to the FDA in the case of an adverse event, or infectious disease data may be sent to the public health department or CDC as permitted by HIPAA.

HIPAA also permits researchers to analyze records containing PHI for the purpose of designing a research protocol when authorized by an internal review board (IRB). However, most releases of secondary data for purposes *other than TPO* consist of de-identified data or aggregated data:

- *De-identified data* is data that has had the PHI elements removed such that an individual cannot be personally identified from the data. Such data can then be used by external users such as researchers for studies and trend analysis.

- *Aggregate data* is data that does not contain PHI because by definition it does not consist of individual records. Aggregate data is the sum of records containing data matching certain criteria. For example, the case mix index described later is derived from the count of patients in each diagnosis-related group (DRG).

### Clinical Trials Research

Clinical trials, introduced in Chapter 8, are conducted to test new drugs, treatments, and medical devices. Clinical trials present several exceptions to what we have just discussed.

First, patients volunteer to participate in a clinical trial. Among the several documents they sign is a HIPAA authorization to use and report PHI as necessary to the clinical trial.

Second, the clinical trial protocol describes the procedures of the trial and the type of data to be collected. However, the clinical trial database is not secondary data but often a separate primary database. That is, data may need to be entered twice; once in the patient's health record and again using special software or a database to capture the clinical trial data. In some cases, EHR data can be transferred electronically to the clinical trials database, but frequently the clinical trial requires manual entry in a separate system. Figure 11-1 shows Clinipace Tempo, a brand of Internet-based clinical trial software.

**FIGURE 11-1**

**Clinipace Tempo registry screen.**

(Courtesy of Clinipace, Inc.)

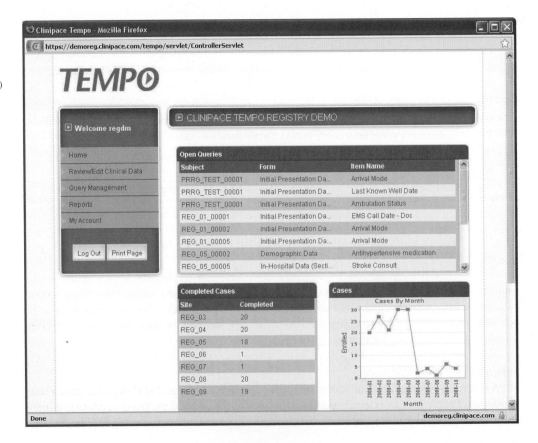

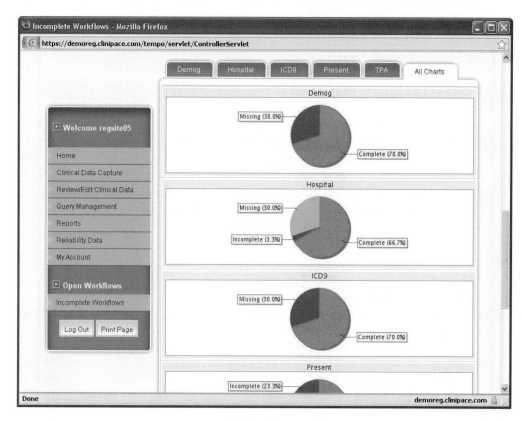

**FIGURE 11-2**

**Aggregate clinical trial report graphs.**

(Courtesy of Clinipace, Inc.)

In addition, to the primary data collected on the clinical trial patient, secondary data is created. Aggregate data is analyzed and reported. De-identified data may be reported to the sponsor of the clinical trial. Figure 11-2 shows graphs created from aggregate clinical trial data.

## Using and Reporting Secondary Health Records

Healthcare providers collect data daily. Beyond the uses of data for treatment are the many uses of data for operations, quality improvement, and research. We will now look at several additional examples where secondary data is created and reported.

### HEDIS

A majority of private health insurance is provided through employer-sponsored plans. Whereas a manufacturer might require suppliers to meet quality standards for the materials the manufacturer purchases, how can an employer measure the quality of the healthcare it purchases for its employees? Though employers have no direct influence over the healthcare provider, at one point they realized that their health insurance plans did. This was especially true of managed care plans.

The National Committee for Quality Assurance (NCQA) created a tool by which it could compare the quality of care patients receive under various health plans. The Health Plan Employer Data and Information Set (HEDIS) consist of 71 measures across eight domains of care. Employers can use the results of NCQA reports derived from HEDIS data to select the best plan for their employees. NCQA has an accreditation program for health plans and audits their processes, quality of providers, quality improvement processes, utilization management (UM), and preventive health initiatives.

NCQA collects HEDIS data directly from managed care HMO and PPO organizations. Plans transfer data to the NCQA Interactive Data Submission System (IDSS). The data consists of secondary records and does not contain PHI. The data is in XML format (illustrated in Figure 11-3).

**FIGURE 11-3**

**Abridged sample of HEDIS data in XML format.[3]**

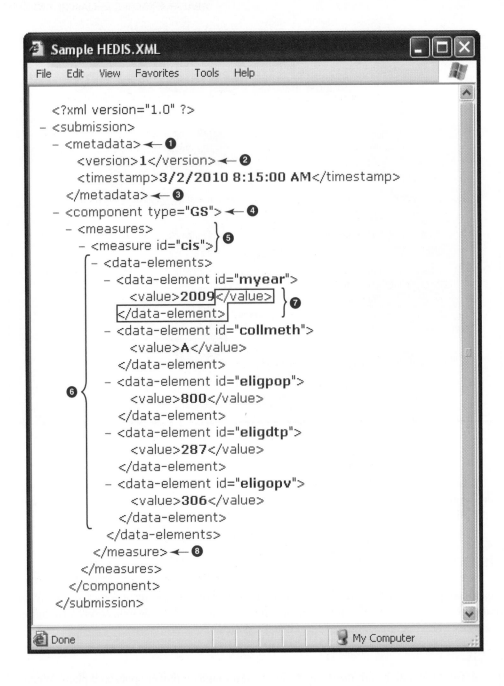

NCQA also allows researchers to use HEDIS data to study trends and collaborates with academic centers. Because about 90 percent of managed care plans submit HEDIS data and because the NCQA includes Medicare and Medicaid data as well, the database is a vast resource of population-based data. Topics of two such studies are the delivery of childhood immunizations by managed care organizations[1] and the importance of early screening for chlamydia.[2]

---

[1]B. Bardenheier, Y. Kong, A. Shefer, et al., "Managed Care Organizations' Performance in Delivery of Childhood Immunizations," *American Journal of Managed Care* 13 (2007):193–200.

[2]John Douglas, Jr., Stuart Berman, and Cathleen Walsh, *Improving Chlamydia Screening* (Washington, DC: National Committee for Quality Assurance, 2008).

[3]Note that the XML in this figure has been abridged and a significant number of HEDIS fields have been eliminated to simplify the example.

## Explanation of Numbered Points Shown in Figure 11-3

Each segment begins with a *tag* or name of the segment surrounded by the characters < >.

**(1)** For example, the general file information at the top of the file begins with the tag <metadata>.

**(2)** The tag on the next line, <version>, begins the field that will identify what version of the HEDIS standards was used. The numeral **1** is the data. The closing tag, </version>, indicates the end of the version field. Closing tags are the same as the opening tag except that the tag is preceded by a slash, </version>.

**(3)** The process repeats until all of the fields in the current segment have been reported. A segment closing tag, </metadata> indicates the end of the metadata segment.

**(4)** The next segment, component type, begins. In many cases the data can be sent *within* the tag by using the equal sign <component type="GS">.

**(5)** Within that component several different measures are going to be reported. Each time a new measure is reported it will start with the tag <measure>. This figure shows an abridged sample of childhood immunization data. The tag <measure id="cis"> identifies this as the childhood immunization status measure segment.

**(6)** The <data-elements> tag begins each field of data. The <data-element id="myear"> provides the field name; in this case "myear" is the measurement year for which data is reported. The tag <value> is followed by the actual data; in this example the year 2009.

**(7)** The </value> tag indicates the end of the value data and the </data-elements> tag ends that data element.

**(8)** The <data-elements> will repeat until all of the data for the childhood immunization status measures have been reported. When all of the data elements in that measure have been reported, the closing tag </measure> will be used to indicate the end of that measure segment. The next <measure> will start and the process repeat until all of the data for all of the measures has been reported.

## XML DATA

XML stands for eXtensible Markup Language. XML differs from the data formats discussed in Chapter 4. Instead of using commas or quotes to separate fields, it uses *tags* to identify and name each piece of fielded data. Refer to Figure 11-3 for more information on each of the tags.

As a database design, XML would be a horrible waste of space, but as a communication format it has several advantages:

- An XML file can be opened and reviewed using an ordinary browser such as Internet Explorer. This means that no special programs are required to view the contents.
- New fields can be added to the specification at anytime without disturbing the structure. For example, in the HEDIS format shown in Figure 11-3, additional immunizations could be reported in the "cis" measure segment by adding new data elements without altering the "cis" measure or affecting the other measures.

Other standards organizations, ANSI X12n and HL7 (discussed in previous chapters), both have workgroups developing XML versions of their standards. Someday the HL7 data exchange standards and the HIPAA transactions may evolve into XML formats.

## Case Mix

Another example of useful secondary data is the case mix, mentioned in Chapter 9. An inpatient hospital's case mix can be a factor in utilization of the hospital's resources and ultimately the hospital costs. Because a prospective payment system pays the same amount for all routine cases of a given DRG, it is important for the hospital to know what types of cases they are treating.

- The total weight of each DRG can be calculated by multiplying the relative weight of the DRG by the number of patients discharged for that DRG.
- The case mix index (CMI) is determined by dividing the sum of the DRG total weights by the number of patients discharged by the hospital as a whole.

The overall financial prospects for a hospital can be monitored and compared to other hospitals by calculating the CMI. This work is performed by a person called the DRG coordinator (discussed in Chapter 2).

CMS publishes a yearly report of the CMI comparing all hospitals that file Medicare A claims. The case mix index figure can be used by hospital administrators in several ways:

- The CMI is a relative measure of the hospital's average cost per case relative to the average cost per case for all hospitals for the year.
- If the CMI is substantially less than that of other hospitals of the same type, it may indicate a problem in the coding or billing department.
- The DRG total weights can be analyzed to determine if the hospital's capacity to handle certain types of cases is being underutilized. For example, a hospital has a new cardiac wing, but the total weights for cardiac DRG codes do not indicate that the hospital is serving enough patients with cardiac problems.
- DRG codes also provide geometric mean length of stay (LOS) and arithmetic mean LOS data. If hospital stays for certain DRGs are averaging longer than normal, the hospital will lose money. Either the hospital is seeing more outlier cases for which it is not billing, or the clinical pathways used to care for patients need to be improved.

The case mix data published by CMS reflects claims filed for CMS patients. Hospitals' inpatients have many other health plans and therefore hospitals perform their own internal calculations to determine an all-payer case mix.

# Using Data for Quality Improvement

The goal of every healthcare organization should be to provide the highest quality healthcare and to improve constantly. The NCQA offers a straightforward formula for improvement: measure, analyze, improve, repeat.

The role of primary and secondary health records in quality improvement is invaluable. Previous chapters have shown how complete, accurate, and timely patient health records can improve the quality of care provided to individual patients. A study of multiple patients' records who are treated for the same condition can reveal which providers or treatments have the best outcome.

Primary records can be studied based on a random sample of patients, or selected for study based on criteria such as principal diagnosis or a range of admission dates. Larger population-based studies might use aggregate data (secondary health records) and statistical analysis to identify areas for improvement. Measurement methods could then be developed to allow further study to find effective treatment protocols and improved processes. One example of this is ORYX®, a series of hospital quality measures that were developed by the Joint Commission.

## ORYX—National Hospital Quality Measures

The Joint Commission's ORYX initiative was designed to integrate outcomes and other performance measurement data into the accreditation process and support healthcare organizations in their internal quality improvement efforts. These measures were standardized with CMS, allowing the facility to collect and report the same data set for the Joint Commission and CMS initiatives. These are called the National Hospital Quality Measures (NHQM).

**GENERAL ORYX REQUIREMENTS FOR HOSPITALS**    Hospitals are required to collect and transmit data to The Joint Commission for a minimum of four core measure sets or a combination of applicable core measure sets and non-core measures as described in the following table[4]:

| Applicable Core Measure Sets | Core Measure Sets Required | Non-core Measures Required |
| --- | --- | --- |
| Four core measure sets | Four core measure sets | None (data not accepted) |
| Three core measure sets | Three core measure sets | Three non-core measures |
| Two core measure sets | Two core measure sets | Six non-core measures |
| One core measure set | One core measure set | Nine non-core measures |
| No core measure sets | No core measure sets | Nine non-core measures |

The measure sets currently available for selection are:

- Acute myocardial infarction (AMI)
- Heart failure (HF)
- Pneumonia (PN)
- Pregnancy and related conditions (PR)
- Hospital-based inpatient psychiatric services (HBIPS)
- Children's asthma care (CAC)
- Surgical Care Improvement Project (SCIP)
- Hospital outpatient program quality measures (HOP).

Future measure sets are anticipated to include:

- Venous thromboembolism (VTE)
- Nursing-sensitive care
- Stroke.

## Understanding Data Analysis and Statistics

Data analysis and statistics are used to understand and predict trends with all types of data, not just healthcare. Because nearly all inpatient hospitals prepare and submit NHQM data, we will use the acute myocardial infarction (AMI) measure set to provide practical examples for some of these concepts. Acute myocardial infarction is commonly referred to as a "heart attack."

### Sampling

The first step is to determine how many records will be used in the study. This is called the *sample size*. If the sample size is too small, the study can result in inaccurate conclusions. For example, if you had 1,000 cases, but examined only 2, you cannot infer that the other 998 cases had the same results. However, mathematicians can predict what size sample would produce statistically meaningful results.

For each measure set, the Joint Commission and CMS have determined the minimum number of cases that would produce statistically valid samples. When a hospital does not have enough cases to meet the minimum, then the sample must include all of the cases meeting the criteria. For example, for the acute myocardial infarction measure sets, the minimum sample size is 20 percent of the inpatient population admitted for AMI per quarter. Therefore, if there were 1,500 cases, the sample size would be 300. Where there are fewer than 78 cases per quarter, the sample size must be 100 percent of the cases. To be valid, the minimum AMI sample must be at least 35 cases.

[4]*General ORYX Requirements for Hospitals* (the most recent data available at time of publication) (Oakbrook Terrace, IL: The Joint Commission, August 8, 2008).

**Order of Data Flow/Process Steps**

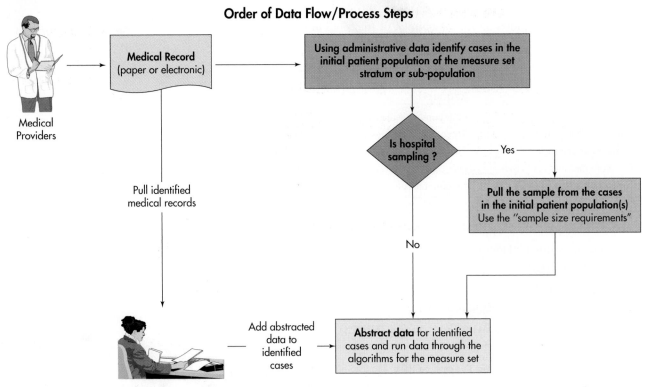

FIGURE 11-4    **Steps for sampling NHQM data.**

Figure 11-4 illustrates the steps used to sample cases for the National Hospital Quality Measures.[5]

## Algorithms

How are sample cases selected? Each measure set's initial patient population and associated measures are described by a unique algorithm. An *algorithm* is a predefined set of rules that helps to break down complex processes into simple, repetitive steps.

The first step is to evaluate and identify which episode of care records are in the measure set's population and are eligible to be sampled. This is called the *initial patient population* from which 20 percent of the cases will be selected. The algorithms serve two purposes:

1. Eliminate episode of care records contain missing and/or invalid data that would be required in the measure set.

2. Determine if:

   For *rate-based measures*, the patient's record belongs in the measure population described by the denominator, and if the patient experienced the event described in the numerator.

   For *continuous variable measures*, the patient's record belongs in the patient population described in the measure's statement and, if so, to define and calculate the measurement value.

A flow diagram can be used to illustrate the flow of logic used in an algorithm. Figure 11-5 shows the flow of the algorithm to select AMI sample cases.[6]

Follow the flow of Figure 11-5. The first thing the algorithm does is make sure the case has not already been processed and previously rejected. Next it determines if the patient's diagnosis is in the range we are looking for (ICD-9-CM 410.00–410.91). If it is not, the case is rejected.

[5]Adapted from *Specifications Manual for National Hospital Inpatient Quality Measures, Version 2.5, for Discharges 10-01-08 through 03-31-09* (Baltimore, MD: Center for Medicare and Medicaid Services, 2009).
[6]Ibid.

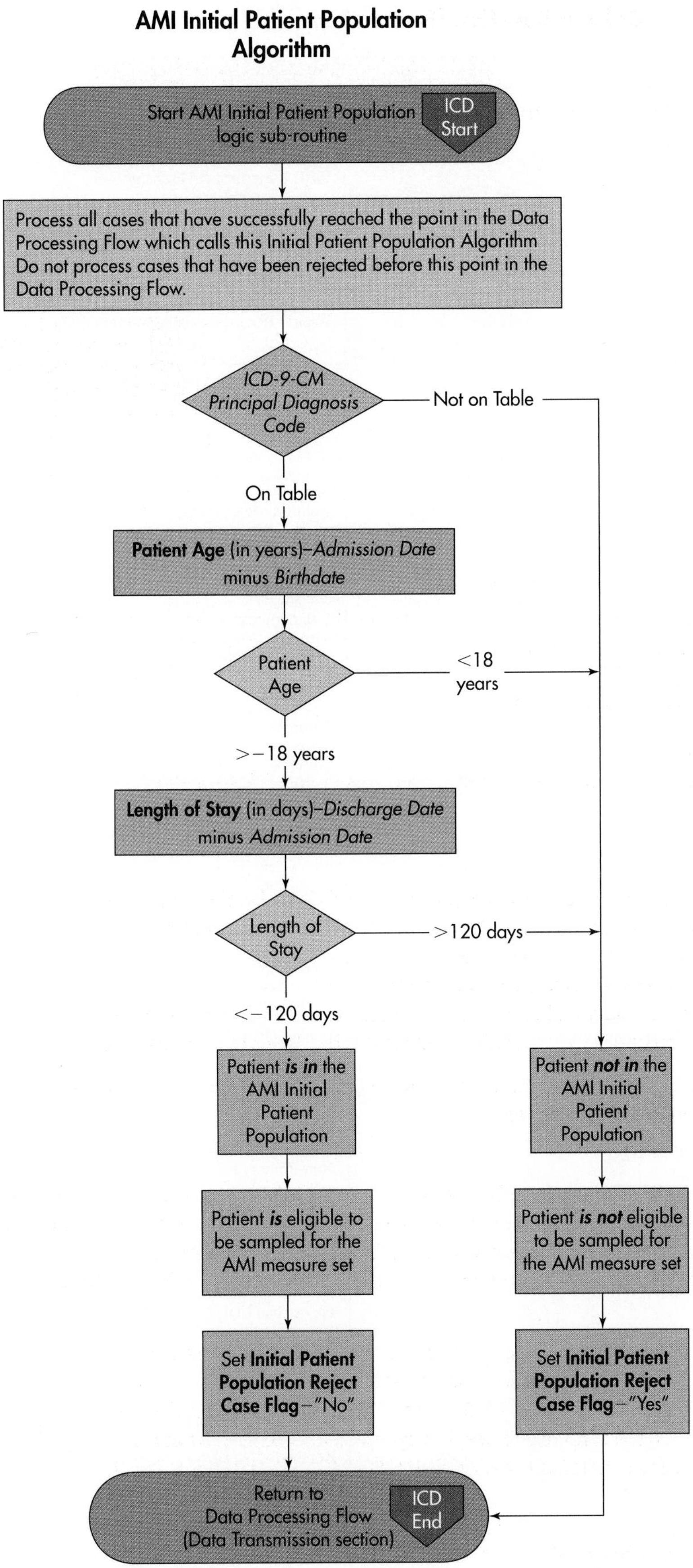

**AMI Initial Patient Population
Algorithm**

**FIGURE 11-5**

**Flow of algorithm
for acute
myocardial
infarction measure
set.**

**FIGURE 11-6**

**Data elements in the acute myocardial infarction measure set.**

| General Data Elements | AMI Data Elements |
|---|---|
| Admission Date | ACEI Prescribed at Discharge |
| Birthdate | Adult Smoking Counseling |
| Discharge Date | Adult Smoking History |
| Discharge Status | ARB Prescribed at Discharge |
| First Name | Arrival Date |
| Hispanic Ethnicity | Arrival Time |
| Hospital Patient Identifier | Aspirin Prescribed at Discharge |
| ICD-9-CM Other Diagnosis Codes | Aspirin Received Within 24 Hours Before or After Hospital Arrival |
| ICD-9-CM Other Procedure Codes | Beta-Blocker Prescribed at Discharge |
| ICD-9-CM Other Procedure Dates | Beta-Blocker Received Within 24 Hours After Hospital Arrival |
| ICD-9-CM Principal Diagnosis Code | Clinical Trial |
| ICD-9-CM Principal Procedure Code | Comfort Measures Only |
| ICD-9-CM Principal Procedure Date | Contraindication to Aspirin at Discharge |
| Last Name | Contraindication to Aspirin on Arrival |
| Patient HIC # (for patients with Medicare) | Contraindication to Beta-Blocker at Discharge |
| Payment Source- Medicare | Contraindication to Beta-Blocker on Arrival |
| Physician 1 | Contraindication to Both ACEI and ARB at Discharge |
| Physician 2 | Fibrinolytic Administration |
| Point of Origin for Admission or Visit | Fibrinolytic Administration Date |
| Postal Code | Fibrinolytic Administration Time |
| Race | First In-Hospital LDL-Cholesterol Qualitative Description |
| Sample indicator; if data has been sampled or represents all cases | First In-Hospital LDL-Cholesterol Value |
| Sex | First PCI Date |
|  | First PCI Time |
| Measurement Category | In-Hospital LDL-Cholesterol Test |
| Measurement Value (output from continuous variable measure algorithms) | Initial ECG Interpretation |
|  | Lipid-Lowering Agent Prescribed at Discharge |
|  | LVSD |
|  | Non-Primary PCI |
|  | Plan for LDL-Cholesterol Test |
|  | Pre-Arrival LDL-Cholesterol Qualitative Description |
|  | Pre-Arrival LDL-Cholesterol Test |
|  | Pre-Arrival LDL-Cholesterol Value |
|  | Pre-Arrival Lipid-Lowering Agent |
|  | Reason for Delay in Fibrinolytic Therapy |
|  | Reason for Delay in PCI |
|  | Reason for No LDL-Cholesterol Testing |
|  | Reason for No Lipid-Lowering Therapy |
|  | Transfer From Another ED |

If the diagnosis is correct, the algorithm proceeds to calculate the patient's age at the time of admission and rejects underage patients. If the patient was at least 18 years old, then the length of stay is calculated. The study does not want patients who were hospitalized for more than 120 days because these would be outlier cases.

## Abstracting

Once the patients for the data sample have been identified, certain fields are abstracted from their records to create the secondary data. Each measure set defines certain elements that are specific to that quality measure, and also includes general elements that are collected for most of the measure sets, such as date of admission, date of discharge, date of birth, and diagnosis codes. Many of the elements can be exported automatically from the hospital information systems. Others may be available from electronic health records if the system has fielded codified EHR data. Otherwise, an HIM professional must manually abstract the data elements.

Manual abstraction involves pulling the selected patient charts and reviewing documents such as physician orders, nursing notes, admission, operative, and discharge reports to locate the information. Data is then manually entered into a secondary database that will be used for the study.

Figure 11-6 lists the data elements used.[7] The general data elements in the left column are used for most of the measure sets. The data elements specific for AMI are listed in the right column.

All of the general elements listed in Figure 11-6 could be abstracted automatically by a computer program. Assuming the hospital has computerized the lab and medication orders, the cholesterol tests and drugs ordered may also be abstracted automatically.

However, elements such as "Reason for Delay . . ." and "Reason for No . . ." drug or therapy must be manually abstracted from the chart. The abstractor may have to search multiple source documents. Here are several examples:

**Patient's Allergy Record:**

- "Intolerant of lipid lowering agents."

**Admission History and Physical:**

- "Hx muscle soreness to statins in past."

**Attending Physician's Notes:**

- "Lipid lowering therapy contraindicated."

# Healthcare Statistics

Once the secondary data has been abstracted, it can be used for analysis to calculate results and measure improvement. Statistics can be used in several different ways to describe the population of our samples and to show us the outcome measurement in relation to the population. Descriptive statistics are used in healthcare for many purposes.

In our example, evidence-based medicine has suggested a number of therapies and interventions that when used within a designated period of time can produce better outcomes for patients suffering acute myocardial infarctions. These are:

- Aspirin at arrival
- Aspirin prescribed at discharge
- ACEI or ARB for LVSD
- Adult smoking cessation advice/counseling
- Beta-blocker prescribed at discharge
- Beta-blocker at arrival
- Fibrinolytic therapy received within 30 minutes of hospital arrival

---

[7]Ibid.

- Median time to fibrinolysis
- Primary PCI received within 90 minutes of hospital arrival
- Median time to primary PCI
- LDL cholesterol assessment
- Lipid-lowering therapy at discharge
- Inpatient mortality (for AMI).

## Ratios, Proportions, and Rates

Healthcare statistics are often stated as ratios, proportions, or rates. Examples include birth rate, mortality rate, bed occupancy, and case mix. These formulas help us compare the relationship between two counts or numbers. For example, the AMI measure sets help hospitals by showing them how quickly and effectively known methods of treating heart attack patients are being applied. These figures are reported as rates per quarter. For most of the AMI measures, an increase in the rate indicates an improvement in performance; note, however, that for three measures (median time to fibrinolysis, median time to PCI, and the mortality rate) a decrease indicates improvement.

To understand this you may wish to think of each of these concepts as fractions. Each calculation begins with a numerator that is divided by a denominator. For example:

$$\frac{\text{Number of AMI patients who were given aspirin (numerator)}}{\text{Number of AMI patients who could have been given aspirin (denominator)}}$$

**FIGURE 11-7**

**Miles per gallon is a ratio of two different things.**

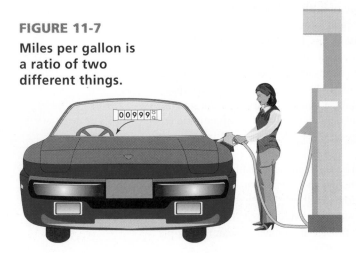

**RATIOS** Ratios can be used to show us the relationship between two different things. For example, the mileage of your automobile is expressed as miles per gallon. While miles and gallons are two different measures, by dividing the miles you have driven (the numerator) by the number of gallons of gasoline your car has used (the denominator), you will know how many miles you get from one gallon of gasoline (see Figure 11-7).

In most cases, ratios are mathematically reduced until either the numerator or denominator is one. Ratios are usually written as two numbers separated by a colon. For example, if the hospital gave 90 AMI patients aspirin, but missed giving aspirin to 10 patients, the ratio would be 9:1.

The formula to calculate a ratio is $x/y$ = ratio.

Though ratios can be used to compare two different measures, they do not have to be about different things. In the example of the ratio of *patients given aspirin: patients not given aspirin,* both measures were the same thing (patients).

**FIGURE 11-8**

**Proportion of patients given aspirin to a whole set of AMI patients.**

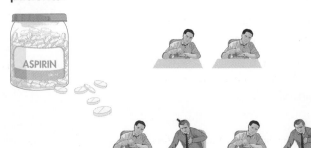

**PROPORTIONS** A proportion is a type of ratio, but there are two differences. The numerator is always a portion of the whole (subset) and the denominator is always the whole set. Therefore, proportions always express the relationship between two counts of the same thing. In Figure 11-8 both the numerator and denominator are patients.

Using the aspirin example, if the nominator was the number of patients given aspirin ($x$), the denominator would be the sum of patients given aspirin ($x$) plus those not given aspirin ($y$); thus, the formula would be $x/(x + y)$ = *proportion:*

AMI patients given aspirin: 90

Patients not given aspirin: +10

Total patients in the set: 100

Calculate the proportion: *90/100 = 0.9*

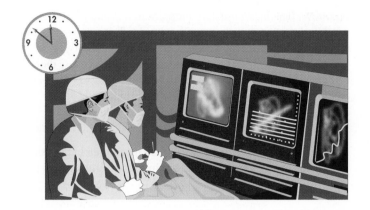

**RATES**   Rates are used to measure events occurring over a period of time or to express a ratio or proportion as a percentage. The National Hospital Quality Measures are reported quarterly. Most AMI measure sets report an aggregate data measure in which the value of each measurement is expressed as a proportion.

For example, national guidelines recommend the prompt initiation of primary percutaneous coronary intervention (PCI), also known as angioplasty, for patients presenting with ST-elevation myocardial infarction or left bundle branch block (LBBB) (see Figure 11-9). One of the AMI sets measures the hospital's rate at getting the angioplasty done quickly.

Numerator:          30 AMI patients for which a primary PCI was done within 90 minutes.

Denominator:     48 Total AMI patients who received a primary PCI

$$30/48 = 0.625$$

To convert the rate to a percentage, multiply by 100

$$0.625 \times 100 = 62.5\%$$

Rates can be used to standardize proportions or ratios for comparison to each other. For example, a researcher wants to study which of several treatments has been most effective, but the therapies have not been used in equal numbers of cases so the comparison is not straightforward. One way hospitals do this is to report data as *rate per 100 cases*.

## Measures of Central Tendency: Mean, Median, and Mode

Two of the AMI measure sets discussed earlier involve time. The value reported is the central tendency as the median time. A *central tendency* is the distribution of a variable, measured by statistics such as the mean, median, and mode.

In the AMI measure sets, the hospital reports number of minutes until an AMI patient either received fibrinolytic therapy or a PCI was performed. If we continue with the PCI example, we know we had 30 patients who received PCI within the desired time frame. However, the number of minutes is a *continuous variable,* that is, it could be any number from 1 minute to 90 minutes. To find the central tendency in this range of time, let us begin with the distribution of data in the secondary health records for this data set as illustrated in Figure 11-10.

Looking at Figure 11-10, you will see a variance of time ranging from 17 to 90 minutes. When the data is sorted by the number of minutes (as shown in Figure 11-10) we can see the *frequency of distribution,* that is, what the range of minutes was and how many cases had the same "minutes until PCI."

A measure of central tendency is a measure of the typical value of a frequency distribution. This typical value may be determined in three ways: mean, median, or mode.

**MEAN**   The *mean* is the sum of the values (minutes) divided by the frequency (number of patients). Another way of saying it is that the mean is the *average*. In our PCI example, the sum of minutes in Figure 11-10 is 1,650; the number of patients is 30.

$$1,650/30 = 55$$

Though the mean is straightforward to calculate, the result can be easily skewed by outlier cases. If several cases had lower or higher values, the mean might be a substantially different result.

| Patient | Minutes Until PCI |
|---------|-------------------|
| Jones, J | 17 |
| Smith, T | 20 |
| Williams | 25 |
| Green | 30 |
| Brown | 30 |
| Garcia | 35 |
| Smythe | 37 |
| Snyder | 39 |
| Franks | 45 |
| Lee | 45 |
| Harris | 45 |
| Meyer | 45 |
| Anders | 47 |
| Karl | 47 |
| Wyozk | 59 |
| Baker | 59 |
| Taylor | 60 |
| Jones, B | 60 |
| Dodd | 61 |
| Roberts | 63 |
| Gold | 64 |
| Todd | 68 |
| Bettes | 68 |
| Close | 71 |
| Ghan | 75 |
| Marsh | 78 |
| Smith, J | 87 |
| Wilson | 90 |
| Bass | 90 |
| Dell | 90 |

**FIGURE 11-10**

**Table of AMI patients' "Time Until PCI" sorted by minutes.**

**MEDIAN** The *median* is the midpoint in a group of ranked values that divides the data into two equal parts. Simply stated, if we sort the cases by number of minutes (as we have in Figure 11-10), then count halfway down the list, we will find the median. If there are an odd number of cases, then the median is the value at the center of the list. If the list has an even number of cases, then the median is the average of the center two values.

Figure 11-10 has 30 cases. The median value is 59.

Median is not influenced by extreme values and outlier cases.

**MODE** The *mode* is a value that occurs most often in the frequency distribution. If we count the number of cases in Figure 11-10 we see:

- 45 minutes—four cases
- 90 minutes—three cases
- 68 minutes, 60 minutes, 59 minutes, 47 minutes and 30 minutes—two cases each

All of the remaining times, 17 to 87 minutes, each occurred once. The most frequently occurring time is 45 minutes; the central tendency expressed as a mode is 45.

Although mode is not influenced by extreme values and outlier cases, it may not be unique. The sample could contain several values for which there were an equal number of cases.

Figure 11-11 illustrates the mean, median, mode, and range for our PCI example.

## Measures of Variability

In addition to calculations of central tendency, it may be useful to know how widely the values vary from the typical value of central tendency (the mean, median, or mode). There are three ways to describe how the data points are spread out: the range, the variance, and standard deviation.

**RANGE** Range is simply the measure of spread between the smallest values and the largest values in a frequency distribution. Figure 11-11 shows a time line for the PCI cases that were listed in Figure 11-10. If we look at Figure 11-11, we see that the shortest time before a PCI was performed was 17 minutes and the longest was 90 minutes. The formula for calculating range is:

$$maximum - minimum = range$$

The range for the PCI measure set is $90 - 17 = 73$.

**VARIANCE** *Variance* is another way to show the variability in the frequency distribution. In Figure 11-11, we also see that there are fewer cases in the 17–55 minute range than in the 55–90 minute range; however, the range would be the same if there were only one case at each end of the timeline. Variance, however, will give us the average variation from the mean.

Variance is calculated in several steps. First, the mean is determined; in the previous section we determined that the mean was 55. Next, the mean is subtracted from each item in the frequency distribution, and the result is squared (multiplied times itself). For example:

$$(90 - 55)^2 = 1,225$$

This is repeated for each case in the set. When we have the results from every case, the totals are summed. For our PCI measure set, the sum of our results is 12,812. To determine the variance, the sum is divided by the number of cases minus one. The variance in our PCI set is calculated as follows:

$$12,812/(30 - 1) = 441.7931$$

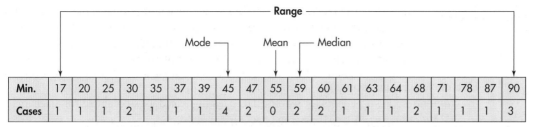

| | Range | | | | | | | | | | | | | | | | | | | |
|---|---|---|---|---|---|---|---|---|---|---|---|---|---|---|---|---|---|---|---|---|
| **Min.** | 17 | 20 | 25 | 30 | 35 | 37 | 39 | 45 | 47 | 55 | 59 | 60 | 61 | 63 | 64 | 68 | 71 | 78 | 87 | 90 |
| **Cases** | 1 | 1 | 1 | 2 | 1 | 1 | 1 | 4 | 2 | 0 | 2 | 2 | 1 | 1 | 1 | 2 | 1 | 1 | 1 | 3 |

**FIGURE 11-11    Timeline showing distribution of AMI cases receiving PCI**

**STANDARD DEVIATION**    It is not easy to apply the variance to the original data because the original values were lost when they were squared. The variability of our data can be better understood by converting the variance back into the same type of values used in our measure set. This will tell us what the *standard deviation* of values from the mean is. Because we squared each value while calculating the variance, all we have to do to calculate the standard deviation is to calculate the square root of the variance:

$$21 = \sqrt{441.7931}$$

In the example the standard deviation is rounded to 21. The graph in Figure 11-12 shows the distribution of "Minutes until PCI" cases and the standard deviation intervals.

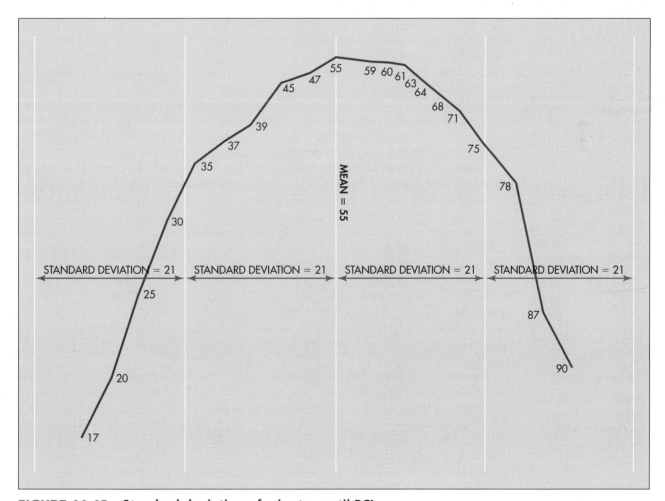

**FIGURE 11-12    Standard deviation of minutes until PCI.**

MEANINGFUL STATISTICS    If statistics are to be useful, they must not be misleading. One way to make statistics meaningful is to clearly state the case to which they apply. Using the NHQM examples, each measure set lists which patients are to be included and excluded in the aggregate data calculated. Compare the following two examples from the AMI measures:

- **LDL cholesterol assessment:**
     *Numerator:* AMI patients for whom LDL-c testing was done or planned for discharge
          *Denominator:* All AMI patients

This measure shows the proportion of AMI patients who are being tested. Because the guidelines recommend this test for all AMI patients, it is valid to rate the hospital based on all AMI admissions.

- **Beta-blocker prescribed at discharge:**
     *Numerator:* AMI patients who are prescribed a beta-blocker at hospital discharge
          *Denominator:* Only AMI patients without beta-blocker contraindications

While drugs known as beta-blockers have been shown to be effective, it would not be wise to give them to patients who cannot take the drug. Therefore, this measure is designed to compare the patients given beta-blockers with those who could have been given beta-blockers. It omits from the calculation those who should not have been given beta-blockers.

When relying on the validity of any statistical information, it is important to consider whether the primary records and the abstraction are accurate, whether the sample was large enough, and whether only cases relevant to the study were included.

## Keeping Data Valuable

Data has become an important product of healthcare facilities. Not only is it used for patients' longitudinal care, but as we have discussed in this chapter, it is also used for research. Many evidence-based medical studies are not new clinical trials, but instead consist of researchers reviewing large numbers of previous cases to study their outcomes.

Paper records once made such research studies laborious and the retention of old records costly. As facilities shift to computerized records, researching of old records is not only easier, but the data can be retained indefinitely at very low costs. This fact is making many facilities rethink their record retention polices (discussed in Chapter 6).

However, to be useful for future research, the data must not only be protected, it must be maintained. One aspect of this involves conversion. Each time a database is redesigned and new fields are added, the database must be converted. For example, if a patient file used to have 20 fields in the record and the new design has 40 fields per record, then a software conversion program is used to read each of the existing records and write the data into the new database records. Hospitals and their vendors rigorously test the conversion program against duplicate or "test" databases to ensure everything will copy correctly.

But what if the data within the records actually needs to be changed? For example, a hospital recorded its patients' race using a proprietary set of codes the hospital made up. In the new version, the codes are being modified to match HIPAA standards and to make it easier to interface with other software the hospital uses. In that case, the data is not only being copied, but is being modified as well. This is not difficult if the translation is straightforward; for example, if the old data for a particular race was a "2" and the new data is a "C."

However, when the new field definition has nuances that were not available previously, then the converted data will not have the same meaning for future researchers as the data entered thereafter. Continuing with the example of race, suppose the old HIS registration only offered 4 choices from which the registration person could select. In the new version, the field is relabeled "Ethnicity" and there are now 10 choices. All existing patients will be in one of the 4 previous categories, whereas new patients will be assigned one of 10 categories. Hereafter, research that includes an ethnic factor will have data that is skewed toward the original 4 categories.

In several earlier chapters we discussed the proposed change of diagnosis and billing codes from ICD-9-CM to ICD-10. One of the paramount issues with that change is what will happen to

## You Never Know What You Don't Know

### *By Thomas Rau*

*Thomas Rau is division chair for information technology at the Mayo Clinic in Rochester, Minnesota.*

In terms of record retention, something that Mayo is challenged with today is that we are spending a lot of money on electronic storage. Our tendency is to keep everything. Our record retention policy is simple—keep it all.

Dr. Christopher Chute likes the quote "You never know what you don't know"—a true researcher right? There is a practical lesson we learned about that.

Early on at Mayo, a pathologist, Dr. Louie B. Wilson, created a program to keep tissues from operations. He stored them in jars over in the medical science building. Well the value of keeping those specimens declined over time, and the space required grew.

Then after many, many years, guess what happened? DNA was decoded. Suddenly, Mayo had a vast tissue collection that we can still get DNA information from. We have the test results of people who were suffering; it is of great value. So it is true that you never know what you don't know.

Today, the field that I think is ripe for a similar leap forward is images. In the last couple of years we have developed something called the Mayo Digital Archive, although archive may not be the best description of it. It was designed to meet some of radiology's needs for storing images long term.

A lot of radiology is pattern recognition. Can't computers do that pretty well? I think so. Are we going to learn more about what patterns mean? I think so. So while there is the negative aspect of the cost of storing large-size radiology files, they may turn out to be a positive research tool in a future time.

The challenge of retaining electronic medical records—making sure they are still there and have integrity—is one thing, but the other challenge is changing technology. We have nearly a petabyte (1,000 terabytes) of storage. When we change technology, we can't covert it all over in a weekend. We have to use a strategy of doing portions of it over time and ensuring its integrity at the same time.

historic data. There are almost twice as many ICD-10-CM codes as ICD-9-CM codes, and in many cases there is not a straight translation between them. Refer back to Chapter 9, Figure 9-8, where you will notice that diagnosis 599.7 could map to four different ICD-10-CM codes. What will happen to the data during this conversion is a topic still under discussion.

Because we don't know what directions medical knowledge will take in the future, we don't understand how valuable what we are building today might be in the future. This point is illustrated in the real-life story.

## Pay for Performance

One of the direct effects of the NHQM data is its application to new reimbursement models. In an effort to improve quality of care, CMS and other payers are developing pay-for-performance (P4P) programs that tie reimbursement to improvements in quality.

The CMS's Hospital Quality Initiative links reporting of the National Hospital Quality Measures described earlier to the payments the hospitals receive for each discharge. Hospitals that submit the required data receive the full payment update to their Medicare DRG payments. As of 2009, 98.3 percent of the hospitals eligible to participate were complying with the program.

In addition to the initiatives for hospitals, CMS is also developing pay-for-performance programs for physicians and physician groups and nursing home care. Recognizing that many of the best opportunities for quality improvement are patient focused and cut across settings of care, CMS is pursuing pay-for-performance initiatives to support better care coordination for patients with chronic illnesses.

CMS also developed a three-year pay-for-performance project for physicians to promote the adoption and use of health information technology to improve the quality of care for Medicare patients who are chronically ill. The focus is on small and medium-sized physician practices.

Doctors who meet or exceed performance standards established by CMS in clinical delivery systems and patient outcomes receive bonus payments.

The goal of pay-for-performance programs is to counteract a tendency that other payment systems have to create a disincentive for quality improvement. Support for pay for performance has been growing rapidly. As of 2009 more than 150 P4P programs existed, many using the NCQA measures we have studied in this chapter.

Margaret O'Kane, president of NCQA, has said:

"The challenge for those organizations that are developing pay for performance initiatives is to ensure that the programs they introduce will help to correct some of the flaws inherent in the current payment system.

This opportunity is about getting the best value for the money for society, making it rewarding to be in the delivery system, allowing those who work in the delivery system to use their ingenuity, their deep knowledge, and their incredible smarts to deliver value for all of us."[8]

# Chapter 11 Summary

## Secondary Health Records and Indexes

Secondary health records are useful for improving quality and performance. They are used internally within the facility and reported to external users for research, statistical analysis, and pay-for-performance incentives. Secondary data may take several forms:

- Indexes, which can be separate files or pointers to data within the primary health records
- Registries, which are usually separate databases created to track specific types of data; for example, cancer tumors, implanted devices, or childhood immunizations
- Custom data sets for reporting performance such as HEDIS or the NHQM measure sets.

## Processing and Maintaining Secondary Data

Meaningful measurements, statistics, and reporting depend on the quality of the primary health record. The following are criteria for ensuring quality data:

- *Validity* or accuracy of the data
- *Reliability* and consistency of the data
- *Completeness* of the data
- *Timeliness* of the data
- *Security* of the data.

Maintenance of data for the long term means converting data when databases are upgraded or modified. In some cases, conversion means translating some coded fields from an old coding standard to a new one. Secondary data may or may not contain PHI. For example, claims, adverse events

reported to the FDA, and infectious disease data reported to the CDC contain PHI. This is allowed by HIPAA.

In other situations, the secondary data does not contain PHI. For example:

- *De-identified data* is data that has had the PHI elements removed such that an individual cannot be personally identified from the data. Such data can then be used by external users such as researchers for studies and trend analysis.
- *Aggregate data* is data that does not contain PHI because by definition it does not consist of individual records. Aggregate data is the sum of records containing data matching certain criteria. For example, the case mix index is derived from the count of patients in each diagnosis-related group (DRG).

HIPAA also makes an exception that permits researchers to examine data containing PHI for the purposes of developing a test protocol or sampling methodology. An internal review board (IRB) monitors and approves the use of data containing PHI for research.

Clinical trials have the patients' permission to use data containing PHI. Clinical trials are not necessarily secondary heath records, but are sometimes another form of primary health record data.

## Using and Reporting Secondary Health Records

The Health Plan Employer Data and Information Set (HEDIS) consists of 71 measures across eight domains of care. Employers use the results of reports derived from HEDIS data to select the best plan for their employees.

---

[8]Margaret E. O'Kane, *Pay for Performance: A Critical Examination*, NCQA 2006 Policy Conference Monograph (Washington, DC: National Committee for Quality Assurance, 2006).

XML is a format that is becoming popular for transferring secondary data from the provider to a central registry or database. XML stands for eXtensible Markup Language. Fields are defined by label *tags* that mark the beginning and end of each field of data as well as groups of data called segments. The format is useful because the data can not only be imported by a computer, but can also be easily viewed by a person using a browser such as Microsoft Internet Explorer. HEDIS data is transmitted in XML format.

The case mix is the statistical distribution of the type of cases that have been treated by the hospital. It is determined from the DRGs of discharged patients. A case mix index is created by CMS from Medicare claims data. Hospitals study the case mix data from Medicare as well as their own internally developed case mix studies because the case mix can be a factor in utilization of the hospital's resources and ultimately hospital costs.

## Using Data for Quality Improvement

The goal of every healthcare organization should be to provide the highest quality healthcare and to improve constantly. The NCQA offers a straightforward formula for improvement: measure, analyze, improve, repeat.

The role of primary and secondary health records in quality improvement is invaluable.

The Joint Commission's ORYX initiative was designed to integrate outcomes and other performance measurement data into the accreditation process and support healthcare organizations in their internal quality improvement efforts. These measures were standardized with CMS, allowing the facility to collect and report the same data set for the Joint Commission and CMS initiatives. These are called the National Hospital Quality Measures (NHQM).

Pay-for-performance programs are being developed to provide incentive to hospitals and physicians alike for improving the quality of care. One way they do this is for the provider to report data using specific measure sets. These measures are related to scientific studies that showed patients did better when certain therapies or procedures were used within specific time frames. The NHQM sets report data on the rate the provider is following the guideline. For most of the measures, an improvement in rate results in improved outcome for the patients.

## Understanding Data Analysis and Statistics

Data analysis includes applying mathematical formulas to produce statistical studies. Not every record has to be included, but for the statistics to be meaningful, the number of records (called the sample size) must have enough cases to be representative of the whole. The data must also include the type of cases that apply to the measure, but exclude those that are not applicable.

An algorithm consists of logical steps to process the data to arrive at the desired result. In the case of sampling, an algorithm is used to select the initial population for the measure set.

Once the sample is selected, data that cannot be imported from the hospital's computer system is abstracted and entered manually from the patient's records.

## Healthcare Statistics

When all the data for the samples has been collected and entered, certain mathematical formulas are used to generate statistics. This chapter discussed several formulas commonly used in healthcare.

### Ratio

Ratios can be used to show us the relationship between two measures. Ratios can be applied to two different things, such as miles and gallons; or to two of the same thing, such as patients who received a therapy and those who did not. The ratio fraction is often mathematically reduced until either the numerator or denominator is one. Often ratios are written as two numbers separated by a colon. An example of a ratio is 10:1. The formula for a ratio is:

$$x/y = \text{ratio}$$

### Proportions

Proportions are ratios, but the numerator is a subset of the denominator; therefore, both parts of the equation must be measures of the same thing. The formula for proportion is:

$$x/(x + y) = \text{proportion}$$

### Rates

Rates are used to measure events occurring over a period of time or to express a ratio or proportion as a percentage.

### Continuous Variable

When values such as time are being measured, they are said to be continuous variables. How frequently the data occurs at given points along the continuous variable is called the frequency of distribution.

### Central Tendency

The central tendency is the distribution of a variable, measured by statistics such as the mean, median, and mode.

### Mean

The mean is the average; that is, the sum of the values divided by the frequency.

### Median

The median is the midpoint in a group of ranked values that divides the data into two equal parts.

### Mode

The mode is a value that occurs most often in the frequency of distribution.

### Measures of Variability

When using data of central tendency, it may be useful to know how widely the values vary from the value of central tendency. There are three statistics of variability: range, variance, and standard deviation.

### Range

The range is the difference from the highest value in the frequency distribution to the lowest.

### Variance

Variance is the average variation from the mean. The variance is calculated as follows:

1. Calculate the mean.
2. Then for each value in the set, subtract the mean from the value and multiple the result times itself.
3. Sum the total of all the calculations
4. Divide the total by the number of values minus 1.

### Standard Deviation

Standard deviation reduces the variance back to the same units as the original values. Once the variance has been calculated, the standard deviation is the square root of the variance.

## Critical Thinking Exercises

1. Ask 10 people their height. Make a list and arrange it in order by height.
2. Find the mean, median, and mode on your list from Exercise 1. Does the list contain outliers (such as children or basketball players) that are much shorter or taller than most of the others on the list?

## Testing Your Knowledge of Chapter 11

1. Name the five factors that affect the quality of primary data.
2. How does coded, fielded primary data help in the creation of secondary data?
3. The text listed nine types of data in a cancer registry. Name three of the types.
4. What does the acronym XML stand for?
5. What is the common name for acute myocardial infarction (AMI)?
6. Which type of statistic discussed in this chapter can be used to compare two different things?
7. What is de-identified data?
8. What code set is used to determine the case mix index?
9. What is sampling?
10. How is an algorithm defined in this chapter?
11. Thirty AMI patients who smoked were counseled against smoking; two were not. What is the *ratio* of AMI smokers who were counseled to those who were not?
12. Ninety AMI patients were given LDL-cholesterol tests, 10 were not. What is the *proportion* of AMI patients being tested?
13. Fibrinolytic therapy should be used for appropriate AMI patients within 30 minutes of arrival. Last quarter, a hospital's quickest time was 17 minutes; its longest time was 29 minutes. What is the *range* of variability in the data?
14. What does the acronym HEDIS stand for?
15. What is the difference between the central tendency values *mean* and *median*?

# Management and Decision Support Systems

## ACRONYMS USED IN CHAPTER 12

Acronyms are used extensively in both medicine and computers. The following acronyms are used in this chapter.

| | | | |
|---|---|---|---|
| **ADT** | Admission, Discharge, Transfer | **HIPAA** | Health Insurance Portability and Accountability Act |
| **AP-DRGs** | All-Patient Diagnosis-Related Groups (severity adjusted) | **HL7** | Health Level 7 |
| **A/R** | Accounts Receivable | **HMO** | Health Maintenance Organization |
| **CAP** | College of American Pathologists | **MCAP** | Medical Care Appropriateness Protocol |
| **CAT** | Computerized Axial Tomography | **MRI** | Magnetic Resonance Imaging |
| **CDC** | Centers for Disease Control and Prevention | **NHQM** | National Hospital Quality Measures |
| **CFO** | Chief Financial Officer | **NPDB** | National Practitioner Data Bank |
| **CMI** | Case Mix Index | **OSHA** | Occupational Safety and Health Administration |
| **CMS** | Centers for Medicare and Medicaid Services | **PCE** | Potentially Compensable Event |
| **EFT** | Electronic Funds Transfer | **PHI** | Protected Health Information (HIPAA) |
| **EHR** | Electronic Health Record | | |
| **EPHI** | Protected Health Information in Electronic Form | **QM** | Quality Management |
| | | **RAC** | Recovery Audit Contractor |
| **FTE** | Full-Time Equivalent Employee | **RN** | Registered Nurse |
| **GL** | General Ledger | **SNF** | Skilled Nursing Facility |
| **HIM** | Health Information Management | **TB** | Tuberculosis |

# Information Systems for Managerial Support

Thus far the emphasis of this book has been on primary and secondary patient health records. Healthcare facilities, however, have many other aspects involved in their operation and nearly all of them are computerized.

This chapter introduces additional information systems that support healthcare operations but are not clinical records. That is not to say the systems do not contain PHI, many of them do; it is that the purpose of these systems is to support the management of the healthcare organization.

As you study this chapter you will realize that there are opportunities to work with information systems other than HIM and EHR systems. These systems are vital to the management and operation of healthcare facilities. The information provides managerial support and is the basis for operational, strategic, and executive decisions.

## Interfaced or Integrated

Depending on the vendor, the management and decision support systems discussed in this chapter are either interfaced systems or integrated systems. Interfaced systems are prevalent in hospitals; integrated systems are prevalent in medical offices (called practice management systems):

- *Interfaced systems* consist of separate software and databases that are linked into the computer network. They exchange information with other healthcare systems using HL7 or a proprietary transaction standard. The software may be from the same or a different vendor.

- *Integrated systems* share a common database. Data records are read and updated without the need for HL7 transactions. Though programs such as registration and billing use separate software modules, they are supplied by the same vendor and work together seamlessly.

# Administrative Systems

In previous chapters we have already discussed two administrative systems, the patient registration system and the billing system. In a hospital, the registration system is also called the admission, discharge, transfer (ADT) system. The billing system is sometimes called the patient accounts or accounts receivable (A/R) system.

These two systems may be thought of as the beginning and end of an episode of care. The ADT system registers patients before they are treated or scheduled for treatment, and the A/R system follows the episodes until the patients' account balances are zero.

Just as there are many uses of secondary health records data for research and operational support, there are many secondary uses for administrative data. In some cases, reports are generated from the primary administrative data. For example, an aged accounts receivables report shows managers how long unpaid balances have been outstanding. In other cases, administrative data is abstracted and exported into a secondary database. For example, patient registration data could be subtotaled by zip code and the totals exported to Excel. In Figure 12-1, a pie chart shows the demographic distribution of patients by zip code.

**FIGURE 12-1**

**Pie chart created from secondary administrative data.**

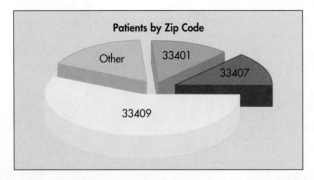

## Financial Information Systems

Financial information systems are used in all types of businesses to track income, expenses, assets the business owns, and liabilities owed by the business. These systems include:

- An overall accounting system called the general ledger (GL)
- Accounts receivable
- Purchasing
- Accounts payable
- Inventory and materials management

- Payroll
- Budgeting
- Cost accounting.

Each type of business has aspects that make its financial systems unique: builders buy materials, lawyers bill by minutes, and realtors are paid by commission. The healthcare business is unique as well. Hospitals and medical practices use financial software uniquely suited to healthcare operations.

## General Ledger

In other lines of business, the general accounting system might include detailed records of daily business, which are then summed for *general ledger* reports. Because of the vast quantity of detailed records in healthcare operations, this is not done. For example, hundreds of thousands of supplies are purchased; thousands of patient encounters are billed to multiple insurance plans. Therefore, separate accounting systems or modules are used to maintain and manage various aspects of healthcare financial operations. Those systems then send only summary information to the GL.

The general ledger is used to produce financial statements and monitor the overall financial health of the organization. The general ledger for a healthcare facility typically includes only the daily, monthly, or quarterly totals from the other financial systems. For example:

- The patient accounting system might send the total amount of charges posted for each department, the total amount of contractual write-down adjustments, and the total of payments posted to the GL system daily.

- The payroll system might send the gross payroll, withholding amounts, employer taxes, employer 401(k) contributions, and so on semimonthly when employee paychecks are printed.

- The accounts payable system might send the amount of each check to the GL in real time as each batch of checks is printed.

| Public Hospital Balance Sheet | | |
|---|---|---|
| **Assets, Liabilities, and Net Assets** | | |
| | | (In thousands) |
| | | 2009 |
| **Assets:** | | |
| Current assets | $ | 35,339 |
| Capital assets, net | | 38,305 |
| Other noncurrent assets | | 18,513 |
| Total assets | $ | 92,157 |
| **Liabilities:** | | |
| Current liabilities | $ | 27,637 |
| Long-term debt outstanding, net | | 36,621 |
| Other long-term liabilities | | 6,496 |
| Total liabilities | $ | 70,754 |
| **Net assets:** | | |
| Invested in capital assets, net of related debt | $ | (3,731) |
| Restricted: | | |
| For debt service | | 8,109 |
| Expendable for specific activities | | 450 |
| Unrestricted | | 16,575 |
| Total net assets | $ | 21,403 |

**FIGURE 12-2**

**Sample balance sheet from a nonprofit hospital.**

There are four principal aspects to a general ledger in a double-entry bookkeeping system:

- *Income:* money that has been received; also called *revenue*
- *Expenses:* money that has been spent
- *Assets:* cash, property and things of value that are owned by the business
- *Liability:* amounts that are owed, but not yet paid.

The income and expenses are compared with each other on a report called an income statement or profit and loss report. If the total income is greater than the total expenses, then the business has made money. If the expenses have exceeded the income, then the business has lost money.

The assets and liability are compared with each other on a report called the balance sheet or statement of financial position. The difference between the assets and liabilities is the *net worth*. This is sometimes called the *net assets*. An example of a balance sheet is shown in Figure 12-2.

The board of directors, executives, and officers use these reports to monitor the facility's financial health and to make decisions about its future. If the facility is a for-profit organization, investors and owners use these reports to make investment decisions. Banks and others use these reports to determine creditworthiness. Federal, state, and accreditation organizations use GL information to determine the facility's financial stability and tax liability.

## Accounts Receivable

The *accounts receivable* is the money that is owed to a business. In healthcare, the principal system is the patient accounting system. Chapters 9 and 10 described the various reimbursement methods by which healthcare facilities are paid. Most of the reimbursement methods involved treating the patient, then being paid at a later date after billing the payers and patients. Therefore, in all practice management systems and most hospitals, the patient accounting system and the billing system use the same data records.

Because patient and insurance billing are the main source of revenue for healthcare organizations of all sizes, a great deal of attention is paid to this. A/R and billing data are used, reported, and analyzed by individuals in billing or collections, managers, supervisors, department heads, executives, and officers.

Because of the unique nature of healthcare billing, A/R reports often separate or subtotal amounts due from insurance from those due from the patient. Summary aging reports may be used by executives or managers to monitor the collection rate. Detailed insurance aging reports may be used by insurance specialists to identify claims that should have been paid but have not. Patient-due aging reports may be used to identify patient accounts that are overdue and to identify which insurance has already made payments.

Analyzing the accounts receivables by separately aging open items that are due from patients and those items due from insurance can provide an overview of money due in different categories. Figure 12-3 divided the A/R into six aging categories; items due in 30 days or less, items

**FIGURE 12-3**

**Aging summary analysis.**

### GOOD HEALTH ASSOCIATES

**Summary Aging Analysis Report**
(for current period)

| Days | 0–30 | 31–60 | 61–90 | 91–120 | 120–150 | 151+ |
|------|------|-------|-------|--------|---------|------|
| Patient | 3414.67 | 4750.11 | 120.01 | 160.50 | 400.00 | 0.00 |
| Insurance | 18559.94 | 2672.00 | 3985.19 | 105.60 | 560.26 | 0.00 |
| Totals | 21974.61 | 7422.11 | 4106.20 | 266.10 | 960.26 | 0.00 |

| | | |
|------|------|------|
| Total Patient Due | 8846.29 | 25.4% |
| Total Insurance Due | 25948.83 | 74.6% |
| Total A/R | 34795.12 | 100% |

# GOOD HEALTH ASSOCIATES

04/15/2009

## DETAILED AGING REPORT BY ACCOUNT BASED ON DATE OF PATIENT RESPONSIBILITY

### (Includes Payments Posted Through 04/14/2009)

| Account | Guarantor /Patient | Doctor | Date of Service | Procedure | Diagnosis | Date Pat Responsible | Date Ins Billed | 0–30 Days | 31–60 Days | 61–90 Days | 91–120 Days | Over 121 Days |
|---|---|---|---|---|---|---|---|---|---|---|---|---|
| 1009 | Patel, Raj | (404) 555-7890 | | | | | | | | | | |
| | Patel, Raj | Dr. Smith | 10/31/08 | 35001 | 441.4 | 01/03/09 | 11/10/08 | | | | 88.00 | |
| | Patel, Raj | Dr. Smith | 10/31/08 | 99233 | 428.0 | 01/03/09 | 11/10/08 | | | | 0.90 | |
| | Patel, Raj | Dr. Green | 11/22/08 | 99214 | 428.0 | 03/16/09 | 01/03/09 | 6.80 | | | | |
| | Patel, Raj | Dr. Green | 11/22/08 | 82465 | 428.0 | 03/16/09 | 01/03/09 | 1.20 | | | | |
| | Patel, Raj | | 03/31/09 | Interest | Interest | 03/31/09 | | 0.95 | | | | |
| | | | | | | | Balance: | 8.95 | | | 88.90 | |
| 1257 | Natel, Gloria | (404) 555-1234 | | | | | | | | | | |
| | Natel, Gl | Dr. Good | 09/02/08 | 99214 | V22.2 | 01/03/09 | 11/22/08 | | | | 4.00 | |
| | Natel, Gl | Dr. Good | 09/02/08 | 81000 | V22.2 | 01/03/09 | 11/22/08 | | | | 2.80 | |
| | Natel, Gl | Dr. Good | 09/02/08 | 85014 | V22.2 | 01/03/09 | 11/22/08 | | | | 1.80 | |
| | Natel, Gl | Dr. Good | 10/18/08 | 99211 | V22.2 | 01/03/09 | 12/01/08 | | | | 2.50 | |
| | Natel, Gl | Dr. Good | 11/30/08 | 99211 | V22.2 | 01/03/09 | 12/01/08 | | | | 2.50 | |
| | Natel, Gl | Dr. Good | 12/02/08 | 99212 | V22.2 | 01/03/09 | 12/02/08 | | | | 4.00 | |
| | Natel, Gl | Dr. Good | 01/03/09 | 99215 | V22.2 | 02/01/09 | 01/03/09 | | | 10.00 | | |
| | Natel, Gl | Dr. Good | 01/03/09 | 81000 | V22.2 | 02/01/09 | 01/03/09 | | | 7.60 | | |
| | Natel, Gl | Dr. Good | 01/03/09 | 85014 | V22.2 | 02/01/09 | 01/03/09 | | | 3.60 | | |
| | | | | | | | Balance: | | | 21.20 | 17.60 | |
| 1938 | Baker, Harold | (404) 555-6354 | | | | | | | | | | |
| | Baker, Ha | Dr. Smith | 11/10/08 | 99212 | 460 | 01/03/09 | 11/10/08 | | | | 20.00 | |
| | Baker, Ke | Dr. Smith | 02/27/09 | 99212 | 461.1 | 04/04/09 | 03/07/09 | 20.00 | | | | |
| | Baker, Ke | Dr. Green | 04/15/09 | 90642 | 783.2 | 04/15/09 | | 28.50 | | | | |
| | | | | | | | Balance: | 48.50 | | | 20.00 | |

**FIGURE 12-4  Detailed aging report.**

due 31 to 60 days, items due 61 to 90 days, items due 91 to 120 days, items due 121 to 150 days, and items due more than 151 days.

In this example, patient-due items are aged from the date the patient became responsible. For patients with health insurance, that is the date the payment from the insurance plan was posted and a balance was due from the patient.

On the next line, the insurance-due items are aged in the same aging categories, but the items are aged from the date the insurance claim was generated.

The totals of the patient-due and insurance-due amounts are given under each category. Then at the bottom of the report, the total A/R and the percentage of the receivables due by responsible party is listed.

Detailed aging reports are used to analyze or work on specific problem areas. Reports can typically be limited to patient-due or insurance-due responsibilities, and filtered to report only items that are within a certain range of days overdue. The example in Figure 12-4 shows procedure and diagnosis code details for every item on the report. Such detail is useful when attempting to collect overdue payments.

**NON-CARE-RELATED A/R**    Healthcare organizations may also have revenue or accounts receivable that is not related to patient care. For example, consider a medical group that owns its building and rents a suite to another doctor's practice, or a hospital that owns a subsidiary transcription service and receives payments from doctors. The patient accounting system is not used for these types of transactions. If there are very few of them, they may be posted directly into the general accounting system or another A/R system may be used.

## Purchasing

Although it is important for providers to track and collect the money they are owed, it is equally important for them to contain costs. One of the ways they do that is through computerized *purchasing* systems.

Purchasing systems are used to order supplies, drugs, and equipment. They keep records of vendors, part numbers, prices, purchase orders, and the amount each department spends. They can track the historical prices the facility has previously paid and the current prices for multiple vendors.

Large hospitals may have more than one purchasing system. The pharmacy, in particular, may order separately through a pharmacy ordering system especially suited to ordering drugs. Certain other departments may also order independently, though ultimately all purchases must go through the central purchasing department system to be assigned a purchase order number.

A *purchase order* is a vendor's assurance that the order is authorized and will be paid by the facility. It is also the control system by which the accounting department knows how much is being spent, by whom, and how much the business will ultimately owe.

When the ordered items arrive, they are compared to the purchase order to verify that the correct items and quantities have been received. When the vendor's invoice arrives, it is matched to the purchase order to verify that the costs quoted on the order match what the vendor charged. The invoice is then sent to the accounts payable system to be paid.

## Accounts Payable

*Accounts payable* systems manage the disbursement of payments for purchases the facility has authorized. They may also be used to manage payments for recurring expenses such as rent, utilities, and insurance and for nonrecurring expenses such as maintenance or repairs.

Accounts payable systems control the outflow of money for expenses (except payroll). They are used to print checks or authorize electronic funds transfers (EFTs) to pay bills and invoices.

Accounts payable reports include not only payments that have been made, but also outstanding purchase orders and forecasts of upcoming disbursements for which funds have already been committed.

## Inventory and Materials Management

All types of healthcare facilities must keep enough supplies on hand to treat patients without overstocking. When quantities on hand are too little, a doctor or nurse may not have a necessary item or drug. When quantities on hand are too large, too much of a healthcare organization's capital may be tied up unnecessarily.

*Inventory and materials management* systems work in conjunction with purchasing systems. Inventory control involves deducting from the quantity on hand supplies that are used, and adding to the system the quantity received as purchase orders are filled.

In addition to tracking the quantity on hand, inventory systems track quantities on order to prevent duplicate purchases. Users can also set minimum and maximum quantity thresholds. These can be used to generate alerts so that supplies can be reordered before they run out. Maximum quantity thresholds can be used to identify items that are overstocked. Inventory systems can also indicate the quantity to reorder.

Inventory can be tracked across multiple locations or facilities. If, for example, a healthcare organization operates multiple clinics, the quantity on hand can be tracked at each clinic. This allows an overstock of supplies at one facility to be transferred to another facility rather than making a new purchase.

Hospitals may have inventory modules within the departmental software; for example, a hospital pharmacy might maintain drug inventory through the pharmacy system instead of the inventory system used by other departments.

Inventory data is not only used for monitoring and reordering supplies; it is also useful for measuring historical usage and predicting future needs. If, for example, a hospital uses 50,000 pairs of latex gloves per year, they may realize savings by purchasing in larger quantities.

## Payroll

*Payroll* is distinctly separate from accounts payable. Payroll has two major aspects, *payroll administration* and *payroll accounting*.

Payroll administration deals with the managerial aspects of maintaining a payroll, including these tasks:

- Managing employee personnel and payroll information.
- Complying with federal, state, and local employment laws.
- Generating reports payroll activities.
- Keeping records. Federal and state laws require that employers keep certain payroll records for specified periods of time. For example, the IRS W-4 form (on which employees indicate their tax withholding status) must be kept on file for all active employees and for four years after an employee is terminated.

Payroll accounting consists of these tasks:

- Determining which federal, state, and local tax coverage rules apply to each employee.
- Computing an employee's taxable wages.
- Calculating the amount of employment taxes to be withheld and paid by the employer.
- Depositing the correct amount of employment taxes with the government agencies.
- Filing employment tax returns.
- Calculating and withholding other amounts such as 401(k), 529 medical savings, and the employee's share of health, dental, and vision insurance.
- Printing and distributing paychecks and/or generating direct deposits.
- Printing and distributing W-2 forms to employees and 1099 forms to contract workers at the end of each year.

Because of its complexity, payroll accounting for hospitals and medical practices is often performed by an outside company such as ADP, Paychex, or the medical group's accountant. The healthcare organization must still perform the administrative functions of obtaining W-4 forms and managing employee information.

## Budgeting

A *budget* is an organization's principal tool for financial planning. Budgets typically forecast revenue and expenses for the next fiscal year. Often budgets are based on analysis of historical data, which is then adjusted for inflation. For example, data from the inventory and accounts payable system allow managers to measure the quantity of supplies used in previous years, adjust the costs to allow for price increases, and estimate the dollars that will be necessary to provide the same level of service in the coming year.

Similarly, payroll data can be analyzed to determine how many and what type of full-time equivalent employee (FTE) hours were used. The number of FTEs at various pay grades can be multiplied by wage and benefit costs to predict labor costs for the coming year.

Finally, planned expansions or new services that can potentially increase costs or increase revenues can be factored into a budget. For example, if a hospital is opening a new cardiac wing or a group medical practice has entered into an HMO contract that guarantees fixed payments for a year, a budget allows managers to anticipate revenue and expenses associated with those situations.

For hospitals, budgeting typically begins at the departmental level, with each manager or department head preparing a list of goals for the coming year and estimating the costs of achieving those goals. These are then evaluated and included in the overall budget by the CFO.

### Cost Accounting

One managerial tool useful for budgeting is *cost accounting*. At a departmental level, the costs of supplies, materials, and labor directly used are attributed to the department by the hospital's accounting system. These are direct costs. To this, indirect costs or overhead, such as rent, insurance, utilities, managers' salaries, and so on, are added.

The items we have discussed so far make up the operating budget for one year. Healthcare organizations also have a capital budget, which covers items whose value extends beyond one year, for example, the purchase of a multimillion dollar MRI system, or a building program for creating an addition to the facility.

Once the budget is completed and reviewed, it is then presented to senior management and finally to the board of directors for approval.

# Human Resources Management Systems

In healthcare, 60 to 70 percent of the budget consists of personnel costs. Human resource managers use computers to maintain personnel records and to create management reports that track staff productivity, absenteeism, and vacation time; monitor turnover rate; and analyze labor expenses.

### Evaluations

Employee retention, promotions, and incentives are based on employee performance evaluations by managers and self-assessments by employees. Increasingly, human resource departments are using online forms and tools to conduct and manage employee evaluations and annual reviews.

### Training

Healthcare employers must train employees in procedures, policies, security, and a vast array of skills ranging from using the EHR to using a point-of-care testing device. Accreditation by the Joint Commission and CAP requires employee training and certification. Employee attendance and completion of training programs can now be tracked by computer.

### Education and Continuing Education

Virtually all care providers must hold qualified degrees for their field and must be licensed by state regulatory agencies. In addition, care providers must complete a required number of hours of continuing education each year. In healthcare, human resource departments track the credentials and licenses of all employees who work with patients.

### Employee Health

The unique environment of healthcare requires regular tuberculosis (TB) tests for all employees. Employee health records track immunizations and tests and generate reminders to employees (typically a month before they need to be retested or have another vaccine). The human resources department as well as the quality management and legal departments track and monitor the occurrence of on-the-job injuries and subsequent workers' compensation claims.

# Scheduling Systems

Another type of administrative system is scheduling systems. Scheduling systems allow for the orderly examination and treatment of patients. They are found at the departmental level, where patients are scheduled for diagnostic testing, therapy, or surgery. They are also found at the facility level, such as the patient appointment schedule for a group medical practice.

Essentially appointment systems have these fields in common:

- Patient
- Provider
- Scheduled start time
- Reason
- Estimated time it will take.

Additional factors are involved in different types of schedules. For example:

- Surgery departments maintain their own schedules for operating rooms. Surgery scheduling must factor in preparation and transport of the patient (preop), surgery, and recovery (postop). Time must also be allotted between surgeries for the operating room to be cleaned and sterilized.
- Home nursing visit schedules must allow for travel time between patients' homes.
- Physician office schedules often overlap patient appointments, relying on the fact that a nurse or medical assistant will attend to patients before the doctor sees them.

Scheduling systems not only provide an order to the flow of patients, but the scheduling system data can be studied to identify bottlenecks, improve workflow, and add efficiencies to the department or medical practice. The volume and type of patients scheduled can also be used to predict labor and resource needs. Busy medical group practices and hospitals with multiple outpatient clinics often have several employees dedicated to scheduling patient visits, tests, and procedures.

**SCHEDULING PATIENTS**    Medical schedules are not blank calendars. Schedule templates are used to show the user the type and length of appointments that should be scheduled (see Figure 12-5). Empty appointment slots are preset for number of minutes and/or certain types of appointments. Appointment reason codes are used to record why patients are coming. The use of reason codes not only make it faster for the staff to schedule the appointment, but also can determine the number of minutes required for the appointment based on reason for the appointment.

The job of scheduling appointments is an important one. The allied health professional who performs this job is often the first contact the patient has with the medical practice or clinic. A pleasant demeanor, an understanding of the providers' scheduling wishes, and the ability to work under pressure are required. The scheduling person often does a minimum amount of triage to determine the reason for the appointment and the urgency. The scheduler must also be familiar with and communicate to the patient the requirements for certain types of

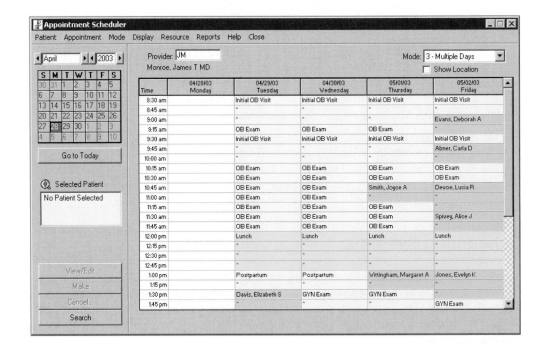

appointments. For example, an MRI cannot be scheduled for patients with pacemakers or metal in their bodies. The scheduling person must be aware of this and question the patient before scheduling the appointment.

Inpatient scheduling is slightly different. A schedule coordinator may handle several different departments. When a physician orders a test that requires moving patients to another department, the coordinator schedules a time for the test and arranges for someone to transport patients from their room to the test and back.

Another type of scheduling is more event oriented rather than time oriented. It may be thought of as task management scheduling. For example, patients who are not being sent home may be discharged to a SNF or rehabilitation hospital. In such a case, the scheduler must arrange with the SNF for the transfer, coordinate the medical transportation, and, finally, confirm that the patient has arrived at the intended facility.

**STAFF SCHEDULING**  A completely different type of schedule is used to manage employees and providers. Because hospitals are open 24 hours a day, it is necessary to have sufficient personnel working at all times. Employees are scheduled to work in shifts and may rotate days of the week they work. For example, some RNs work four consecutive days, then have four days off. The human resources department also tracks and manages vacation schedules, employee sick days, and holidays.

Similarly, group medical practices must block a physician's schedules so that patients are not scheduled on days when the doctor is away. They also must designate another physician to see that doctor's patients while he or she is away. This doctor is called the *covering* physician. Doctors must also be available during off hours if needed. This is known as being "on call." Usually doctors in a group practice take turns being on call. The office manager or office administrator maintains the on-call schedule, keeping track of which doctor is on call each day and ensuring that there is a fair distribution of on-call days among the doctors on the schedule.

# Facility and Equipment Maintenance Systems

A number of administrative systems are used to maintain facilities and equipment. These include systems to track requests for repairs and upgrades to the building, rooms, or various departments. Automated systems are used to control heat, air, and energy usage. Repair orders for systems that require outside service, such as large refrigeration units, are tracked and reported to purchasing and account payable similar to the process used for materials purchases.

Biomedical, surgical, radiological, laboratory, and other medical equipment must be serviced and tested regularly. Maintenance records must be maintained for Joint Commission and CAP audits and regulatory agencies. These testing and maintenance records are usually the responsibility of the respective departments and may be a function of the departmental software system; for example, the laboratory information system described in Chapter 8.

Fire control and facility security systems are also almost entirely computerized as are employee tracking and timekeeping systems.

# Quality Management Systems

Quality management (QM) covers a number of different areas related to the operation of the hospital and the care provided to patients. The main product of quality management is data and reports used for risk analysis and decision support, by which the appropriateness and effectiveness of medical care are evaluated. These include case management, utilization management, physician peer review, NHQM data, incident reports, and hospital mortality and autopsies. Quality management systems not only track and maintain data entered by the QM department, but also use and analyze data abstracted from patient health records and other departmental systems.

Quality management can be used to identify indications for intervention, assess functionality after intervention, analyze undesirable outcomes of treatment, and identify opportunities for improvement. Quality management can also be used by providers to uncover opportunities for improvement and for monitoring their progress over time.

Quality management frequently targets specific areas of concern. For example, surgical complications, transfusions, critical care, obstetrics, or neonatal care are areas that expose the hospital to particular risk. Figure 12-6 shows a quality management screen for a patient who had a cardiac arrest following knee surgery.

## Case Management

Case management systems begin by documenting the patient assessment and utilization management. The case manager identifies appropriate levels of care and considers alternative therapies and resource usage. Utilization management evaluates the case using standard criteria and seeks authorization from the payer. Case management tracks certification, authorization, and concurrent

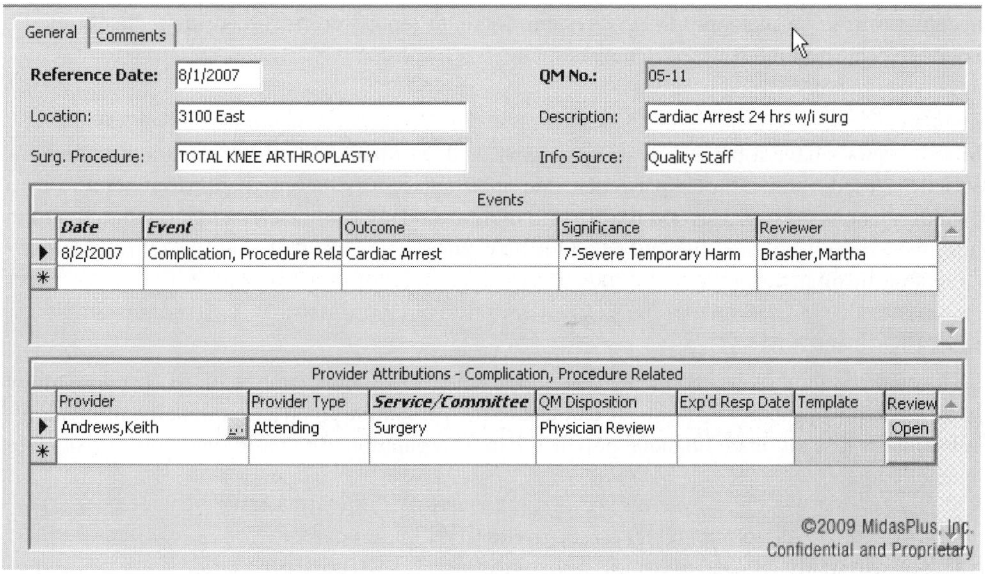

**FIGURE 12-6**

**MIDAS+ quality management screen.**

(Courtesy of MidasPlus, Inc.)

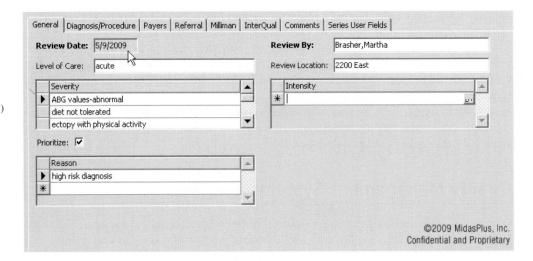

review of the case. It also tracks avoidable days, denials, and appeals. A case management concurrent review is shown in Figure 12-7.

A standard tool is the Interqual® criteria tool, which addresses admissions, continued stay, and discharge planning with evidence-based criteria that is used and accepted by CMS and third-party payers. Other criteria standards include the Medical Care Appropriateness Protocol (MCAP) and the Millman® guidelines used by managed care plans.

### Infection Control

Infections are tracked and reported by QM. These include patients admitted with communicable diseases, hospital-acquired infections, and diagnoses that must be reported to the CDC.

### Incident Tracking

Incident reports are entered for both patient and nonpatient incidents. Examples of patient incidents include medication errors, slips or falls, surgical mistakes, or adverse results. Examples of nonpatient incidents include slip or falls by visitors, volunteers, or employees; accidental exposure to toxic or medical waste; and security problems in or around the facility. In Figure 12-8 the incident of a patient falling from bed is recorded.

Incidents that can result in financial loss or lead to litigation are called *potentially compensable events* (PCEs). Incident reports are always filed and maintained separately from the patient health record in an incident tracking system. Incident reports are recorded immediately by the employees most familiar with the incident.

### Patient Relations

Most hospitals have a patient relations person or department. Whether the patient complains about the food, the care, or a particular doctor or nurse, it is recorded and responded to by a patient relations person. The QM department reviews and analyzes each patient relation report to improve care and patient satisfaction and identify patterns or cases that could present a risk to the patient or hospital.

### Risk Management

Risk can be thought of as any incident or circumstance that might result in a loss. The loss might be to a person's property or rights or damage to the person physically, emotionally, or mentally. A hospital's loss might be financial or damage to its reputation. The basic functions of risk management are:

- Risk identification
- Risk analysis

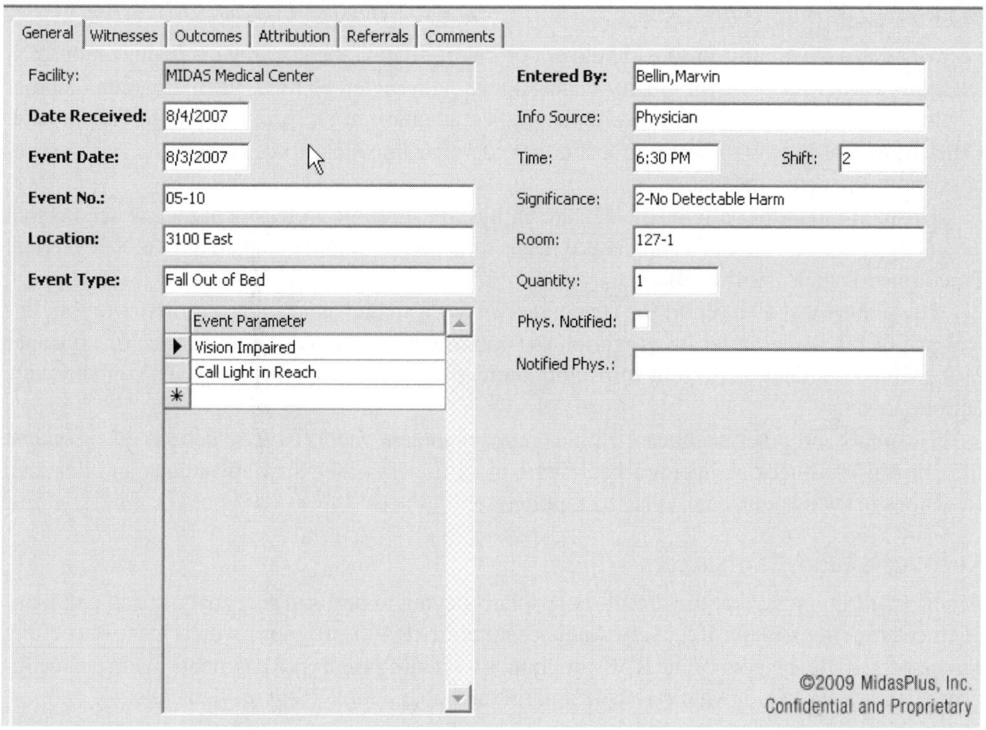

**FIGURE 12-8**

**MIDAS+ risk management screen records a patient fall.**

(Courtesy of MidasPlus, Inc.)

- Loss prevention or reduction
- Claims management.

Risk assessment involves analyzing processes and measuring statistical data with the goal of identifying preventable losses and minimizing their occurrences. One example, discussed in Chapter 3, involves risk assessment of computer security to minimize security risks to EPHI data. In the example of PCE, incident reports are assessed to determine the healthcare organization's liability for the occurrence.

The goal of risk management programs is to minimize loss by reducing risk through preventive policies and measures. For example, the policy of immediately filing incident reports allows management to conduct an immediate investigation of facts surrounding the incident. These facts can significantly improve the legal department's ability to defend the case should it be necessary to do so.

Risk management also provides the organization with the information needed to proactively improve performance and processes and provide a safer environment for employees, patients, volunteers, and visitors.

**CLAIMS MANAGEMENT**    Claims management does not refer to the third-party payer claims for reimbursement discussed in Chapters 9 and 10, but rather to claims against the healthcare organization for incidents, occurrences, or malpractice. It is the legal and administrative management of injury claims against the organization. Claims management usually involves the following steps:

- Reporting of claims to the risk manager, upper management, and the facility's insurance company
- Initial investigation of claims
- Sequestering of primary and secondary health records
- Negotiation of settlement of claims out of court
- Management of litigation (if settlement was not reached)
- Use of case outcomes for performance improvement or to create policies to prevent or reduce future risk.

## Peer Review

Peer review in the context of QM should not be confused with the peer review organizations discussed in earlier chapters. In quality management, peer review is used when a patient, another employee, or an audit of health records has called attention to an issue relevant to patient care. Other providers review the case, procedures, orders, or treatment to determine the appropriateness and make recommendations.

Hospitals and other eligible healthcare entities must report professional review actions that adversely affect a physician's clinical privileges for a period of more than 30 days to the National Practitioner Data Bank (NPDB).[1]

Hospitals must also report the acceptance of a physician's surrender or restriction of clinical privileges while under investigation for possible professional incompetence or improper professional conduct, or in return for not conducting an investigation or professional review action.

Hospitals and other healthcare entities may voluntarily report adverse actions taken against the clinical privileges of licensed healthcare practitioners other than physicians and dentists. Revisions to such actions must also be reported.

## Recovery Audit Contractors

A new CMS initiative that may result in hospitals having to perform risk analysis and risk management functions is the Recovery Audit Contractor (RAC) program, which went into effect January 1, 2010. The goal of the RAC program is to identify improper payments made on healthcare claims provided for Medicare beneficiaries and obtain repayment to Medicare.

Healthcare providers may receive either a request for medical records or a letter requesting that an overpayment be repaid for claims that were submitted to and paid for by Medicare. Healthcare providers subject to review under the RAC program include hospitals, physician practices, nursing homes, home health agencies, durable medical equipment suppliers, and any other provider or supplier that bills Medicare Parts A and B.

A key difference between the RAC program and earlier efforts by CMS to audit claims is that the recovery audit contractors are private companies, paid a percentage of what they recover; therefore, they have a stronger incentive to identify and recoup overpayments. This makes the risk of financial loss to the hospital or provider more substantial.

In forming a RAC risk management strategy, a hospital might consider taking these steps:

- Establish a committee to handle RAC issues.
- Set up a procedure or computer system to track RAC requests and ensure they are handled within the timelines permitted.
- Conduct an internal assessment to ensure that submitted claims meet the Medicare rules.
- Prepare and provision the HIM department to comply with RAC requests.
- Create policies and procedures for deciding which RAC denials to appeal.

Although the RAC program appears promising in terms of saving CMS money by recouping unnecessary overpayments, it can also create a burden on HIM departments and even the finances of the healthcare organizations. The best strategy for dealing with RAC requests is to ensure that claims are as accurate as possible when first submitted and that requests from the recovery audit contractor are handled efficiently, effectively, and according to procedures and policies that have been put in place well ahead of the RAC requests.

## Comparative Performance Measure Systems

Quality management also involves comparing performance measures to those of other similar facilities. In addition to the NHQM and CMI information available from Medicare, hospitals can also download data from vendors who contractually provide this service to hospitals. By using

---

[1] *Fact Sheet on the National Practitioner Data Bank*, NPDB-00921.04.00 (Washington, DC: U.S. Department of Health and Human Services, July 2008).

## Functions of a Quality Management Department

*By Jayme Stewart*

*Jayme Stewart works in the Department of Quality Management for a large hospital in the Midwest.*

Our quality management department serves decision support, handles our physician peer review process, and performs chart abstraction for core process and hospital quality measures. We use two software systems, MIDAS+ and Premier Clinical Advisor.

Case management electronically documents the patient assessment in MIDAS+; that is, the demographic, social, and psychological patient information. They do the utilization review using an interface we have to Interqual to determine if the patient meets the criteria to be in the hospital. We can then fax directly from MIDAS+ to most of our payers.

Case management also does a chart audit; they monitor case managers to see if they are fulfilling the requirements of the assessment. They also enter discharge planning information. We are then able to run a lot of utilization-type reports out of MIDAS+.

We use another module of the system for physician peer review. When there is an issue about a physician, it is entered into MIDAS+. We then can track where it is in the process; for example, if it goes to the chief of the department for review and then goes back to the physician in question for comment.

Preparing Joint Commission core process measures is one of the functions of our department. For accreditation, we are required to collect data on high-volume conditions or procedures and submit that data. From this we calculate our compliance. Collecting the data involves a significant amount of chart abstraction. We have nurses perform that function because much of the clinical information in a chart is interpretive. They enter the data in MIDAS+.

We can compare our core measure data with national and state performance measure data. We also report it to CMS, because you receive a 2 percent reduction in your payments if you don't. On the other hand, our Blue Cross Blue Shield plan has incentives that link to their pay-for-performance program. If we meet their performance thresholds, we actually receive an incentive.

We also use a comparative performance measure system from our vendor that has about 150 different statistics that benchmark us with other MIDAS+ clients. We can look at it by teaching/nonteaching hospital, by bed size, by region, or nationally. We take a lot of indicators from the system to report on our hospital-wide balance scorecard. We report our hospital-wide mortality rate, admission rate, and other things using our data and the benchmarks from them.

Risk management and patient relations use MIDAS+ as well. All types of risk management events are entered in the MIDAS+ system. Events include medication errors, assessment errors, patient falls, hazardous spills, safety issues, and security issues. We have an online application that allows any employee in the hospital to enter reportable events.

We have a reporting mechanism with hospital-wide distribution set up, so that if a manager's department is involved in one of the reports they receive automatic notifications via e-mail.

Claims management uses MIDAS+ as well; our attorneys document any potential claims through the point where the risk of a claim or the claim itself is resolved.

As I mentioned, Patient Relations also uses MIDAS+. We enter both complaints and compliments in the patient relations module. We also enter any HIPAA complaints there so that our HIPAA compliance officer can track data in the system.

Other data our department tracks includes infection control data, employee vaccinations, TB tests, committee-specific studies, and employee injuries. Our workers' compensation department uses it; also, any report that state or federal OSHA laws require us to generate comes right out. We also track mortality, autopsies, cardiac arrests, and conscious sedations.

We use Premier Clinical Advisor in addition to MIDAS+. It is a severity adjustment clinical benchmarking system. It uses the 3M AP-DRGs (all-patient diagnosis-related groups). It allows us to compare our data with that of other hospitals in their database by disease. So we can compare, for instance, pneumonia length of stay, complications, readmissions, or mortality rates for hospitals our size. They also have best performers criteria that allow us to do physician profiling using the severity adjusted data. From that data you can support why a physician has a higher length of stay or higher mortality rate. Severity adjustment adjusts for risk factors and severity of illness.

We are also able to analyze utilization information out of the system to compare utilization to different peer groups. For example, if we had a stroke patient who had CAT scans every day, but the best performers only have two CAT scans per stay and the evidence shows that is effective, then that can impact utilization.

We also utilize a decision support system for clinical cost accounting. With it we analyze financial information, billing data, and utilization information, such as the length of stay for a specific patient population and cases by attending physician.

QM involves a lot of process analysis, trying to determine how to make things more efficient and how to bring systems into that. My recommendation for students interested in QM is to develop analytical and auditing skills; accounting is very helpful in terms of developing that knowledge. Classes such as applied managerial statistics, performance improvement techniques, and, of course, medical terminology and information systems are helpful.

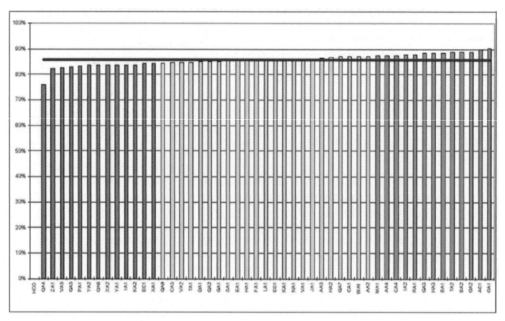

**FIGURE 12-9**  **High scores on hospital quality measures.**

performance data from similar size institutions, hospitals can benchmark themselves against the best performers.

Figure 12-9 shows an example of a facility performance report based on the quality indicators discussed in Chapter 11. The hospital's quality improvement measures are compared to other similar hospitals to generate the comparative report.

# Chapter 12 Summary

## Information Systems for Managerial Support

In addition to HIM and EHR systems, other types of information systems are vital to the management and operation of healthcare facilities. These systems provide managerial support and are the basis for operational, strategic, and executive decisions.

Practice management systems have separate functional modules that are *integrated;* that is, they share a common database and are produced by the same vendor. Hospital systems are often *interfaced;* that is, the systems use disparate systems from different vendors with separate databases. These systems exchange data using HL7 or proprietary transactions.

## Administrative Systems

Administrative systems include financial, human resource, scheduling, and quality management systems.

## Financial Information Systems

Financial accounting systems in healthcare typically consist of the following:

- An overall accounting system called the general ledger is used to produce financial statements and monitor the overall financial health of the organization.

A standard accounting practice called the double-entry method divides the GL into four categories: income, expenses, assets, and liabilities. Income and expenses are reported on an income statement or profit and loss statement. Assets and liabilities are reported on a balance sheet or statement of financial position.

- Accounts receivable is the money that is owed to the business.
- Purchasing systems are used to order supplies and services.
- Accounts payable is the money the business owes to its suppliers and others.
- Inventory is material goods and supplies that have been purchased.
- Payroll deals with the administration of employee payroll information and the payment of wages, employer taxes, and employee benefits.
- Budgeting is used to predict expected income and expenses, usually for one year.
- Cost accounting is used to attribute direct and indirect costs to various departments.

## Human Resources Management Systems

Human resource systems maintain personnel records, employee evaluations, and records of training and continuing education credits, employee immunizations, TB tests, and work-related health issues.

## Scheduling Systems

Several different types of scheduling systems are used in healthcare:

- Outpatient scheduling allows for the orderly examination and treatment of patients. Patient scheduling involves making appointments for a length of time appropriate to the reason the patient has scheduled an appointment.
- Inpatient scheduling consists of processing doctors' orders for tests or services, coordinating with the respective department, and arranging for an orderly or other assistant to transport patients from their rooms to the department and back.
- Employee scheduling systems are used to schedule which employees are working at what time each day.
- Vacation and leave schedules are used by human resources and department managers to know when employees will be gone so that others can be scheduled to perform their duties.
- Provider scheduling in a medical practice includes blocking the doctor's appointment schedule for times they will not be in the office and arranging for another doctor to "cover" their patients. Doctors must also be available after hours. Physicians in group practices take turns being "on call." The practice administrator maintains the on-call schedule.
- Surgery scheduling must factor in preparation and transport of the patient (preop), surgery, and recovery (postop). Time must also be allotted between surgeries for the operating room to be cleaned and sterilized.

## Facility and Equipment Maintenance Systems

Facility and equipment management systems are used to operate various aspects of the facility, such as air conditioning, energy usage, fire control, and security. Other systems track the repair and maintenance of rooms, equipment, and the grounds.

## Quality Management Systems

The main product of quality management is the data and reports used for risk analysis and decision support. Quality management can be used to identify indications for intervention, assess functionality after intervention, analyze undesirable outcomes of treatment, and identify opportunities for improvement. Quality management can also be used by providers to uncover opportunities for improvement and for monitoring their progress over time.

Quality management systems cover a number of different areas related to the operation of the hospital and the care provided to patients. These include:

- Case management and utilization management
- Infection control
- Incident tracking
- Patient relations
- Risk management
- Peer review
- Comparative performance measures.

The basic functions of risk management are:

- Risk identification
- Risk analysis
- Loss prevention or reduction
- Claims management

The basic steps of claims management are:

- Reporting of claims to the risk manager, upper management, and the facility's insurance company
- Initial investigation of claims
- Sequestering of primary and secondary health records
- Negotiation of settlement of claims out of court
- Management of litigation (if settlement was not reached)
- Use of case outcomes for performance improvement or to create policies to prevent or reduce future risk

# Critical Thinking Exercises

A hospital risk management department has received an incident report that a visitor slipped on ice in the hospital parking lot and was injured.

1. Is this a PCE?
2. What steps should be taken immediately?
3. What structures and processes in the facility should be examined?
4. What improvements should be made to prevent such accidents in the future?
5. What changes should be made to limit liability for similar events in the future?

# Testing Your Knowledge of Chapter 12

1. Explain the difference between interfaced and integrated systems.

2. What general ledger report discussed in this chapter shows income and expenses?

3. Describe the purpose of an aging report.

4. Which of the financial systems is used to track a purchase order?

5. Name three types of information tracked by human resource systems.

6. Patient scheduling systems have at least five data elements in common; what are they?

7. What does the acronym PCE stand for?

8. Name four basic functions of risk management.

9. Name at least three types of reportable incidents.

10. What department abstracts and reports National Hospital Quality Measures?

11. What is the term for a doctor who must answer calls after hours?

12. Administrative systems do not contain PHI.

    *True      False*

13. What is a GL asset?

14. What is a GL liability?

15. How long must a hospital retain copies of the W-4 form?

# Comprehensive Evaluation of Chapters 9-12

This comprehensive evaluation will enable you and your instructor to determine your understanding of the material covered so far.

1. Which Medicare plan pays for professional services?
   a. Part A
   b. Part B
   c. Part C
   d. Part D

2. In which HMO model are the doctors employed by the insurance plan?
   a. group model
   b. staff model
   c. EMC model
   d. IDN model

3. RBRVS is used for determining:
   a. length of stay
   b. central tendency
   c. payment schedule
   d. capitation

4. What does comorbidity mean?
   a. the patient died
   b. the patient developed an infection after being admitted
   c. the patient developed a complication
   d. the patient had more than one condition when admitted

5. What is a standard method of calculating PCP capitation payments?
   a. per patient treated
   b. per diem
   c. per member per month
   d. none of the above

6. A participating provider charges $80.00, but the Medicare allowed amount is $70.00. What is the amount of the write-down adjustment?
   a. $80.00
   b. 80 percent
   c. 10 percent
   d. $10.00

7. Which of the following hospital types is exempt from IPPS?
   a. children's hospitals
   b. cancer hospitals
   c. critical access hospitals
   d. all of the above

8. Which central tendency value is the midpoint in a group of ranked values that divides the data into two equal parts?
   a. mean
   b. mode
   c. median
   d. none of the above

9. Which paper form was designed for institutional claims?
   a. Part A
   b. UB-04
   c. CMS-1500
   d. W-4

10. Which of the following EDI transactions is **not** required by HIPAA?
   a. remittance advice
   b. report of first injury
   c. consent
   d. eligibility

11. Which number identifies the provider on a claim?
   a. NPI
   b. group number
   c. member number
   d. PSI

12. What is the common name for acute myocardial infarction (AMI)?
   a. pink eye
   b. pulmonary embolism
   c. stroke
   d. heart attack

13. What code set is used to determine the case mix index?
   a. ABC
   b. CPT-4
   c. DRG
   d. SNOMED

14. What type of statistic can be used to compare two different things?
    a. rate
    b. ratio
    c. mean
    d. median

15. Twenty AMI patients who smoked were counseled against smoking, 10 were not. What is the ratio of AMI smokers who were counseled to those who were not?
    a. 10 percent
    b. 30:1
    c. 20:1
    d. 2:1

16. What is a standard formula for calculating proportion?
    a. $x/(x + y)$
    b. $x/y$
    c. $x^2/y$
    d. none of the above

*Write the full name represented by each of the following acronyms:*

17. EOB _____

18. DRG _____

19. PCE _____

20. FTE _____

21. EMC _____

22. What is meant by payment floor?
    a. the minimum amount a plan will pay
    b. the maximum amount a plan will pay
    c. the delay before a plan will pay
    d. the last date a provider can file a claim

23. Software systems that share a common database are:
    a. interfaced
    b. integrated
    c. indexed
    d. regulated

24. What department abstracts and reports National Hospital Quality Measures?
    a. billing department
    b. utilization management
    c. quality management
    d. utility department

25. A general ledger is used to report income and expenses.
    T. true
    F. false

26. Aging reports are used to determine immunization schedules.
    T. true
    F. false

27. Fibrinolytic therapy should be used for appropriate AMI patients within 30 minutes of arrival at the hospital.
    T. true
    F. false

28. Medicare pays most types of inpatient hospitals using IPPS.
    T. true
    F. false

29. The first step in preparing a claim is to calculate the DRG.
    T. true
    F. false

30. You should use ICD-10 to code insurance claims.
    T. true
    F. false

**ABC**  Acronym for alternative billing codes, which are used to bill for alternative medicine such as acupuncture, behavioral health, and homeopathy.

**ABN**  Acronym for Advance Beneficiary Notice, a form that provides information in advance to the patient that a particular test or procedure will not be covered by Medicare or insurance. The same acronym is sometimes uses as the abbreviation for abnormal.

**Abstracting**  Creating a brief summary of a document, or the process of extracting elements of a source document for data entry such as a patient's condition, illness, treatments, and outcome.

**Access control (HIPAA)**  Technical policies and procedures to allow access only to those persons or software programs that have been granted rights to access EPHI.

**Accession number**  A unique number assigned to a lab test, radiology study, or a case in a cancer registry.

**Accreditation**  An acknowledgment by a recognized authority that a person or institution complies with applicable standards such as the Joint Commission, CARF, or CAP.

**ACE inhibitors**  A drug used for people who have had heart attacks or heart failure to block production of a hormone that constricts the blood vessels.

**ACEI**  Acronym for angiotensin converting enzyme inhibitor.

**Acute**  Severe, but of short duration.

**Acute self-limiting**  Problems that normally resolve themselves over a short period of time.

**Administrative safeguards (HIPAA)**  Administrative functions that should be implemented to meet the standards of the HIPAA Security Rule. These include assigning security responsibility to an individual and security training requirements.

**Administrative Simplification (HIPAA)**  The Administrative Simplification Subsection of HIPAA covers providers, health plans, and clearinghouses. It has four distinct components: Transactions and Code Sets, Uniform Identifiers, Privacy, and Security.

**ADT**  Acronym for "admission, discharge, and transfer," a component of hospital information systems usually related to patient registration or a transaction between a departmental system and the registration computer system.

**Aggregate data**  Data that is the summation of other data records matching certain criteria.

**AHIMA**  Acronym for American Health Information Management Association, the leading organization for HIM

professionals and a trusted source for education, research, and professional credentialing.

**AHRQ**  Acronym for Agency for Healthcare Research and Quality, a Public Health Service agency in the U.S. Department of Health and Human Services. This agency supports research designed to improve the quality, safety, efficiency, and effectiveness of healthcare for all Americans.

**AIS**  Acronym for Abbreviated Injury Scale, an anatomical scoring system that provides a reasonably accurate way of ranking the severity of injury using a scale of 1 to 6, with 1 being minor, 5 severe, and 6 an unsurvivable injury.

**Alert**  A warning, message, or reminder automatically generated by EHR systems based on logical rules.

**Algorithm**  A series of logical steps used to process data to consistently arrive at the desired result.

**Allowed amount**  An amount for a medical service that the provider has contractually agreed to accept from an insurance plan. It is usually less than the provider's normal fee.

**ALOS**  Acronym for average length of stay. The sum of the length of stay for all patients discharged in a given period, divided by the number of patients discharged.

**Alphanumeric**  A field type permitting both letters and numbers; a filing system in which chart numbers are a combination of a few letters of the patient's surname followed by a unique number.

**AMA**  Acronym for American Medical Association when referring to the national nonprofit organization of doctors. Acronym for against medical advice, when used in a chart. It means a patient chooses to be discharged against the advice of the medical staff.

**Ambulatory**  A healthcare treatment or facility that does not involve an overnight stay; often used interchangeably with the term *outpatient*.

**AMI**  Acronym for acute myocardial infarction. Commonly referred to as a heart attack, an AMI is a life-threatening condition that occurs when blood flow to the heart is stopped. The lack of blood and oxygen causes the heart to die.

**Angina pectoris**  A disease marked by brief, recurrent pain, usually in the chest and left arm, caused by a sudden decrease of the blood supply to the heart muscle.

**Angiogram, angiography**  An x-ray (roentgenogram) of the flow of blood after injecting a contrast material.

**ANSI**  Acronym for American National Standards Institute, a private, nonprofit organization that administers and creates product and communication standards in the United States. ANSI uses a voluntary consensus process to arrive at and maintain standards not only in healthcare but in many diverse areas of industry and manufacturing. The organizational hierarchy that develops and maintains the HIPAA transactions, which in this book are referred to simply as ANSI transactions, is as follows: American National Standards Institute (ANSI) Data Interchange Standards Association (DISA) Accredited Standards Committee (ASC) X 12n.

**AP DRG** Acronym for all-patient diagnosis-related groups, which is severity-adjusted data from 3M Corporation that hospitals use to compare performance measures with other hospitals. It provides a case mix index of non-Medicare discharges.

**APC** Acronym for ambulatory payment classification, a prospective payment system used for reimbursement of hospitals for outpatient services provided to Medicare and Medicaid beneficiaries.

**Application software** Computer programs that perform functions. Examples include word processing, e-mail, billing, and electronic health records.

**ARB** Acronym for angiotensin receptor blocker, a drug sometimes used as an alternative for patients who cannot be given ACE inhibitors because ARB has the similar effect of blocking a hormone that constricts blood vessels.

**ASC** Acronym for Accredited Standards Committee, a group within ANSI that oversees the development and publication of standards.

**ASCII character** The computer standard for the letters of the alphabet, punctuation, and numeric and primitive graphic characters using a single byte of data per character.

**Assessment (chart)** The diagnosis or determination arrived at by a clinician after reviewing medical examination subjective and objective findings and test results.

**Assignment of benefits** A patient's authorization for a payer to send a remittance directly to the provider.

**Asthma** A generally chronic disorder often caused by an allergic origin, characterized by wheezing, coughing, labored breathing, and a suffocating feeling.

**Authorization (HIPAA)** HIPAA authorization differs from HIPAA consent in that it *does* require the patient's permission to disclose PHI. Under the HIPAA Privacy Rule, authorization is required for most disclosures of PHI other than for treating the patient, seeking payment, or operation of the healthcare facility.

**Authorization (insurance)** Some situations and health plans require providers to get prior authorization before performing certain services for patients of those plans. This is also called a healthcare services review, preauthorization, or precertification.

**Balance forward statement** A balance forward statement lists the balance from the previous statement, new charges that have occurred, payments that have been received, and accounting adjustments that have been posted in the current period.

**Batch posting** Entering data in batches rather than in real time. Charges and payments are grouped by date or provider and posted as a batch; batches are totaled and verified. Batch posting is common in hospitals as well as group practices that use billing services.

**Bed count** The number of hospital beds set up and staffed for patients.

**Best of breed** A health information system created by selecting systems that best meet each department's needs regardless of the vendor. This ensures maximum software functionality for the individual departments, but such systems may not work with the EHR or each other.

**Biomedical devices** Monitoring devices and instruments that attach to the patient or are intended for the patient to touch. Examples include telemetry devices for measuring vital signs, cardiac function, or arterial blood gas.

**Bit** The smallest unit of data in a computer. It represents one or zero. Bits are combined in groups to create larger units such as bytes or pixels.

**BLOB** Acronym for binary large object, a format for storing images and other nonfielded data in a database.

**Business associate agreement** The HIPAA Privacy Rule requires covered entities that use the services of other persons or businesses to obtain a written agreement that the business associate will comply with the protection of PHI under the Privacy Rule.

**Byte** A basic unit of computer data consisting of eight bits and capable of representing numbers or characters from 0 to 255.

**CAC** Acronym for children's asthma care.

**CAP** Acronym for College of American Pathologists, an organization of board-certified pathologists and the accrediting organization for reference laboratories.

**Capitation** A managed care reimbursement model in which a health plan pays a provider a flat amount per member based on the number of enrolled plan members selecting that provider instead of the actual number of member encounters or procedures.

**Cardiac catheterization** A test to evaluate the heart and arteries. A thin flexible tube is threaded through a blood vessel into the heart, then a contrast material is injected to trace the movement of blood through the coronary arteries.

**Cardiovascular** The heart and the system of blood vessels.

**Care plan** A statement of treatment goals and planned outcome that is amended as the patient's condition changes and further assessment dictates.

**CARF** Acronym for the Commission on Accreditation of Rehabilitation Facilities, which provides accreditation for organizations offering behavioral health, physical, and occupational rehabilitation services as well as assisted living, continuing care, community services, employment services, and others.

**Case management** Ongoing concurrent review of the necessity and effectiveness of the clinical services being provided to a patient; the development of a care plan for a patient; the coordination of a patient's care and transfer to multiple facilities over time.

**CAT scan**   Computerized axial tomography uses multiple x-rays and a computer to generate images of cross sections of the body.

**CBC**   Acronym for complete blood count, a lab test that includes separate counts for both white and red blood cells.

**CC**   Acronym for chief complaint; also acronym for comorbidity/complication.

**CCOW**   Acronym for Clinical Context Object Workgroup and the standard developed by them. The standard is designed to allow software from different vendors to retain the selected patient and provider when switching among applications.

**CD**   Acronym for compact disk, an optical disk capable of storing about 700 megabytes of data. It is frequently used in radiology to send copies of diagnostic images to another provider.

**CDA**   Acronym for Clinical Document Architecture, an HL7 standard for incorporating clinical text reports or other information in a claim attachment.

**CDC**   Acronym for the Centers for Disease Control and Prevention, a division of the U.S. Department of Health and Human Services.

**CDISC**   Acronym for Clinical Data Interchange Standards Consortium, an organization that has created standards that enable sponsors, vendors, and clinicians to acquire and exchange data used in clinical drug trials. CDISC has become part of HL7.

**CDR**   Acronym for clinical data repository, a database that stores data from multiple systems.

**Central tendency**   The distribution of a variable, measured by statistics such as the mean, median, and mode.

**CEO**   Acronym for chief executive officer, the head of all business and administrative divisions of an organization.

**CF**   Acronym for conversion factor, used in a formula for calculating reimbursement schedules such as the Medicare allowed amount.

**CFO**   Acronym for chief financial officer, the person responsible for financial and accounting matters.

**CHAMP-VA**   Acronym for the Civilian Health and Medical Program–Veterans Affairs, a program to provide healthcare for dependents and survivors of veterans with disabilities and those killed in the line of duty.

**Chargemaster**   A table of procedure codes, descriptions, and fees a facility charges.

**Chief complaint**   A concise statement describing the symptom, problem, condition, diagnosis, or other factor that is the reason for the encounter, usually stated in the patient's words.

**Chief of staff**   A doctor who is head of the hospital medical board and medical staff.

**Chronic**   Disease or problem that lasts a long time or recurs often.

**CIO**   Acronym for chief information officer, the person responsible for all computer, telephony, and information services and infrastructure in a business.

**Claim attachment**   Supplemental documents providing additional medical information to the claims processor that cannot be accommodated within the paper or electronic claim format; for example, a laboratory report to justify medical necessity of a treatment.

**Claim scrubber**   A software program that analyzes electronic claims before they are created or sent; it compares them to claim edits used by the health plan computers to identify billing errors that might cause a claim to be denied.

**Claim status**   A query to a health plan about a claim for which the provider filed but has not received payment or denial.

**Clearinghouse**   *See* Healthcare clearinghouse.

**Client/server**   A software configuration in which only a portion of the application software (the client) is installed on a desktop computer; the remainder (database, principal applications) is located on a networked computer called the server.

**Clinical chemistry (pathology)**   Tests for various components of blood and urine, including the use of chemicals, enzymes, and light (spectrometry). Today most clinical chemistry is performed by automated laboratory devices.

**Clinical microbiology (pathology)**   Pathology tests for the presence of microorganisms and pathogens such as bacteria, viruses, fungi, or parasites.

**Clinical terminology**   An organized list of medical phrases and codes. *See* Nomenclature.

**Clinical trials**   The testing of a new drug, device, or procedure on human subjects. The FDA divides clinical trials into four phases. Phase I tests a very small group to see if the product is safe and tolerated by a healthy person. Phase II is tested on a group of patients for whom the treatment is intended to prove the treatment works. Phase III uses a larger group of test subjects, some of whom are given the treatment and some a placebo. Phase IV trials are conducted after the treatment has been approved, to survey its interaction once it is in general use.

**Clinical vocabulary**   An organized list of medical phrases and codes. *See* Nomenclature.

**CMI**   Acronym for case mix index, which is calculated by dividing the sum of the DRG total weights by the number of patients discharged by a hospital as a whole during a given time period. CMS publishes a yearly report of the CMI comparing all hospitals that file Medicare A claims.

**CMN**   Acronym for certificate of medical necessity.

**CMS**   Acronym for the Centers for Medicare and Medicaid Services (formerly HCFA), a division of the U.S. Department of Health and Human Services.

**CMS-1500** A paper health insurance claim form for professional services.

**CNO** Acronym for chief nursing officer, the person who has administrative responsibility for all nurses and to whom all nurse supervisors report. Some facilities call this position the vice president of nursing.

**COB** Acronym for coordination of benefits. When a patient is covered by more than one health insurance plan, the plans involved determine how much each plan is to pay. A HIPAA transaction permits the plans to do this electronically.

**Code of ethics** The professional standards by which we conduct ourselves are called *ethics*. A code of ethics provides guidance on how to act in a professional capacity and helps to guide those who create policies and procedures for their facilities.

**Codified data (chart)** EHR data with each finding assigned a standard code; use of codified data ensures uniformity of medical records, eliminates ambiguities about the clinician's meaning, and facilitates communication between multiple systems.

**Coinsurance** The portion of a medical bill that a health plan beneficiary must pay after the deductible has been met; usually a percentage of the allowed amount. *See also* Allowed amount.

**COLD** Acronym for computer output to laser disk, a method of outputting reports directly to disk instead of printing them to paper and then scanning them.

**Comorbidity** A diagnosed condition that coexists with the principal reason for hospitalization and will affect the treatment or length of stay.

**Consent (HIPAA)** Under the revised HIPAA Privacy Rule, a patient gives consent to the use of their PHI for purposes of treatment, payment, and operation of the healthcare practice by acknowledging that they have received a copy of the office's privacy policy. HIPAA privacy consent should not be confused with consent to perform a medical procedure.

**Consent (treatment)** A document signed by patients or their guardians giving consent to be treated. Additional consent called *informed consent* is required for surgery and specific procedures.

**Contingency plan** Strategies for recovering access to EPHI should a medical office experience an emergency, such as a power outage or disruption of critical business operations. The goal is to ensure that EPHI is available when it is needed.

**Continuous variable** A series of values that increment evenly, for example, time.

**COO** Acronym for chief operating officer, an executive responsible for most functional aspects of running a facility (except medical staff, accounting, and information services).

**COP** Acronym for conditions of participation, the agreement and rules for Medicare participating providers.

**Copay** The amount a health plan patient must pay for an office visit; usually a flat rate.

**Covered entity (HIPAA)** HIPAA refers to healthcare providers, plans, and clearinghouses as covered entities. In the context of this book, think of a covered entity as the medical practice and all of its employees.

**COW** Acronym for computers on wheels, portable wireless computers on movable carts that are taken from room to room in a hospital.

**CPOE** Acronym for computerized physician order entry; also computerized provider order entry.

**CPR** Acronym for cardiopulmonary resuscitation, a life-saving procedure used when a person's heart and breathing have stopped.

**CPRI** Acronym for Computer-based Patient Record Institute, formed to promote the universal and effective use of electronic healthcare information systems to improve health and the delivery of healthcare; was merged into HIMSS in 2002.

**CPT-4** Acronym for Current Procedural Terminology, Fourth Edition. CPT-4 codes are standardized codes for reporting medical services, procedures, and treatments performed for patients by the medical staff. CPT-4 is owned by the American Medical Association.

**CPU** Acronym for central processing unit, the main processing chip in a computer.

**CR** Acronym for computed radiography, an x-ray using existing x-ray equipment but replacing film with a reusable phosphor plate to capture the image.

**CRNA** Acronym for Certified Registered Nurse Anesthetist, a nurse licensed to provide anesthesia service under the supervision of an anesthesiologist.

**Cross-walk (codes)** A reference table for translating a code from one set to a code with the same meaning in another code set. For example, the ICD-9-CM and the ICD-10-CM codes.

**CT scan** Acronym for computerized tomography scan. *See* CAT scan.

**Cytology (pathology)** The study of cells in terms of structure, function, cellular change, and the diagnosis of cellular disease.

**Data elements** A definition of the standard types of information that health systems should keep for a particular purpose. The concept of data elements applies to both paper and electronic health records.

**Data set** A list of data elements collected for a particular purpose.

**Database** A file or group of files that store related data in a computer.

**Decision support** *See* Medical decision support.

**Decryption** A method of converting an encrypted message back into regular text using a mathematical algorithm and a string of characters called a *key*. *See also* Encryption.

**DEEDS** Acronym for Data Elements for Emergency Department Systems; its use by hospital emergency departments is optional.

**Deemed status** A facility accredited by the Joint Commission, CARF, or CAP is "deemed" to be in compliance with the CMS conditions of participation.

**De-identified data** Data from which the PHI elements have been removed, such that an individual cannot be personally identified from the data.

**Diabetes mellitus** A chronic form of diabetes; characterized by an insulin deficiency, an excess of sugar in the blood and urine, and by hunger, thirst, and gradual loss of weight.

**Diagnosis** A disease or condition, or the process of identifying the diseased condition. Generally codified using the ICD-9-CM code set.

**DICOM** Acronym for Digital Imaging and Communication in Medicine, a standard for communication and a file structure for transfer of digital images between various types of equipment and computer systems.

**Dictation/transcription** In medicine, the process of creating portions of the patient chart by dictating findings and observations into a recording device. The recording is later typed into a word processor by a nonclinical allied health professional known as a transcriptionist.

**Digital images (chart)** EHR data in image format. This includes diagnostic images, digital x-rays, and documents scanned into the EHR. Image data usually requires specific software to view the image. *See also* Scanned images.

**Digital pathology** Digital pathology uses imaging systems to replace the microscope capturing the image of the specimen slide in a digital file, which can then be electronically manipulated or enlarged.

**DISA** Acronym for Data Interchange Standards Association, a component within ANSI that develops and maintains electronic transaction standards including the healthcare transactions.

**Discrete data (chart)** Discrete data, either fielded or codified. Fielded data identifies the type of information by its position in the EHR record. Codified data pairs each piece of information with a code, which identifies the information in a uniform way.

**DME** Acronym for durable medical equipment, such as wheelchairs, crutches, or medical devices, that is rented or sold to patients for home use.

**DNA** Acronym for deoxyribonucleic acid, the basic material of chromosomes containing the genetic code of our hereditary traits.

**DNR** Acronym for do not resuscitate, which is an order in the chart of a patient who has requested not to be given CPR. The DNR order is one of the options of a patient's advance directive (also known as a living will).

**Document image management** A computer system or component of the EHR for organizing, retrieving, and displaying images of scanned records.

**DR** Acronym for digital radiography, x-ray equipment that directly captures the x-ray in a digital image file.

**DRG, MS-DRG** Acronym for diagnosis-related groups, which are used in calculating a flat rate reimbursement for inpatient stays based on the diagnosis. MS-DRG is an acronym for Medicare severity diagnosis-related groups, which was introduced by Medicare to better factor the severity of the case into the calculation. Both DRG and MS-DRG operate on the theory that patients with the same diagnosis should require about the same length of stay and consume a similar amount of resources.

**Drug formulary** Used to look up drugs by name or therapeutic class; they provide an updated list of the drugs that are available in the inventory, information on costs, indications for use, treatment recommendations, dosage, guidelines, and prescribing information. Health insurance programs use the term *formulary* for plan-specific drug lists.

**DUR** Acronym for drug utilization review, which is the process of analyzing a drug prescription for a given patient to determine contraindications, overdosing, underdosing, allergic reactions, drug/drug interactions, and drug/food interactions.

**DVD** Acronym for digital video disk, an optical disk capable of storing from 4.2 gigabytes to more than 50 gigabytes of data. It is frequently used in medical facilities to back up computer data and image files.

**Dx** An abbreviation for diagnosis (especially in a medical health record).

**E&M (codes)** Evaluation and management codes are CPT-4 codes used to bill for nearly every kind of patient encounter, such as physician office visits, inpatient hospital exams, nursing home visits, consults, emergency room doctors, and scores of other services.

**ECG, EKG** Acronym for electrocardiogram, a graphic recording of the electrical activity of the heart.

**EDI** Acronym for electronic data interchange. Information exchanged electronically as data in codified transactions.

**EEG** Acronym for electroencephalogram, a graphic recording of the electrical activity of the brain.

**EFT** Acronym for electronic funds transfer, the payment or direct deposit of funds to a provider's bank account instead of issuing a check.

**EHR** Acronym for electronic health records, the portions of a patient's medical records that are stored in a computer system as well as the functional benefits derived from having an electronic health record. Also know as electronic medical records, computerized patient records, or electronic chart.

**Electronic signature** A method of marking an electronic record as "signed" that gives the record the same legal authority as a written signature. The electronic signature process involves the successful identification and authentication of the signer at the time of the signature, binding of the signature to the document, and nonalterability of the document after the signature has been affixed.

**Electronic views**   A method of instantly reorganizing data in EHR systems to allow the user to switch between a problem-oriented chart, source-oriented chart, reverse chronological order, or other organizational method without actually altering the EHR data.

**Eligibility**   Communicating by phone, fax, or EDI to determine if a patient's health insurance information is valid, what types of services are covered, and what the coinsurance or copay amounts are.

**EMC**   Acronym for electronic media claims, the process of creating and transmitting claims data in an electronic format instead of paper. HIPAA requires EMC to be in a standard transaction format: 837-I for institutional claims, 837-P for professional claims, 837-D for dental claims, and NCPDP for pharmacy claims.

**EMR**   Acronym for electronic medical record. *See* Electronic health record.

**EMT**   Acronym for emergency medical technician, a medical professional trained for emergency services such as ambulance services.

**Encounter**   The medical record of an interaction between a patient and a healthcare provider.

**Encounter form**   A form frequently used in outpatient settings to communicate billing and diagnosis information from the provider to the person posting charges. The form usually lists the procedure and diagnosis codes frequently used by the practice so the provider can simply circle the codes appropriate to the visit. The form is also referred to as a superbill.

**Encryption**   A method of converting an original message of regular text into encoded text that is unreadable in its encrypted form. The text is encrypted by means of an algorithm using a private *key*. *See also* Decryption.

**ENT**   Acronym for ears, nose, and throat.

**EOB**   Acronym for explanation of benefits; also called remittance advice. This can be a paper document, an electronic file, or a report generated from an ERA file. It is used to post payment from health plans. The EOB informs the provider of the amounts being paid for each claim. Patients also receive an EOB showing what the plan has paid the provider. The patient version may look different from the provider's version.

**EPHI (HIPAA)**   Protected health information in electronic form. *See also* Protected health information.

**ER**   Acronym for emergency room or emergency department, usually located in an acute care hospital. Sometimes the acronym ED is used as well.

**ERA**   Acronym for electronic remittance advice, the transmission of claims payment data in a standard format (ANSI 835) as required by HIPAA.

**Ergonomics**   The study of the physical effect of human/computer interaction on workers with the goal of minimizing or eliminating problems.

**E-visit**   An E-visit is a patient encounter conducted over the Internet, without an office visit. The patient enters symptom, history, and HPI information, which is then reviewed by a clinician who communicates via the Internet to ask additional questions and provide a diagnosis, treatment orders, and patient education. E-visits are used only for nonurgent visits and are reimbursed by a growing number of insurance plans.

**Family numbering**   A method of numbering patient charts in a family or pediatric practice where a family is given a primary account number and each patient chart is numbered by adding a decimal to the family number. For example if a family is assigned the number 777, the head of the household would be assigned number 777.0, the spouse 777.1, the first child 777.2, and the second child 777.3.

**FDA**   Acronym for the Food and Drug Administration, a division of the U.S. Department of Health and Human Services. This federal agency regulates prescription and nonprescription drugs.

**FECA**   Acronym for the Federal Employee Compensation Act, which pays the healthcare costs and lost income from work-related injuries for federal employees.

**Fee-for-service**   Reimbursement based on the encounter or services performed.

**FEIN**   Acronym for federal employer identification number, a number assigned by the U.S. Internal Revenue Service; also known as a business tax ID.

**Field**   Defined units representing a specific type of data in a database, for example, a zip code or a birth date.

**Finding**   A precorrelated combination of terms from the nomenclature or clinical terminology into a clinically relevant phrase.

**Flow cytometry (pathology)**   A study counting, examining, and sorting microscopic particles suspended in a stream of fluid flowing through an optical or electronic apparatus.

**Flow sheet**   A presentation of medical data from multiple dates and times in column format resembling a spreadsheet. Flow sheets allow findings from any previous encounter to be cited in the current note. Flow sheets can be created based on a list, a form, or a problem.

**Formulary**   *See* Drug formulary.

**Free-text**   EHR information that is not codified; may be attached to a codified finding as supplemental notes.

**Frequency distribution**   How frequently data occurs at given points along a continuous variable such as a timeline.

**FTE**   Acronym for full-time equivalent employee, a method of stating the number of full-time people required for a task.

**FTP**   Acronym for File Transfer Protocol, a transmission standard for transferring files over a network or the Internet.

**GL** Acronym for general ledger, the central component of financial accounting systems.

**Glucose monitors** Home device used by patients with diabetes to monitor their glucose levels.

**GPCI** Acronym for geographic practice cost indices, which are used in reimbursement calculations to factor in regional differences in costs.

**H&P** Acronym for the history and physical portion of a medical exam.

**HAC** Acronym for hospital-acquired condition, an infection or other condition acquired by the patient during the hospital stay that is not related to their reason for admission and that could have been prevented through the application of evidence-based guidelines.

**Hanging protocol** The order in which x-rays or diagnostic images are arranged for the radiologist.

**Hard drive** A portion of a computer that stores large quantities of data magnetically on disks inside a sealed unit.

**HBIPS** Acronym for hospital-based inpatient psychiatric services.

**HCFA** Acronym for the Health Care Financing Administration. HCFA has since been renamed CMS. See *CMS*.

**HCPCS** Acronym for Healthcare Common Procedure Coding System. The HCPCS codes are an extended set of billing codes for reporting medical services, procedures, and treatments not listed in CPT-4 codes.

**Health information manager** The person responsible for the health information records and services. A Registered Health Information Administrator (RHIA) has a bachelor or master's degree and has passed an AHIMA certification exam.

**Health information technician** Person who enters medical records data, performs coding for billing departments, works with the cancer registry, or generates reports from patient data to support administrative functions of the hospital. A Registered Health Information Technician (RHIT) has passed an AHIMA certification examination.

**Health maintenance** EHR system component to provide preventive health recommendations.

**Healthcare clearinghouse** A computer system or covered entity that performs the specific function of translating nonstandard EDI transactions into HIPAA-compliant transactions.

**Healthcare services review** *See* Authorization (insurance).

**HEDIS** Acronym for Health Plan Employer Data and Information System, a data set used to measure performance for comparison of quality of care provided by managed care plans.

**Hematology** A medical specialty concerned with the study of blood, the blood-forming organs, and blood diseases. Similarly, the group of laboratory tests referred to as hematology includes those which study the components and coagulation of blood. Examples of hematology tests include

the complete blood count (CBC), prothrombin time (PT), and partial thromboplastin time (PTT).

**HF** Acronym for heart failure, a condition in which the lower chambers of the heart are unable to pump blood effectively.

**HHA** Acronym for home health agency, a provider of nursing, therapy and medical assistance to patients in their homes.

**HHRG** Acronym for home health resource group, which is used to calculate reimbursement based on an OASIS assessment of the patient's condition.

**HHS** Acronym for the U.S. Department of Health and Human Services. HHS includes CMS, the Office of Civil Rights, the Office of Inspector General, and the CDC.

**HIMSS** Acronym for Healthcare Information and Management Systems Society, an organization that provides leadership in healthcare for the management of technology, information, and change through member services, education and networking opportunities, and publications. Members include healthcare professionals, hospitals, corporate healthcare systems, clinical practice groups, HIT supplier organizations, healthcare consulting firms, and government agencies.

**HIPAA** Acronym for Health Insurance Portability and Accountability Act (of 1996). HIPAA law regulates many things. However, it is not uncommon for medical offices to use the term HIPAA when they actually mean only the Administrative Simplification Subsection of HIPAA. *See* Administrative Simplification (HIPAA).

**HIPPS** Acronym for Health Insurance Prospective Payment System code set, a field on UB-04 and ANSI 837-I claims for a billing code that varies by the type of institutional provider. HCPCS is used for outpatient claims, RUG for SNF and long-term hospitals, and the accommodation rate for acute care hospitals.

**HL7** Acronym for Health Level Seven, the leading messaging standard used to exchange clinical and administrative data among different healthcare computer systems.

**HMO** Acronym for health maintenance organization, one of several types of managed care plans.

**Holter monitor** A device worn by a patient to record the heart rhythm continuously for 24 hours. This provides a record that can be analyzed by a cardiologist to uncover any irregular or abnormal activity of the heart. Named for Dr. Norman Holter, its inventor.

**HOP** Acronym for hospital outpatient measures.

**HPI** Acronym for history of present illness, which is a chronological description of the development of the patient's present illness from the first sign and/or symptom or from the previous encounter to the present.

**Hx** An abbreviation for history (patient's past medical, surgical, social, or family history).

**Hybrid record** Patient health records that contain a mix of both paper charts and electronic records, usually occurring during the time a facility is transitioning to an EHR.

**ICD-9-CM**   Acronym for International Classification of Diseases, Ninth Revision, Clinical Modification, a system of standardized codes to classify mortality and morbidity. ICD-9-CM is currently published in three volumes. The first two volumes provide a listing and an index of diagnosis codes, the third volume lists codes for hospital inpatient procedures.

**ICD-10**   Acronym for International Classification of Diseases, Tenth Revision, a revision of the ICD-9 codes; used in the United States only for codifying the cause of death on death certificates until 2013.

**ICD-10-PCS**   International Classification of Diseases, Tenth Revision, Procedure Coding System (but not derived from the ICD-10 codes). This system is intended to replace inpatient procedure codes in ICD-9-CM, Volume 3. The ICD-10-PCS codes are not used for billing at this time.

**ICU**   Acronym for intensive care unit, a special section of the hospital with monitoring equipment and staff for patients who are seriously ill.

**IDN**   Acronym for integrated delivery network, a managed care model in which facilities and physicians form a business arrangement for the purpose of contracting with the HMO to provide both hospital and physician services.

**IDSS**   Acronym for Interactive Data Submission System, a system for electronically submitting HEDIS data to NCQA.

**IHS**   Acronym for Indian Health Service, the division of the U.S. Department of Health and Human Services responsible for providing federal health services to American Indians and Alaska natives.

**Immunology (pathology)**   Pathology tests that analyze body fluids to detect immune system diseases. Sometimes referred to as immunopathology.

**Implant**   Nontissue materials or devices intentionally placed in the patient's body during surgery. Examples include heart valves, pacemakers, breast implants, and artificial joints.

**Implementation specifications**   An implementation specification in the HIPAA Security Rule is an additional detailed instruction for implementing a particular security standard.

**Incidental disclosures (HIPAA)**   HIPAA's Privacy Rule permits incidental uses and disclosures of protected health information when the covered entity has in place reasonable safeguards and minimum necessary policies and procedures to protect an individual's privacy.

**Information system activity review (HIPAA)**   A regular review of records such as audit logs, access reports, and security incident tracking reports. The information system activity review helps to determine if any EPHI is used or disclosed in an inappropriate manner.

**Inpatient**   A hospital patient who stays overnight.

**Integrated record**   A method of organizing a patient's chart that intermingles documents from various sources arranged sequentially in chronological date order or in reverse chronological order (date order, but with the newest documents at the front of folder and the oldest document at the back).

**Integrated system**   A health information system approach that biases decisions toward software compatibility by using a single vendor's systems insofar as possible and where it isn't possible to select systems that have been interfaced with the vendor's systems at other hospitals.

**Internet**   A worldwide public computer network, which can be accessed from nearly anywhere.

**IOM**   Acronym for Institute of Medicine of the National Academies, a nonprofit organization created to provide unbiased, evidence-based, and authoritative information and advice concerning health and science policy.

**IPA**   Acronym for Independent Practice Association, a managed care model in which a number of independent physicians form a business arrangement for the purpose of contracting with an HMO.

**IPF**   Acronym for inpatient psychiatric facility.

**IPPS**   Acronym for inpatient prospective payment system, a method using DRG or MS-DRG by which insurance plans calculate reimbursement for most acute care hospitals.

**IRB**   Acronym for internal review board.

**ISS**   Acronym for Injury Severity Score, an anatomic scoring system that provides an overall score for patients with multiple injuries. Each injury is assigned an Abbreviated Injury Scale (AIS) score. The three most severely injured body regions have their score squared and added together to produce the ISS score.

**IV**   Acronym for intravenous; refers to the introduction of blood, fluids, or medicine directly into the vein.

**JCAHO or Joint Commission**   Acronym for Joint Commission on Accreditation of Healthcare Organizations. The name has been changed to the Joint Commission but the acronym JACHO is still frequently used.

**JPEG**   Acronym for Joint Photographic Experts Group, the standard format for photos and images in which the size of the file is compressed without a significant loss in quality.

**Kiosk**   An unattended computer terminal for use by patients in a medical office's waiting area.

**LAN**   Acronym for local-area network, a network that allows computers to exchange information via wired cables that connect them.

**LDL, LDL-c**   Low-density lipoprotein cholesterol in blood plasma; sometimes referred to as "bad cholesterol," it is often associated with clogged arteries.

**Leapfrog Group**   A coalition of 150 of the largest U.S. employers that created a strategy to tie the purchase of group health insurance benefits to quality care standards and promoted computerized physician order entry and the use of EHRs.

**Licensed practical nurse, licensed vocational nurse** Licensed practical nurse (LPN); also known as a licensed vocational nurse (LVN); a nurse who provides routine care to patients, but is licensed only to work under the direct supervision of registered nurses or physicians.

**LIS** Acronym for laboratory information system, a computer system for managing test orders and test equipment in a medical laboratory.

**Lists (EHR)** A subset of findings (typically) used for a particular condition or type of exam; the list format makes the findings easier to read and navigate.

**Login** The process by which users enter their name (or ID) and password into a computer in order to gain access to the computer's programs; the action of entering a program through such a screen. Note that some systems use the term *log on* for this function.

**LOINC** Acronym for Logical Observation Identifier Names and Codes. LOINC was created and is maintained by the Regenstrief Institute, which is affiliated with the Indiana University School of Medicine. LOINC is an important clinical terminology for laboratory test orders and results.

**Loop** A segment of an EDI format intended to be repeated a number of times. For example, multiple procedures are billed on an EMC claim by repeating the service loop until all of the procedures have been listed.

**Loose sheets** Patient medical documents from internal or external sources that need to be scanned into the EHR or filed in a paper chart.

**LOS** Acronym for length of stay, the number of days a patient is in the hospital from date of admission up to, but not counting, the date of discharge.

**LTCH** Acronym for long-term care hospital. LTCH facilities are used for inpatient stays exceeding 30 days that require less intensive nursing care than acute care hospitals.

**LVSD** Acronym for left ventricular systolic dysfunction, the term used when the lower left chamber of the heart is not contracting with enough force to pump the blood effectively.

**Malicious software** Software such as viruses, trojan horses, and worms that infiltrates computer networks without authorization. Malicious software can damage or destroy data or cause expensive and time-consuming repairs. It is frequently brought into an organization through e-mail attachments and programs that are downloaded from the Internet. One requirement of the HIPAA Security Rule is to protect against malicious software.

**Malpractice** Professional liability of a provider for errors or omissions in the delivery of healthcare.

**Mammogram, mammography** An x-ray of the breast that can be used to detect tumors before they can be seen or felt.

**MCAP** Acronym for Medical Care Appropriateness Protocol, a utilization management tool for assessing the appropriateness of admissions and length of stay in acute care hospitals.

**MCC** Acronym for major complication/comorbidity, which is used in MS-DRG to determine medical severity.

**MDC** Acronym for major diagnostic category, the first level of the DRG system in which ICD-9-CM codes are classified into 25 major diagnostic categories from which they are then grouped into DRG codes.

**MDS** Acronym for minimum data set, which is used with the Resident Assessment Instrument in long-term care facilities and is required by CMS.

**Mean** The average; the sum of the values divided by the frequency.

**Medcin** A medical nomenclature and knowledge base developed by Medicomp Systems, Inc. Recognized as a national standard, MEDCIN is incorporated in many commercial EHR systems as well as the Department of Defense CHCS II system.

**Median** The midpoint in a group of ranked values that divides the data into two equal parts.

**Medicaid** State-operated medical programs that receive federal funding to provide medical assistance to low-income patients with limited financial resources.

**Medical decision support** Computer or Internet-based systems used to improve the process and outcome of medical decisions by delivering evidence-based information to the clinician determining the diagnosis or treatment orders.

**Medicare** Federal health program for persons ages 65 or older and persons of any age with certain disabilities or end-stage renal disease.

**Medication list** A page or screen in a patient chart that provides a list of what medications the patient is currently taking. The medication list is always reviewed before writing new prescriptions.

**Microfilm, microfiche** An older method of archiving paper records by photographing each page of the chart on film. The images are stored on rolls of film called microfilm or on small sheets of film called microfiche. The photographic images are very small, but can be viewed at full size using a projector called a microfilm reader.

**Microscopy** Studies or images of studies performed using a microscope.

**Middle digit filing** A filing method for paper charts that uses the middle set of the hyphenated record number as the primary set for filing. The middle digits correspond to a numbered subsection of the file room shelving. Middle digit filing reduces the chance of filing errors by limiting the number of charts in each subsection, but it is not used in facilities having medical record numbers longer than six digits.

**Minimum necessary standard (HIPAA)** A standard in the HIPAA Privacy Rule intended to limit unnecessary or inappropriate access to and disclosure of PHI beyond what is necessary. The minimum necessary standard does not apply to disclosures to or requests for information used by a healthcare provider for treatment of the patient.

**Mode**   The value that occurs most often in the frequency of distribution.

**Morbidity**   A diseased state, injury, or symptom.

**MOU**   Acronym for memorandum of understanding (between government entities); can be used between government agencies to meet the HIPAA Security rule requirement in lieu of business associate agreements.

**Mouse**   A computer device for moving a pointer or cursor on the screen, selecting items, and invoking actions in computer software.

**MPI**   Acronym for master patient index, which is a file or database index of all patients registered in a healthcare organization. It is used to locate patient records and prevent duplicate registration.

**MRI**   Acronym for magnetic resonance imaging, which uses magnetic fields and pulses of energy to create images of organs and structures inside the body that cannot be seen by x-ray or CAT scan.

**NASA**   Acronym for National Aeronautics and Space Administration.

**NCCI**   Acronym for the National Correct Coding Initiative, a series of claim edits introduced by Medicare to identify incorrect coding practices, such as unbundling a single complex procedure into multiple procedure codes for the purpose of increasing reimbursement.

**NCDB**   Acronym for National Cancer Data Base, a cancer registry.

**NCPDP**   Acronym for the National Council for Prescription Drug Programs and for the pharmacy claim EDI format created by that organization.

**NCQA**   Acronym for the National Committee for Quality Assurance, a nonprofit organization that accredits health plans and that developed and maintains the HEDIS reporting measures.

**NCVHS**   Acronym for National Committee on Vital and Health Statistics, an advisory panel within the U.S. Department of Health and Human Services that selects national standards for HIPAA and recommends standards for the federal government initiatives on electronic health records.

**NDC**   Acronym for National Drug Code. The NDC is the standard identifier for human drugs. It is assigned and used by the pharmaceutical industry.

**NDF-RT**   A nonproprietary terminology being developed by the VA that classifies drugs by mechanism of action and physiologic effect.

**NEC**   Acronym for "not elsewhere classified" (diagnosis codes).

**NHII**   Acronym for National Health Information Infrastructure, a plan to make EHR records available wherever the patient is treated.

**NHQM**   Acronym for National Hospital Quality Measures, specific measure sets developed by CMS and based on the Joint Commission's ORYX initiatives. NHQM data is used to determine how effectively facilities are following evidence-based guidelines that improve patient care. The data is compared to other facilities and used to calculated pay-for-performance–based reimbursement and incentives.

**NMDP**   Acronym for the National Marrow Donor Program.

**Nomenclature**   A system of names created by a recognized group or authority and used in a field of science. An EHR nomenclature is an organized list of medical phrases and codes that helps to standardize the way clinicians record information. These are also referred to as clinical vocabularies or clinical terminologies.

**NOS**   Acronym for "not otherwise specified" (diagnosis codes).

**NPDB**   Acronym for National Practitioner Data Bank, a database operated by the U.S. Department of Health and Human Services to facilitate a comprehensive review of healthcare practitioners' professional credentials, malpractice, and other reportable incidents.

**NPI**   Acronym for national provider identifier, which is used by doctors, nurses, and other healthcare providers. Required for EDI under HIPAA's uniform identifier standards.

**OASIS**   Acronym for Outcome and Assessment Information Set, which is used by home health agencies to assess the patient's condition. It is required by CMS.

**OB**   An abbreviation for obstetrics, which is the medical specialty concerned with pregnancy, childbirth, and the period following delivery.

**Objective (chart)**   The clinician's observations and findings from the physical exam.

**OCR**   Acronym for optical character recognition software, which can convert a scanned image of typed text into computer data.

**OCR**   Acronym for Office for Civil Rights within the U.S. Department of Health and Human Services.

**OIG**   Acronym for the Office of Inspector General within the U.S. Department of Health and Human Services.

**Open item statement**   A statement that lists each charge, how much has been paid by the insurance plan, how much was written down by the provider, and how much is due from the patient. The charges for each visit are reprinted on subsequent statements until they are paid in full.

**Operating system (software)**   Control programs that enable us to work with a computer's hardware to manage the CPU and other control chips that operate the monitor display, memory storage devices, and input/output devices, including the keyboard and mouse.

**OPPS**   Acronym for outpatient prospective payment system, a Medicare prospective payment system used for hospital-based outpatient services and procedures based on ambulatory payment classifications. *See* APC.

**Optical disks** Removable disks such as CD-ROMs or DVDs that use lasers to burn information on a disk for long-term storage.

**OR** Acronym for operating room or surgery room in a hospital or ambulatory surgical center.

**ORYX®** A set of quality measures developed by the Joint Commission and required for accreditation. ORYX measures are used to measure performance and outcomes in acute care hospitals.

**OSHA** Acronym for Occupational Safety and Health Administration, a federal agency and the rules created by that agency for safety in the workplace.

**Outguide** A paper or plastic placeholder that indicates that a paper chart has been removed from the files and usually contains information as to who has the chart.

**Outlier** In a statistical study, outliers are data points at either end of the spectrum that deviate so greatly as to skew the average, mean, median, or mode. In a prospective payment system, outlier cases are those in which the cost of treating a patient greatly exceeds the usual reimbursement for the DRG. In such cases the provider can ask for additional reimbursement.

**Outpatient** A patient who is examined or treated at a healthcare facility but is not hospitalized overnight.

**P4P** Acronym for pay for performance.

**PACS** Acronym picture archiving and communication system, a computer system for storing, retrieving, and displaying medical diagnostic image files.

**Pathology** Clinical pathology uses chemistry, microbiology, hematology, and molecular pathology to analyze blood, urine, and other bodily fluids. Anatomic pathology performs gross, microscopic, and molecular examination of organs and tissues and autopsies of whole bodies. Surgical pathology performs gross and microscopic examination of tissue removed from a patient by surgery or biopsy.

**Payment floor** A period of time during which Medicare and other health plans delay sending the payment for a claim that has been adjudicated and will be paid.

**PCE** Acronym for potentially compensable event, any incident that can result in financial loss or lead to litigation.

**PCI** Acronym for percutaneous coronary intervention; also known as angioplasty. PCI is a procedure to widen an artery or place a stent in an artery to hold it open. It is performed during a cardiac catheterization.

**PCP** Acronym for primary care physician, a physician in a managed care plan that acts as the gatekeeper to medical services such as diagnostic tests or other providers such as specialists.

**PDA** Acronym for portable digital assistant, a small pocket-sized computer.

**PDF** Acronym for Portable Document Format, a standard format for documents and images of documents.

**PE** An abbreviation for physical exam (sometimes Px).

**Pending order** A lab test or diagnostic procedure that has been ordered but for which no results have been received.

**Perioperative** The entire surgical event from surgery scheduling, the arrival of the patient in the presurgery holding area, the actual surgery in the OR suite, and the immediate recovery in the postanesthesia area.

**Personal representative (HIPAA)** The HIPAA Privacy Rule allows a patient to appoint a personal representative and requires covered entities to treat an individual's personal representative as the individual with respect to uses and disclosures of the individual's protected health information and the individual's rights under the Privacy Rule.

**PET** Acronym for positron emission tomography, which combines CT (computerized tomography) and nuclear scanning using a radioactive substance called a tracer, which is injected into a vein. A computer records the tracer as it collects in certain organs and then converts the data into three-dimensional images of the organ, which can be used to detect or evaluate cancer.

**PFSH** Acronym for past history, family history, and social history, which is obtained from a patient or other family member.

**PHI (HIPAA)** Acronym for protected health information, a patient's personally identifiable health information (in any form), which is protected by the HIPAA Privacy Rule.

**Phlebotomist** An allied clinical professional trained to draw blood specimens from patients

**Phonemes** The basic sound units of words. In English there about 50 phonemes made from 16 vowel sounds and 24 consonant sounds.

**PHR** Acronym for personal health record, which is used by patients to maintain their own electronic or paper copy of health records.

**Physical safeguards (HIPAA)** The HIPAA Security Rule requirements to implement physical mechanisms to protect electronic systems, equipment, and EPHI from threats, environmental hazards, and unauthorized intrusion. They include restricting access to EPHI and retaining off-site computer backups.

**Physician assistant** A healthcare provider who works under the supervision of physicians to conduct physical exams, diagnose and treat illnesses, order and interpret tests, counsel patients on preventive healthcare, and write prescriptions.

**PIN** Acronym for personal identification number, a secret number that is used like a password.

**Pixel** The basic unit of a digital image consisting of from 8 to 32 bits that represent the color and luminosity of a single dot of the image.

**PKI** Acronym for public key infrastructure, which is used to secure messages or electronically sign documents.

**Plan of treatment**   Prescribed therapy, medication, orders, and patient instructions for treatment or management of a diagnosed condition.

**PN**   Medical abbreviation for pneumonia.

**POA**   Acronym for "present on admission," which is an indicator that a condition was present at the time of the order for inpatient admission. The POA indicator is required for each primary and secondary diagnosis on an inpatient claim.

**POP3**   Acronym for Post Office Protocol, version 3, a standard e-mail method.

**Posting**   A term used for the act of entering data into one of the HIS systems, for example, entering charges and payments into the patient accounting system.

**PPO**   Acronym for preferred provider organization, a managed care model in which members pay a smaller copay or coinsurance when using providers within the PPO, but pay a larger amount if treated by out-of-network providers.

**PR**   Medical abbreviation for pregnancy and related conditions.

**Preauthorization**   *See* Authorization (insurance).

**Precertification**   *See* Authorization (insurance).

**Privacy officer (HIPAA)**   One individual designated by the healthcare organization as having overall responsibility for implementing the HIPAA Privacy Rule.

**Privacy policy**   A policy that covered entities must implement that meets the requirements of the HIPAA Privacy Rule. A copy of the privacy policy must be made available to each patient.

**Privacy Rule (HIPAA)**   Federal privacy protections for individually identifiable health information.

**Problem list**   Acute conditions for which the patient was recently seen as well as chronic conditions such as high blood pressure or diabetes that are monitored at nearly every visit and can affect decisions about medications and treatments for unrelated illnesses.

**Problem-oriented chart**   A method of organizing a patient's chart by problem or condition with the correlating symptoms, observations, and treatments related to that assessment.

**Prompt (EHR)**   Prompt stands for "prompt with current finding." Prompt is a software feature that generates a list of findings that are clinically related to the finding currently highlighted. *See also* Lists.

**Proportions**   Ratios in which the numerator is a subset of the denominator, allowing measures of the same thing to be compared.

**Protocol (medical)**   Standard plans of tests and therapy used for a disease or condition.

**Protocol (network)**   A set of rules computers use to communicate on a network. The Internet and many hospital networks use TCP/IP, which stands for Transmission Control Protocol/Internet Protocol.

**Px**   Medical abbreviation for physical exam (same as PE), the objective portion of the SOAP exam.

**Radiologists**   Specialists who interpret x-rays, CAT scans, and other diagnostic images.

**RAI**   Acronym for Resident Assessment Instrument, a questionnaire used to assess long-term care patients.

**RAID**   Acronym for redundant array of independent disks, a series of computer hard drives that, working together, maintain duplicate data so that the data is protected and accessible even if one drive of the array is damaged or stops working.

**RAM**   Acronym for random access memory, a computer chip that is used to temporarily store data during processing.

**Range**   A statistical term for the difference between the lowest and the highest values in a frequency distribution.

**Rates**   The measure of events occurring over a period of time or to express a ratio or proportion as a percentage.

**Ratio**   A ratio shows the relationship between two different measures. The measures do not have to be the same thing, for example, miles and gallons.

**Real time**   Entering data at the time an event occurs; for example, entering nursing notes, EHR data, charges, or payments from the patient while the patient is still present. Also, a transaction such as an eligibility verification in which a query is transmitted and the response is received in the same session.

**Record (database)**   A database record is a group of defined fields holding data about a specific thing.

**Record retention period**   The length of time that health records must be retained by state law, contractual obligations, or facility policy.

**Recovery Audit Contractor (RAC)**   Four private companies contracted by CMS to audit Medicare claims and recover from providers any overpayments or amounts that should not have been paid. The RAC is paid a portion of the money they recover.

**Registered nurse**   A healthcare professional licensed to administer medications and perform various medical procedures, nursing assessments, and nursing interventions.

**Relational data**   Records stored in multiple files or database tables that are connected by a common identifier stored in the records of each table. For example, a medical record number stored in different types of patient records is used to link all of the medical records for a given patient.

**Remittance advice**   *See* EOB.

**Remote access**   The ability to access EHRs from outside the medical facility network by using a direct-dial connection or a secure connection through the Internet.

**Revenue code**   A numeric code in the chargemaster used to total the charges of items for Medicare billing.

**Review of systems**   An inventory of body systems starting from the head down. the body systems in a standard ROS are constitutional symptoms, HEENT (head, eyes, ears, nose, mouth, throat), cardiovascular, respiratory, gastrointestinal, genitourinary, musculoskeletal, integumentary (skin and/or breast), neurologic, psychiatric, endocrine, hematologic/lymphatic, and allergic/immunologic.

**RF ID** Acronym for radio-frequency identification, a system in which patient, employee, or equipment ID tags are used to wirelessly identify, locate, and track the person or device.

**RHIA** Acronym for Registered Health Information Administrator. *See* Health information manager.

**RHIO** Acronym for regional health information organization, a network created for the purpose of enabling providers to access their patient's health records from multiple healthcare facilities where the patient has been treated.

**RHIT** Acronym for Registered Health Information Technician. *See* Health information technician.

**RIS** Acronym for radiology information system, which is used to schedule, bill, and track diagnostic tests, which are then interpreted by radiologists.

**Risk analysis** Identify potential risks and determine the probability of occurrence and magnitude of risks.

**Risk management** Making decisions about how to address risks, minimize liability and vulnerabilities, and prevent future occurrences.

**ROM** Acronym for read-only memory computer chips that retain stored data even when the power is off.

**ROS** Acronym for review of systems. *See* Review of systems.

**Router** A computer device, sometimes called a hub or switch, that interconnects all the computers in a network and manages the transfer of data between them.

**RUG, RUG-III** Acronyms for Resource Utilization Groups, third version, a system of 53 groups to which residents of skilled nursing facilities are assigned using MDS data from the Residential Assessment Instrument to calculate the per diem payment to the facility for patient care.

**RVS, RBRVS** RVS is an acronym for relative value scale, which is used to determine the value of a procedure using its relative value units (RVUs). The RBRVS, which is an acronym for Resource-Based Relative Value Scale, factors the provider's work, expenses, and malpractice insurance adjusted for regional wage and cost differences to determine the value of a procedure.

**RVU** Acronym for relative value unit, which is used to compare the value of a procedure to other procedures in terms of difficulty and expense.

**Rx** Medical abbreviation for therapy (including prescriptions); also, the therapy tab in EHR software.

**Rx norm** A nonproprietary vocabulary being developed by the NLM to codify drugs at the level of granularity needed in clinical practice.

**SAN** Acronym for storage area network, a method of distributing database records over a number of computers and disk drives.

**Sanction policy (HIPAA)** An office policy to deter noncompliance so that workforce members understand the consequences of failing to comply with security policies and procedures.

**Scanned images** Exam notes, letters, reports, and other documents that have been converted to an image by use of a scanner, then stored in the EHR. The data is accessible by a person viewing the chart, but the image contents cannot be used as data by the system for trend analysis, health maintenance, or similar purposes.

**SCIP** Acronym for Surgical Care Improvement Project, a national quality partnership of organizations committed to improving the safety of surgical care through the reduction of postoperative complications.

**SDO** Acronym for Standards Development Organization, an organization recognized by ANSI to develop national standards; examples in this book include DISA, HL7, and NCPDP.

**Search (EHR)** A word search used to quickly locate all findings in the nomenclature containing either matching words or synonyms of the search word.

**Secure messaging** A recommended alternative to sending PHI in e-mail messages. Secure messaging uses a secure web page to read and write messages. The only message sent as e-mail is an alert to the receiving party that a message is waiting on the secure site. Copies of the message are stored in a secure server, not in an e-mail system.

**Secured Socket Layer (SSL)** A security protocol to ensure privacy on a public network by encrypting the data.

**Security officer (HIPAA)** One individual designated by the healthcare organization as having overall responsibility for implementing the HIPAA Security Rule; however, specific security responsibilities may be assigned to other individuals.

**Security reminders (HIPAA)** One of the implementation requirements in the HIPAA Security Rule; includes notices, agenda items, and specific discussion topics at monthly meetings, as well as formal retraining about office security policies and procedures.

**Security Rule (HIPAA)** HIPAA security standards requiring implementation of appropriate security safeguards to protect health information stored in electronic form.

**Serial numbering** Chart numbers where hospitals sequentially number their records, assigning a new number for each admission or ER visit. This allows the hospital to easily assemble and track every record and service related to that stay under one number. The disadvantage is that patients who have been in the hospital several times have several different medical chart numbers. *Contrast with* Serial-unit numbering.

**Serial-unit numbering** A numbering method for charts in which a new chart is created each time the patient is admitted, but upon discharge the patient's previous chart is brought forward and merged into one patient chart. *Contrast with* Serial numbering.

**Sig** Instructions for labeling a prescription (from Latin *signa*).

**SMTP** Acronym for Simple Mail Transfer Protocol, a standard for transmission of e-mail.

**SNF** Acronym for skilled nursing facility, a long-term care hospital that provides patients with nursing care that is needed less frequently than an acute care facility.

**SNOMED-CT** A medical nomenclature developed by the College of American Pathologists and United Kingdom's National Health Service. It is a merger of two previous coding systems, SNOMED and the Read codes. SNOMED is an acronym for Systemized Nomenclature of Medicine that had its origins in 1965. (CT is an acronym for Clinical Terms.) The Read codes were a nomenclature developed by Dr. James Read in the United Kingdom. SNOMED CT has been recommended to become the core terminology for codified EHRs in the United States.

**SOAP** A defined structure for documenting a patient encounter by organizing the information into four sections. The acronym SOAP represents the first letter of each of the section titles: subjective, objective, assessment, and plan.

**Soundex** A code used to identify surnames by their phonetic sound. It consists of the first letter of the surname followed by a three-digit numeric code created from the consonants in the name.

**Source-oriented record** Organizes the contents of the chart according to the source of the document. For example, physician notes are grouped in one section, radiology reports in another, lab results in another, nursing notes in another.

**Speech recognition software** Software that recognizes the patterns in human speech as words and turns them into computer text. (See Chapter 8 for a detailed explanation.)

**Spirometer** An instrument that measures how much and how quickly air can enter and leave the lungs. Measurements may include VC (vital capacity), FVC (forced vital capacity), PEFR (peak expiratory flow rate), MVV (maximal voluntary ventilation), and FEV (forced expired volume).

**Spirometry** An objective measurement useful in the diagnosis and management of asthma and other lung conditions. *See also* Spirometer.

**SSL** Acronym for Secure Socket Layer, a protocol that transparently encrypts and decrypts web pages over the Internet.

**Standard deviation** A measure of variability in a frequency distribution in the original units of measure; calculated as the square root of the variance.

**STAT** Medical abbreviation from the Latin term *statim* that means "without delay."

**Stress test** An electrocardiogram performed before, during, and after strenuous exercise to measure heart function.

**Subjective (chart)** Patients describe in their own words what the problem is, what the symptoms are, and what they are experiencing.

**Superbill** *See* Encounter form.

**Surgeon assistant** A healthcare provider who works under the supervision of physicians to assist in surgery.

**Sx** Medical abbreviation for symptoms, which are subjective evidence of disease or physical disturbance; also, the symptom tab in EHR software.

**Table (database)** A database table stores multiple unique records in a database or computer file.

**Tablet PC** A self-contained, battery-operated computer similar to a laptop computer, but utilizing a special stylus and screen to replace the mouse, thus allowing the computer to be used as though the user was writing on a tablet.

**TB** Medical abbreviation for tuberculosis, an infectious, sometimes deadly, bacterial disease that usually attacks the lungs.

**TCP/IP** Acronym for Transmission Control Protocol/Internet Protocol, the basis for nearly all internet transmission and many LAN and WAN networks.

**Technical safeguards (HIPAA)** Primarily automated processes used to protect EPHI data and control access to data. They include using authentication controls to verify that the person signing onto a computer is authorized to access that EPHI, or encrypting and decrypting data as it is being stored and/or transmitted.

**Telemedicine** Delivery of medical care or consultation to a patient by a doctor in another location using modern communication technologies.

**Telemonitor** The transmission of medical data from a patient device to a provider for review and assessment.

**Teleradiology** The transmission of diagnostic images from one location to another. Usually this is for the purpose of having the images "read" by a radiologist at the receiving end.

**Terminal digit filing** A filing method for paper charts that uses the last set of the hyphenated record number (called the terminal digits) as the primary set for filing. The terminal digits correspond to a numbered subsection of the file room shelving. Terminal digit filing reduces the chance of filing errors by limiting the number of charts in each subsection.

**Text data (EHR)** Information stored in the EHR as word processing, blocks of text, or text reports. The data is searchable but neither codified nor standardized and generally not indexed.

**TIFF** Acronym for Tagged Image File Format, a standard format for images that are not compressed.

**Total cholesterol** A blood test that measures the sum of all types of cholesterol in the blood, including both HDL (high-density lipoprotein) and LDL (low-density lipoprotein).

**Transactions and code sets (HIPAA)** HIPAA regulations requiring all covered entities to use standard EDI transaction formats and standard codes within those transactions for claims, remittance advice and payments, claim status, eligibility, referrals, enrollment, premium payments, claim attachments, reports of injury, and retail drug claims.

**Transplants** The replacement of a patient's organs, bone marrow, or tissue with those from a donor.

**Trend analysis** Comparing data from different dates, tests, or events to correlate the changes in the results with changes in the patient's health.

**Triage** The screening of patients for allocation of treatment based on the urgency of their need for care. ER triage is often a simplified, organ-specific review of systems conducted by the triage nurse, based on the presenting complaint.

**TRICARE** A military-sponsored program to provide healthcare for active duty and retired military personnel and their dependents.

**Tx** Medical abbreviation for tests (performed); also, a tab in EHR software.

**UACDS** Acronym for Uniform Ambulatory Care Data Set, which is used by ambulatory care facilities and required by CMS.

**UAMCMDS** Acronym for Uniform Ambulatory Medical Care Minimum Data Set, a standard for the suggested minimum data that should be collected in an ambulatory setting.

**UB-04** A paper universal billing claim form for institutional billing; also known as CMS-1450.

**UCDS** Acronym for Uniform Clinical Data Set, which is used by quality improvement organizations and required in hospitals that participate in Medicare.

**UHDDS** Acronym for Uniform Hospital Discharge Data Set, which is used by acute care hospitals and required by CMS.

**UM, UR** Acronyms for utilization management and utilization review, which is a preadmission or precertification process between the provider and insurance plan to determine if the patient's condition qualifies him or her for inpatient admission or a requested surgery, treatment, or procedure.

**Unbundling** Posting charges for a single complex procedure as multiple procedure codes instead of posting the correct code that represented the procedure as a whole, for the purpose of increasing reimbursement.

**Uniform identifiers (HIPAA)** HIPAA regulations require all covered entities to adopt and use standard identification numbers for plans, providers, and employers in all HIPAA EDI transactions.

**Unit numbering** Process in which hospitals assign a single medical record chart number the first time a patient is registered and the same number is used every time the patient returns.

**UNOS** Acronym for United Network for Organ Sharing, the most prominent registry for organ transplants. UNOS maintains lists of potential recipients to identify the best donor–recipient matches as organs become available.

**Upcoding** Posting procedure or principal diagnosis codes that represent higher payment rates than what is supported by the medical record.

**URI** Acronym for upper respiratory infection, an infection affecting the nose, nasal passages, or upper part of the pharynx.

**U.S. Preventive Services Task Force** An independent panel of experts in primary care and prevention sponsored by AHRQ that systematically reviews the evidence of effectiveness and develops recommendations for clinical preventive services based on the patient's age, sex, and risk factors for disease. These recommendations are published by the AHRQ and are also incorporated in the health maintenance component of EHR systems.

**VA, VHA** Common abbreviations for the U.S. Department of Veterans Affairs, which provides hospitals and healthcare services to military veterans.

**Variance** The average variation from the mean in a frequency distribution.

**VBC** Acronym for visible black character, a relatively new method of calculating the pay rate for a transcriptionist.

**Vital signs** Functional measurements recorded at nearly every visit, including temperature, respiration rate, pulse rate, and blood pressure; most clinics measure height and weight as well.

**Vital statistics** Statistics about the births, deaths, disease states, and health of a population.

**VPN** Acronym for virtual private network. On a VPN, data sent over a public network is encrypted and de-encrypted without user intervention to attain a level of security similar to that of a private network.

**VTE** Acronym for venous thromboembolism, a potentially fatal condition in which blood clots travel through veins.

**WAN** Acronym for wide-area network, a private computer network similar to a LAN except a portion of the network extends over telephone or other cables to more distant facilities.

**WC** Acronym for workers' compensation, which covers healthcare costs and lost income from work-related injuries for employees in most types of businesses. It is funded by premiums that employers pay into a state fund or to private insurance carriers in states that do not operate state WC programs.

**Wellness conditions** Findings that are not disease related but rather used in health maintenance and preventive screening programs to keep healthy patients healthy. Wellness conditions are based on the age, sex, and history of the patient. Examples of preventive recommendations based on wellness conditions include a mammogram for a healthy woman over age 35, immunization vaccines at certain ages in children, and a colonoscopy for a healthy person with a family history of colorectal cancer.

**WEP** Acronym for Wired Equivalent Privacy, a protocol for securing the content of radio signals in wireless network devices.

**WHO** Acronym for World Health Organization, the United Nations' agency for health and the entity responsible for maintaining the International Classification of Diseases coding standards.

**Wi-Fi** An abbreviation for wireless fidelity, a type of wireless computer networking. Wireless networks use radio signals in place of wired network cables. (See a detailed explanation in Chapter 4.)

**WNL** Acronym for "within normal limits" in medical charts.

**X12n** ANSI insurance standards committee responsible for developing and maintaining HIPAA transactions.

**XML** Acronym for eXtensible Markup Language, a format in which fielded data can be transferred between computers, yet easily read by humans.

**X-ray** Traditionally an image made by the passage of short-wave radiation through the body onto photographic film. Digital receptors are now able to replace film, allowing the image to be captured and stored in digital form without photo processing.

**X-ray jacket** A large folder or envelope that holds a patient's x-ray films for transport or storage in a nonelectronic file system.

# Index